INTRODUCTION TO
Health Services Administration

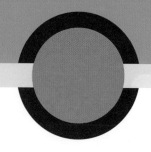

CONTENTS IN BREIF

UNIT I INTRODUCTION TO HEALTH SERVICES ADMINISTRATION

1 THE HEALTH SERVICES ADMINISTRATOR
2 HEALTH CARE PROFESSIONALS AND SETTINGS
3 HEALTH CARE DELIVERY

UNIT II ADMINISTRATIVE MANAGEMENT

4 HEALTH CARE PROCESSES AND WORKFLOW
5 DOCUMENTATION
6 TECHNOLOGY
7 MANAGING SUPPLIES AND INVENTORY
8 BASIC FINANCE AND HEALTH CARE ACCOUNTING
9 THE REVENUE CYCLE
10 QUALITY, PERFORMANCE IMPROVEMENT, AND RISK MANAGEMENT

UNIT III ETHICAL AND LEGAL CONCERNS

11 LEGAL ISSUES AND FRAUD IN HEALTH CARE
12 HEALTH INSURANCE PORTABILITY AND ACCOUNTABILITY ACT (HIPAA)
13 COMPLIANCE

UNIT IV COMMUNICATION

14 BUSINESS COMMUNICATION AND PROFESSIONALISM
15 MARKETING

UNIT V PEOPLE AND ORGANIZATIONAL MANAGEMENT

16 HIRING, TRAINING, AND EVALUATING EMPLOYEES
17 LEADERSHIP, MOTIVATION AND CONFLICT MANAGEMENT
18 PROJECT MANAGEMENT

INTRODUCTION TO
Health Services
Administration

EDITOR

Jaime Nguyen, MD, MPH, MS
Senior Program Director
Medical Assistant and Patient Care Technician Program
Virginia College in Birmingham
Birmingham, Alabama

ELSEVIER

ELSEVIER

3251 Riverport Lane
St. Louis, Missouri 63043

INTRODUCTION TO HEALTH SERVICES ADMINISTRATION ISBN: 978-0-323-46223-5

Notices

Knowledge and best practice in this field are constantly changing. As new research and experience broaden our understanding, changes in research methods, professional practices, or medical treatment may become necessary.

Practitioners and researchers must always rely on their own experience and knowledge in evaluating and using any information, methods, compounds, or experiments described herein. In using such information or methods they should be mindful of their own safety and the safety of others, including parties for whom they have a professional responsibility.

With respect to any drug or pharmaceutical products identified, readers are advised to check the most current information provided (i) on procedures featured or (ii) by the manufacturer of each product to be administered, to verify the recommended dose or formula, the method and duration of administration, and contraindications. It is the responsibility of practitioners, relying on their own experience and knowledge of their patients, to make diagnoses, to determine dosages and the best treatment for each individual patient, and to take all appropriate safety precautions.

To the fullest extent of the law, neither the Publisher nor the authors, contributors, or editors, assume any liability for any injury and/or damage to persons or property as a matter of products liability, negligence or otherwise, or from any use or operation of any methods, products, instructions, or ideas contained in the material herein.

Library of Congress Cataloging-in-Publication Data

Title: Introduction to health services administration.
Description: St. Louis, Missouri : Elsevier, [2018] | Includes bibliographical references and index.
Identifiers: LCCN 2017016818 | ISBN 9780323462235 (pbk. : alk. paper)
Subjects: | MESH: Health Services Administration | Healthcare Financing | Personnel Management
Classification: LCC RA399.A1 | NLM W 84.1 | DDC 362.1068–dc23 LC record available at
    https://lccn.loc.gov/2017016818

Senior Content Strategist: Linda Woodard
Senior Content Development Manager: Luke Held
Content Development Specialist: John Tomedi, *Spring Hollow Press*
Publishing Services Manager: Jeff Patterson
Project Manager: Lisa A. P. Bushey
Design Direction: Maggie Reid

Printed in China

Last digit is the print number: 9 8 7 6 5 4 3 2 1

Working together
to grow libraries in
developing countries

www.elsevier.com • www.bookaid.org

CONTRIBUTORS

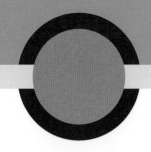

Carol Colvin, EdD, MBA
Director of Financial Aid—Online Operations and Nashville
South College
Knoxville, Tennessee

Pat DeVoy, EdS, LPN, RHIT, CPC, CPPM, CMA
Assistant Professor, Health Information Management
University of Detroit Mercy
Detroit, Michigan

Deborah Proctor, EdD, RN
Adjunct Faculty Member
Butler County Community College
Butler, Pennsylvania

Meredith Robertson, MS, MPP
Instructor
University of Central Florida
Orlando, Florida

Nanette Sayles, EdD, RHIA, CCS, CHDA, CHPS, CPHIMS, FAHIMA
Associate Professor
Health Information Management
East Central College
Union, Missouri

Betsy Shiland, MS, RHIA, CCS, CPC, CPHQ, CTR, CHDA, CPB, EMT
AHIMA-Approved ICD-10-CM/PCS Trainer
Former Assistant Professor
Allied Health Department
Community College of Philadelphia
Philadelphia, Pennsylvania

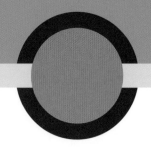

PREFACE

Since 1965, health care expenditures have grown from 6% of the United States gross domestic product to over 17% today. As the health care industry swells to an ever-larger portion of the economy, health services administrators are needed to manage the business of health care. These individuals work in ambulatory care settings, such as urgent care facilities, dialysis treatment centers, and long-term care facilities. They are in charge of hiring and supervising staff, planning and overseeing budgets, and ensuring their facility remains compliant with laws and regulations. They serve as the bridge among clinicians, health information management professionals, vendors, regulators, researchers, payers, and, of course, patients. The work of the health services administrator is central to organized and efficient health care delivery in the modern age.

Introduction to Health Services Administration is a comprehensive, easy-to-understand textbook designed to teach students the role and functions of a health services administrator in the ambulatory care setting. With a friendly tone and a colorful design, this book welcomes all students entering this field, even those with limited experience in a health care or office setting. To that end, the text provides ample visuals and discussions of the real work performed in a variety of ambulatory settings every day. The goal is to make the connection for students between high-quality care of the patient and running a successful, financially-solvent practice.

As such, *Introduction to Health Services Administration* was written to provide a comprehensive overview of the management of many types of medical offices. Its goal is to be as useful to the student who will manage a traditional physician's office as the student who will manage the retail care clinic—and everywhere in between. Students are provided with an overview of health care delivery in the United States and introduced to the concepts, principles, and practices associated with the administration of health care services. The text explores each aspect of the workflow in an ambulatory care facility, from scheduling patients to managing the revenue cycle. In addition, students will be introduced to medical documentation, use of the electronic health record system and practice management software, budgeting for staff and equipment, and inventory management functions. They will learn about quality and performance improvement, risk management, and marketing strategies. Legal and ethical competencies, including HIPAA, regulatory compliance, and civil and criminal law, are also presented. Students will learn how to communicate effectively with patients and professionals, along with skills to manage both people and practice.

The scope of the book is designed to satisfy the competencies for the Certified Medical Manager (CMM) credential from Professional Association of Health Care Office Management (PAHCOM), as well as the Certified Physician Practice Manager (CPPM) credential from the American Academy of Professional Coders (AAPC). In addition, the text is mapped to the Commission on Accreditation for Health Informatics and Information Management Education (CAHIIM) Associate degree curriculum requirements. With its focus on application, however, *Introduction to Health Services Administration* is not written solely for the classroom, but also as a professional resource. Because there is a wealth of practical advice in the text, health services administrators can refer to this book throughout their careers.

KEY FEATURES

Introduction to Health Services Administration offers accessible, easy-to-understand text and includes several features to aid student comprehension. Throughout each chapter, **Takeaway** boxes highlight key points and important concepts. **Learning Checkpoints** generally follow each main heading, giving students time to pause, reflect, and retain what they've learned. A **Current Trends in Health Care** feature discusses concepts in the news, and a **Take Learning to the Next Level** box encourages students to seek out supplemental information.

Each chapter opens with an outline of the material covered, learning objectives, and key terms, and the book includes the definitions of the key terms in the margins for easy understanding. The chapters finish with Review Questions, which are tied to the learning objectives, allowing students to check their understanding of all aspects of topics.

To strengthen this book's "hands-on," practical approach, every chapter includes a series of Case Studies drawn from real-life job situations. These case studies have been woven through the chapters, taking the information presented and applying it to situations encountered by health services administrators every day. The answers to the intratext exercises and Review Questions are in the back of the text.

ORGANIZATION OF THE TEXT

Unit I provides an overview of the job of the health services administrator and a survey of health care as an industry. Chapter 1 focuses on the role of the health services administrator in an ambulatory environment. Chapter 2 illustrates the work of various kinds of professionals and the settings in which they work. Chapter 3 provides a history of modern health care delivery, ending with an overview of the complicated relationship between patients, providers, and payers in existence today.

Unit II walks the student through the day-by-day work of the health services administrator. In Chapters 4 through 6, students are introduced to facility workflow, the importance of documentation, and the use of EHR and practice management software. Chapters 7 through 9 discuss inventory management, budgeting, and the revenue cycle. This unit ends with a survey of the most-up-to-date information on quality, performance improvement, and risk management in outpatient care.

Unit III explores ethical, legal, and compliance concerns.

Unit IV offers students a background in business communications and marketing.

Unit V discusses the management of people and organizational management.

FOR THE INSTRUCTOR

The TEACH Instructor's Resource Manual provides detailed lesson plans, PowerPoint slides, and a test bank. The lesson plans allow instructors to quickly familiarize themselves with the material in each chapter. PowerPoint slides are tailored to each lesson, highlighting the most important concepts from the text. The test bank includes over 750 questions. Each question is tied to a specific objective and mapped to PAHCOM, AAPC, and CAHIIM competencies.

Instructors using this textbook also have access to a full suite of course management tools on Canvas provided by Evolve. Canvas provided by Evolve may be used to publish the class syllabus, outlines, and lecture notes. Instructors can set up email communication and "virtual office hours" and engage the class using discussion boards and chat rooms.

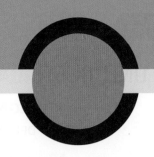

CONTENTS

UNIT I INTRODUCTION TO HEALTH SERVICES ADMINISTRATION

1 THE HEALTH SERVICES ADMINISTRATOR, *3*
PAT DEVOY

2 HEALTH CARE PROFESSIONALS AND SETTINGS, *14*
BETSY SHILAND AND PAT DEVOY

3 HEALTH CARE DELIVERY, *35*
JAIME NGUYEN AND CAROL COLVIN

UNIT II ADMINISTRATIVE MANAGEMENT

4 HEALTH CARE PROCESSES AND WORKFLOW, *75*
BETSY SHILAND

5 DOCUMENTATION, *90*
BETSY SHILAND

6 TECHNOLOGY, *113*

7 MANAGING SUPPLIES AND INVENTORY, *135*
PAT DEVOY AND CAROL COLVIN

8 BASIC FINANCE AND HEALTH CARE ACCOUNTING, *147*
CAROL COLVIN

9 THE REVENUE CYCLE, *160*
NANETTE B. SAYLES

10 QUALITY, PERFORMANCE IMPROVEMENT, AND RISK MANAGEMENT, *182*
CAROL COLVIN

UNIT III ETHICAL AND LEGAL CONCERNS

11 LEGAL ISSUES AND FRAUD IN HEALTH CARE, *209*
DEBORAH PROCTOR

12 HEALTH INSURANCE PORTABILITY AND ACCOUNTABILITY ACT (HIPAA), *238*
CAROL COLVIN

13 COMPLIANCE, *251*
CAROL COLVIN AND JAIME NGUYEN

UNIT IV COMMUNICATION

14 BUSINESS COMMUNICATION AND PROFESSIONALISM, *271*
MEREDITH ROBERTSON

15 MARKETING, *297*

UNIT V PEOPLE AND ORGANIZATIONAL MANAGEMENT

16 HIRING, TRAINING, AND EVALUATING EMPLOYEES, *319*
MEREDITH ROBERTSON

17 LEADERSHIP, MOTIVATION AND CONFLICT MANAGEMENT, *347*
CAROL COLVIN

18 PROJECT MANAGEMENT, *362*
CAROL COLVIN

ANSWER KEY, *373*

GLOSSARY, *403*

INDEX, *417*

INTRODUCTION TO HEALTH SERVICES ADMINISTRATION

1 THE HEALTH SERVICES ADMINISTRATOR

2 HEALTH CARE PROFESSIONALS AND SETTINGS

3 HEALTH CARE DELIVERY

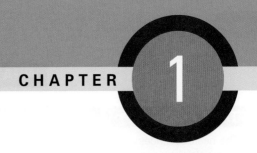
THE HEALTH SERVICES ADMINISTRATOR

Pat Devoy

CHAPTER OUTLINE

WHAT IS HEALTH SERVICES
ADMINISTRATION?
A Routine Visit
THE ROLE OF THE HEALTH
SERVICES ADMINISTRATOR
Duties

A CAREER IN HEALTH SERVICES
ADMINISTRATION
Settings
Education
Internships and
Externships

Certifications and
Credentialing
Continuing Education
Employment Outlook

VOCABULARY

allied health professional
certification

claim
continuing education unit (CEU)

credential
provider

CHAPTER OBJECTIVES

After completing this chapter, the student should be able to do the following:

1. Explain the function of health services administration.
2. Discuss the role of the health services administrator.
3. Discuss the settings in which a health services administrator may be employed.

4. List the educational and credentialing requirements for health services administrators.
5. Discuss the job outlook for health services administrators.

WHAT IS HEALTH SERVICES ADMINISTRATION?

Health services administration is the field relating to the leadership and general management of various health care settings. A health services administrator (HSA) is a medical or health services manager who plans, coordinates, and supervises the operations for an entire facility, a specific clinical area or department, or a medical practice for a group of physicians, as well as the staff who work there. From the moment a new patient walks in the door of a medical office until the time the office receives payment for its services, the HSA works to ensure the health care facility or clinic is efficiently operating on a daily basis, while also ensuring the best delivery of health services to its patients.

The HSA's role at the medical office is multifaceted and critical to the office's successful operation. Depending on the size and type of practice, the HSA may need to be skilled and experienced in policy analysis, finance, accounting, budgeting, human resources, and marketing. They must have strong leadership and supervisory skills because they will need to manage the medical staff, which will include the hiring, firing, and training of new and current staff. They must have a strong and thorough knowledge of clinical practices, health care laws and regulations, and health care policies and procedures to ensure full compliance with all state and federal laws and industry codes and regulations. Health service administrators must have strong ability in accounting, budgeting, finance, and medical billing and coding. Thus to be a successful health care administrator, one must be skilled in a number of multiple fields and have a comprehensive understanding of the operations of a medical office.

The purpose of this text is to explore all facets in preparation for being a successful HSA.

● CASE STUDY

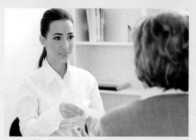

Jennifer is just completing an associate degree in medical assisting and is about to begin her externship at Community Outpatient Services. She is excited to be completing her degree and is anxious to learn and to put her new knowledge into practice. But Jennifer has never worked in a health care facility before and is not quite sure what to expect. She is nervous and is concerned that she will feel out of place.

Jennifer has been introduced to the clinic's office staff and will now be working with the health services administrator, Ms. Diaz. Ms. Diaz has been employed at Community Outpatient Services for 15 years and is very familiar with the staff and flow of the office. Ms. Diaz is also familiar with mentoring new graduates, and she takes an intern student each semester. She is looking forward to acting as a mentor for Jennifer to help her gain more experience and begin her new career.

As we journey through this first chapter, take a moment to think about Jennifer. What will she be learning at her externship site, and how will she be able to apply the knowledge she has learned from school? How will you feel when it is your turn to be the extern? Will you feel comfortable or a little nervous? Will you enjoy being able to apply your new knowledge?

A Routine Visit

To better understand the role of the HSA, think back to the last time you were at a physician's office for yourself or a family member. What processes or steps needed to be in place to make sure you had a good patient visit?

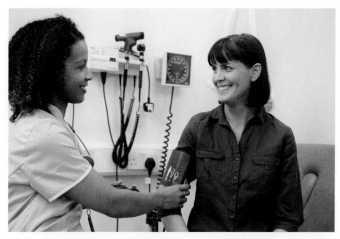

Figure 1.1 A medical assistant takes the patient's blood pressure.

When the patient arrives, the patient registration staff must be welcoming and ensure privacy and confidentiality as the patient is checked in, or *registered*. The patient registration staff obtains pertinent patient information, such as personal data and insurance information. This information is entered into the electronic health records (EHR) system, which is a computerized database system that allows authorized health care facility employees to view and access patient information. During the patient registration process, it is critical that the patient's personal information is protected and that no patient data are disclosed to any other patients also waiting in the lobby. Patient registration personnel are part of the administrative staff in a medical office.

Once the patient registration has been completed, the patient registration staff then notifies the clinical staff that the patient is ready to be seen. The clinical staff member, usually a medical assistant, brings the patient to the back office to obtain his or her height, weight, and vital signs, and then directs the patient to an examination room (Fig. 1.1). There, the medical assistant asks the reason for the visit (chief complaint) and takes a medical history, which includes a list of current medications. All of this information is documented and submitted into the EHR system. When complete, the patient waits to see the **provider**—a physician's assistant, nurse practitioner, or physician.

The provider reviews the information obtained by the medical assistant, examines and assesses the patient, and decides on a treatment plan. Laboratory tests or diagnostic imaging may be ordered to aid in a diagnosis. This can be done either during the patient visit and in the same facility or afterward at another facility. Once completed, test results are then reviewed by the provider, who may then prescribe medication, perform a procedure, or request additional tests be conducted for the patient.

If a medication is prescribed, either the administrative or clinical staff may obtain the patient's preferred pharmacy, and the provider will transmit the prescription electronically, or via e-script, for the patient to pick up later that day. During the patient checkout (Fig. 1.2), a follow-up appointment may be scheduled, and the administrative staff may collect money from the patient for the medical services provided during the visit. After the patient visit, a medical coder reviews the patient chart and billing report and assigns special codes that represent these services. These codes are then submitted to a medical biller who will prepare a medical **claim** to the insurer, who reviews it and pays the provider.

This scenario may seem fairly routine and simple, but it involves many complex, interrelated steps, which must be meticulously followed in order for the entire patient delivery system to function. Fig. 1.3 illustrates the steps making up a patient health care visit, such as the one discussed, following the patient from registration at the medical office until payment is received for the services rendered.

TAKE AWAY
The patient registration staff obtains pertinent patient information, such as personal data and insurance coverage.

TAKE AWAY
Clinical staff collect initial patient health information.

provider an individual or organization that provides health services to patients.

claim a statement of services sent to a health insurer for payment to the provider.

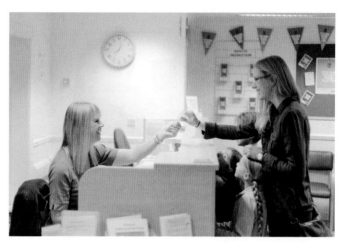

Figure 1.2 Administrative staff may schedule a follow-up appointment during patient checkout.

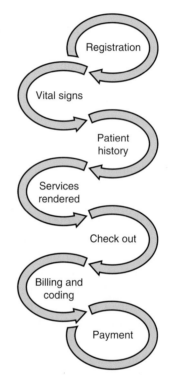

Figure 1.3 Components of a routine patient visit.

Consider all the things that had to be in place for the patient visit to run smoothly. Before the patient visit, there was planning, hiring, training, and budgeting. Staffing and medical supplies were coordinated so that all necessary items and employees were in place to complete the health care service. The patient's data were communicated first to the patient registration staff and medical assistant, then to the provider, and next to the laboratory, pharmacy, and insurance company, all while maintaining the patient's privacy. The coordination of all these systems to produce a patient outcome that is beneficial to both the medical office and the patient is the responsibility and result of the HSA.

THE ROLE OF THE HEALTH SERVICES ADMINISTRATOR

Providing a quality health care experience means coordinating many different moving parts, as discussed in the "routine patient visit" example earlier. You can think of these

CURRENT TRENDS IN HEALTH CARE

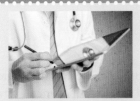

In recent years, digital technology has helped medical practices operate more efficiently and with better controls for patient privacy. Today, many medical offices use computerized practice management (PM) and electronic health record (EHR) systems to schedule and register patients, record the provider's diagnosis and treatment, prescribe medicine, and bill for the service. Chapter 6 explores how computer technology helps the medical office run smoothly.

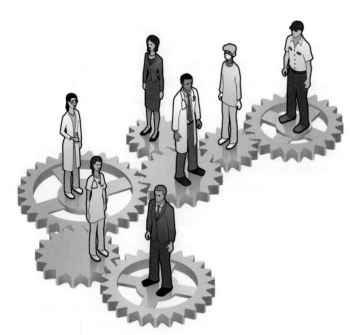

Figure 1.4 The delivery of health care requires many different professionals working together.

components as gears in a machine (Fig. 1.4). If one component is broken, the system as a whole will not work, leading to unsatisfied patients, poor quality of service, or providers who do not receive payments.

Because health care is a service-centered business, patient satisfaction drives income. Thus managing health care as a business in a way that creates a satisfied customer—while controlling costs and securing appropriate payments for services—is essential to remain profitable and in business.

The HSA should have an expansive understanding of the medical practice and business as a whole. They must manage health care personnel, coordinate the daily operations, ensure compliance with health care laws and regulations, and monitor cash flow. An HSA must be knowledgeable of the various areas encompassed within the business, from patient care to medical billing and coding. Although an HSA does not have to be an expert in each area of the business, a healthy knowledge of each area aids in the decision-making process and makes for efficient business operations.

In addition to having a strong business acumen, the HSA must have excellent interpersonal and communication skills. The HSA must be empathetic and have the ability to effectively communicate with administrative and clinical staff, patients, and all others associated with the medical practice. Conflict resolution skills are also a must because the HSA will handle both employee and patient complaints. They are often

TAKE AWAY ●·········

The health services administrator should have an expansive understanding of the medical practice and business as a whole.

the front-line supervisors of employees and must be able to motivate and delegate tasks and responsibilities to the appropriate staff member.

Duties

The role and duties of the HSA depend on the type and size of the health care organization. They may manage an entire facility, a specific clinical area or department, or a medical practice for a group of physicians. Although the HSA should be knowledgeable about all aspects of the business, their level of involvement in the daily activities and operations varies by setting. At larger organizations, such as a hospital, an HSA may have broader functions and may be responsible for longer-term planning and implementing the organization's vision. The HSA may have to interact with a governing board, medical staff, and department heads. They may have to plan the budgets and set rates for health services. They may be involved with fundraising and planning community events.

At a smaller health care facility or clinic, the HSA may consult with the providers (Fig. 1.5), manage patient relations, assist in billing, hire and train staff members, manage inventory, and perform a wide array of administrative duties as necessary. An HSA at these facilities may also be referred to as a medical office administrator or manager.

Some of the most common duties of the HSA include:

- Educating and training providers in operational practices and regulations
- Liaising among medical personnel, department leaders, and governing boards
- Participating in the development of quality assurance, patient services, and community outreach
- Recruiting, hiring, and evaluating assistant administrators, nurses, office staff, and providers
- Fundraising and community health planning
- Acting as a compliance manager for the purpose of internal audits
- Serving as a facilities and maintenance manager
- Acting as a privacy and security officer, ensuring the health care facility is in compliance with all Health Insurance Portability and Accountability Act (HIPAA) regulations, which protect patient information
- Acting as a utilization manager to optimize the use of the facility's health care resources
- Obtaining and maintaining appropriate facility licenses and credentials
- Overseeing the compliance of all staff members with proper licensing and professional credentials as needed for their job

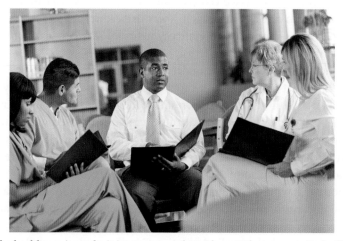

Figure 1.5 The health services administrator consults with providers at a medical office to discuss the health of the business.

The daily activities of an HSA also vary greatly depending on the type of facility. There are numerous types of health care facilities, including physicians' offices, urgent care centers, hospitals, clinics located within hospitals, retail care centers, surgery centers, imaging centers, nursing homes, and assisted living facilities. Some practices may have two administrators: one over the administrative practice and the other over the clinical practice. For the administrative practice, the HSA may be called an office manager or practice manager and oversees such duties as patient scheduling, patient and insurance billing, overall facility budgeting, and staff training. Clinic or clinical managers have a more concentrated area of management, which is based on their clinical experience and expertise and may include the coordination of treatment and rehabilitation services. Smaller to mid-sized health care facilities will have either a clinical or administrative HSA. However, in larger health care organizations, it is more common to have multiple HSAs who oversee different aspects of the business and work together to coordinate a more fluid and efficient health care delivery.

LEARNING CHECKPOINT 1.1
What Is Health Services Administration?

1. Patient registration personnel are part of the _____ staff in a medical office.

2. Another name for a physician, physician's assistant, or nurse practitioner is a(n) _____.

3. A(n) _____ is a statement of services sent to a health insurer for payment to the provider.

A CAREER IN HEALTH SERVICES ADMINISTRATION

Settings

HSAs are employed in many different types of health care facilities. An outpatient clinic, such as a physician's office or clinic, is one such facility. Others include ambulatory surgery centers, urgent care centers, imaging and diagnostic facilities, and retail care clinics. Each of these settings will be discussed in detail in Chapter 2.

Education

HSAs are considered **allied health professionals**, a term describing those individuals who work in health care but who are not doctors or nurses. Allied health professionals work in health care teams to provide their expertise and knowledge to support the health care provider in the care of the patient.

allied health professional a health care professional who provides a supporting function in health care delivery.

Because of the growth in the health care industry, more institutions of higher education are offering various programs in allied health. Certificates, diplomas, and degrees are offered in fields such as health services administration and management, health information technology, health information management, medical billing and coding, medical office administration, and medical assisting.

Take Learning to the Next Level················

Other allied health professionals include dieticians, social workers, phlebotomists, audiologists, paramedics, and respiratory therapists, just to name a few.

Depending on the type of health care facility, a medical office may require the HSA to have at least a certificate or degree such as medical assisting, medical office administration or management, or medical billing and coding, along with a number of years of experience. To manage a hospital or large medical facility, the HSA may need to have a bachelor's or master's degree, such as in health or business administration and management.

Internships and Externships

Most allied health certificate programs and degrees include an internship or externship as part of the curriculum. During this experience, students get to work "hands on" in a medical facility. In most cases, the student will shadow a working administrative professional for a period of 4 weeks or more. This allows individuals to put their classroom learning into practice, preparing them for an actual job in the field.

Certification and Credentialing

Certification is becoming an important factor in the health care industry. More and more employers are looking at certification as a way to assess whether an individual possesses the skills and knowledge required for successful performance in a particular job role. **Certifications** are provided through a formal process that validates an individual's ability to complete a task or job. Many medical careers, such as medical assistants and medical billers and coders, have a certification program that can be obtained after completion of a certain level of education.

Certifications can differ from state to state, and not being certified in some medical careers in some states may prevent an individual from working in that field. The process of acquiring and maintaining certifications varies depending on the certifying agency and the specific certification. Some agencies or associations require a certain number of years of work experience before sitting for the certification examination. Other certifying agencies require candidates to complete an accredited educational program. After completing the program, the candidate must then successfully pass an exam in order to be certified.

Credentials provide an employer with proof that an individual has obtained education and training to a certain level of qualification or competence within a field. Most credentials are issued by a university or professional association. Many positions held by health care professionals demand both certifications and credentials, whereas some expect one or the other.

Several credentialing bodies are available to the HSA who wants to demonstrate their knowledge and competency. The American Academy of Professional Coders offers the Certified Physician Practice Manager (CPPM) credential for HSAs who are employed in a physician's medical office. The CPPM credential focuses on the health care business workflow of an outpatient setting and financial duties, such as medical office accounting, reimbursement, and the revenue cycle. The candidate should also have knowledge in HIPAA regulations, human resources, quality control, compliance, medical records management, and emergency and disaster planning. To sit for the CPPM exam, it is recommended that the candidate have at least an associate's degree, as well as some physician practice management experience.

The Professional Association of Healthcare Office Management (PAHCOM) offers the Certified Medical Manager (CMM) credential, which is a nationally recognized

certification the verification that an individual or entity has met certain professional standards.

credential a professional qualification, represented by the abbreviation a qualified individual may list after their name.

TAKE AWAY ●··········

The Certified Physician Practice Manager (CPPM) and the Certified Medical Manager (CMM) are two credentials for health services administrators.

professional certification for managers of solo providers and small group physician practices. This credential requires knowledge in revenue management, risk management, human resources, finance, technology, practice marketing, and provider licensing and credentialing. The CMM credential is an advanced certification and requires both experience and education. To qualify to sit for the CMM exam, a candidate must have at least 12 college credit hours in health care or business management and two years of experience in a patient care or clinical setting.

Continuing Education

Health care practices are constantly changing. Thus learning must continue long after graduation. There is a constant need for continued training and education in the health care field to stay up to date on industry regulations, innovations, and trends. As a result, most health care professionals, especially those with certifications, require the completion of a specific number of **continuing education units (CEUs)**. CEUs are credits earned when completing a course for certification, license, or a profession. Almost all certifications require completion of a number of CEUs for renewal, which is usually a one-, two-, or three-year period of time. The number of CEUs required varies by state, licensure, and profession.

CEUs can be earned in a number of ways. They may be offered or taken as a seminar (Fig. 1.6), courses, workshop, tutorial, or self-study course. Health care professionals can also attend webinars and participate in industry events, as well as be guest lecturers, to earn more CEUs. Each activity is allotted a specific number of credits, depending upon the hours attended or participated.

In addition to keeping one's certification active, it is imperative to stay current in one's own discipline. Allowing a certification to lapse or expire without renewal may lead to a loss of employment. Reacquiring or reactivating a certification may require the individual to have to go through the entire process all over again, including retesting and covering all of the associated costs.

Employment Outlook

More people need health care services today than ever before because of several factors. First, a large demographic of people known as the *baby boomers*—the generation born between 1946 and 1964—are now in their 50s, 60s, and 70s. This means that, as a whole, the American population is getting older. At the same time, new approaches to treatment, new technology, medical discoveries, and better access to information have

continuing education unit (CEU) a measure of the amount of education an individual has acquired after a degree or credential, which is required to stay current in the field.

TAKE AWAY ●·········

More people need health care services today than ever before.

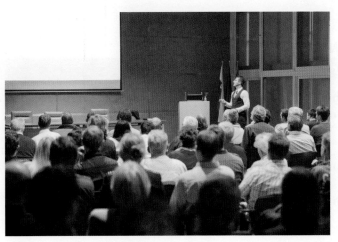

Figure 1.6 Health services administrators attend a seminar to stay current on trends in their field and earn CEUs to maintain their certification.

led to better quality care and, in turn, longer lifespans. With the population getting older and living longer, the demand for health services will be far greater.

Adding to the demand for health care services is preventative medicine, which seeks to avoid the disease process before it becomes a costlier problem to the payer, such as a health insurer, or a life-threatening problem to the patient. Screenings for heart disease, diabetes, and different types of cancers all seek to prevent the onset of disease. Although preventative medicine saves on the costs and resources it would take to treat diseases in the long term, it results in younger populations accessing health care more often than they have in the past.

These trends have created a dramatic and significant demand for physicians, nurses, and the allied health professionals who support them. Thus the need for health services administrators will continue to grow. According to the Bureau of Labor Statistics, employment of medical and health services managers is projected to grow 17% from 2014 to 2024, much faster than the average for all occupations.[1]

As the industry evolves, so does the need for specialized health services administrative positions. For example, federal government incentives encouraging the use of EHRs have led to new positions for HSAs, as providers find it necessary to implement new technology to remain compliant and in business. Technology-specific compliance positions have also surfaced, as health care businesses strive to ensure the safety and security of protected health information and that they are compliant with stringent HIPAA regulations regarding data exchange.

◉ CASE STUDY

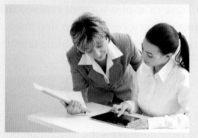

At the end of her first day of shadowing Ms. Diaz, Jennifer wonders why she felt nervous at all. She knows she is lucky to have Ms. Diaz as a mentor, because Ms. Diaz is not only skilled at her job as an HSA, she also takes time to make sure Jennifer is learning how the facility works.

Jennifer decides that to get the most out of her externship, she should treat her learning experience as if it were her job. She will stay focused, professional, and polite and ask plenty of questions. This will be the only medical experience on her resume, so she wants to make sure she leaves a great impression with Ms. Diaz. And who knows? Maybe Community Outpatient Services will have a position for her once she finishes her degree!

▪ LEARNING CHECKPOINT 1.2
A Career in Health Care Administration

1. Health services administrators, medical billers, and medical coders are all types of _____ health professionals.

2. To be _____, a candidate must complete an accredited educational program and pass an examination.

3. Which credential is offered by PAHCOM? _____

---

[1](http://www.bls.gov/ooh/management/medical-and-health-services-managers.htm).

1. True or False: A health services administrator plans, coordinates, and supervises the operations for an entire facility.

2. List three duties of a health services administrator in a smaller facility.

3. List three types of facilities that employ a health services administrator.

4. What is the difference between a credential and a certification?

5. List two professional credentials available to health services administrators.

6. Why is the health care field growing?

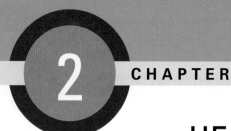

CHAPTER

HEALTH CARE PROFESSIONALS AND SETTINGS

Betsy Shiland and Pat Devoy

CHAPTER OUTLINE

INTRODUCTION
HEALTH CARE PROFESSIONALS
  Credentialing
  Licensing
  Physicians
  Nurses
  Physician Assistants (PAs)
  Medical Assistants
  Medical Billers and Coders
  Other Health Professionals

AMBULATORY CARE SETTINGS
  Physician's Office
    Organization
    Ownership
  Clinic
  Diagnostic Facility
  Ambulatory Surgery
    Center (ASC)
  Urgent Care Clinic
  Retail Health Clinic

ACUTE CARE SETTINGS
  Hospital
OTHER SETTINGS
  Long-Term Care and Skilled
    Nursing Facilities
  Home Health Care
  Hospice Care

VOCABULARY

acute care
advanced practice registered nurse
  (APRN)
ambulatory care
ambulatory surgery center (ASC)
assisted living facility
care plan
certification
clinic
continuing medical education (CME)
  unit
continuity of care
credential
encounter

gatekeeper
home health care
hospice care
hospital
inpatient
intermediate care facility (ICF)
licensed practical (vocational) nurse
  (LPN, LVN)
licensing
long-term care facility (LTC)
medical assistant (MA)
nurse
outpatient
palliative care

physician
physician assistant (PA)
physician's office
primary care
primary care provider (PCP)
privileges
registered nurse (RN)
referral
retail health clinic
scope of practice
skilled nursing facility (SNF)
urgent care clinic
visit

CHAPTER OBJECTIVES

After completing this chapter, the student should be able to do the following:

1. Explain the roles of credentialing, certification, and licensing in quality health care.
2. Differentiate among the roles of physicians, nurses, and physician assistants.
3. Explain the roles of medical assistants in a medical practice.
4. Discuss the roles of a medical biller and a medical coder in a medical office.
5. List the health care professionals who support the physicians and nurses in the delivery of patient care.

6. Understand the difference between acute care and ambulatory care.
7. Differentiate among the different types of outpatient health care facilities, including the physician's office, ambulatory care center, urgent care center, retail clinic, home health care, and hospice care.
8. Discuss the various types of inpatient care, including acute care hospitals, long-term care facilities, skilled nursing facilities, and assisted living facilities.
9. Explain the functions of home health care and hospice care.

INTRODUCTION

When patients need medical services, how do they know where to go? Do they go see their provider at a clinic or hospital? Should they see a physician or a nurse practitioner?

Most people understand that hospitals are for patients who are seriously ill or injured, whereas the doctor's office is for less critical or non-urgent medical care. For example, you would not go to the office of your family physician for heart surgery, just as you would not go to the hospital for an earache. The distinction, however, is not always so clear, especially because so many different health care settings offer many different services and specialties. This chapter will describe the various types of health care facilities and professionals and how they work together to offer different services and levels of care to meet patients' health care needs.

○ CASE STUDY

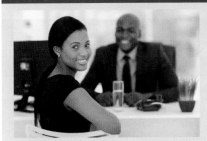

Amala has been looking forward to starting her externship at one of the community medical practices in her city. Today, she will visit the Healthy Hearts Cardiology Practice, a group of seven cardiologists affiliated with one of the city's university hospitals.

On the first day of her externship, she arrives 15 minutes early. As she enters the building, she steps into a waiting room filled with patients busily filling out forms, flipping through magazines, and watching a local television news program. She sees the receptionist at the far end of the room, waits for him to finish processing a patient, and steps forward. She introduces herself, explaining why she is there and asks for the clinic's administrator, Christopher Saardi. Mr. Saardi welcomes her and invites her on a quick tour of the facility. As they make their way through the maze of exam rooms and offices, Amala tries to memorize all of the faces, names, titles, and credentials on each of the staff members' name tags, but she knows that it will take a while to learn them all. "MD" and "RN" were familiar abbreviations, but she wishes she could have taken notes so that she could decipher all of the other abbreviations she saw.

Mr. Saardi finishes the tour with a stop in his office, where he informs Amala that he is currently working on checking the progress of the staff's continuing education.

HEALTH CARE PROFESSIONALS

The health services administrator is just one member of an entire medical team composed of specialists and support staff. Because there are so many different functions and roles in a medical team, there are differing levels of education and training for each provider and staff member.

The clinical side of medical care is involved in diagnosing and treating patients, whereas the non-clinical or administrative staff is instrumental in receiving and scheduling patients, coordinating the practice's daily activities and operations, and billing for visits. Depending on the size of the practice, a variety of qualified professionals are needed to fill both clinical and nonclinical staff roles. This section will describe the various members in a health care team and their education, training, credentials, roles, and in which health care settings they can be found (Fig. 2.1).

Credentialing

As discussed in Chapter 1, **credentials** verify an individual's professional qualifications. Almost all medical staff will need to be credentialed in one form or another, especially

○ credential a professional qualification, represented by the abbreviation a qualified individual may list after his or her name.

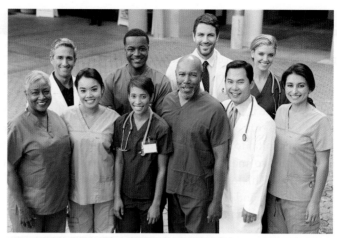

Figure 2.1 A variety of health professionals work to provide quality health care.

TABLE 2.1

SUMMARY OF HEALTH SERVICES OFFICE PROFESSIONALS, THEIR CREDENTIALS, AND THEIR ACCREDITING AGENCIES

Professional	Credential	Accrediting Agency
Physicians		
Medical Doctor	MD	Federation of State Medical Boards (FSMB) and the National Board of Medical Examiners® (NBME®)
Doctor of Osteopathy	DO	National Board of Osteopathic Medical Examiners (NBOME)
Physician Assistant	PA	National Commission on Certification of Physician Assistants (NCCPA)
Nurses		
Advanced Practice Registered Nurse	APRN	State Board of Nursing, National Council of State Boards of Nursing (NCSBN)
Registered Nurse	RN	State Board of Nursing, National Council of State Boards of Nursing (NCSBN)
Licensed Practical Nurse/Licensed Vocational Nurse	LPN or LVN	State Board of Nursing, National Council of State Boards of Nursing (NCSBN)
Medical Assistants	CMA	American Association of Medical Assistants (AAMA)
	RMA	American Medical Technologists (AMT)
	CCMA	National Healthcare Association (NHA)
	NCMA	National Center for Competency Testing (NCCT)
	NRCMA	National Association for Health Professionals (NAHP)
Medical Biller/ Coders	CCS, CPC, CPB	American Health Information Management Association (AHIMA)
	CPC	American Association of Professional Coders (AAPC)
	CPB	American Association of Professional Coders (AAPC)

certification the verification that an individual or entity has met certain professional standards.

if they are providing direct patient care. Table 2.1 summarizes the different kinds of health professionals and their qualifications. In addition to credentials, almost all health care professionals will have some kind of **certification**, which verifies the competence of professionals and, in some cases, legally allows them to work in their field.

Licensing

licensing an official permission to practice or operate.

Licensing is an official permission to perform certain duties. Some, but not all, of the medical staff in a clinic will require licenses according to state statutes and laws. For example, physicians and nurses must be licensed by the state in which they are employed. Medical billers, however, do not require a license, but may have a form of certification. The difference is that licenses are legal requirements, whereas certifications are not legally required for employment. However, some employers may prefer or even require certification. Whatever the level of required credentials your facility has chosen for each of the positions, the health services administrator needs to confirm that each staff member is current and compliant with the respective state and federal laws or accrediting body.

Physicians

Physicians are doctors who are licensed by their state medical boards and who are trained to diagnose and treat illnesses and disorders and to provide preventive care. After completing their bachelor's degree, which includes premedical coursework, they complete an additional four years of advanced training at medical school to receive their medical degree. Depending on the kind of medical school attended, the physician will either be a Medical Doctor (MD) or Osteopathic Doctor (DO). Traditionally, when we think of a physician, we think of a Medical Doctor or Doctor of Medicine (MD), who graduated from an allopathic medical school accredited by the Liaison Committee on Medical Education. Conversely, an Osteopathic Doctor or Doctor of Osteopathy (DO) is a graduate of an osteopathic school of medicine accredited by the American Osteopathic Associate Commission within the Commission on Osteopathic College Accreditation. Although the curricula are fairly similar at both medical schools, students attending osteopathic schools receive 200 hours of training on manipulation techniques of the musculoskeletal system, or osteopathic manipulation techniques.

physician a health care professional trained and licensed to diagnose and treat illnesses and disorders and to provide preventive care.

Both MDs and DOs can be fully licensed in all 50 states and must meet the same requirements to practice medicine by the Federation of State Medical Boards. To be licensed, osteopathic medical students must take the Comprehensive Medical Licensing Examination, whereas allopathic medical students must take the United States Medical Licensing Exam. Although you may find both types of physicians in all medical specialties, such as cardiology, orthopedics, and surgery, osteopathic physicians are more commonly found as primary care physicians.

Once they complete their medical education, physicians must complete a residency, which is a graduate level of medical training, to be licensed to practice medicine. Medical residency provides the physician specialized training in a specific branch of medicine, such as internal medicine, pediatrics, surgery, psychiatry, or obstetrics and gynecology. Currently, there are more than 9000 accredited residency programs and 24 different medical specialties in the United States. Residency training may be followed by a fellowship, or "subspecialty" training, such as child psychiatry, interventional cardiology, or sleep medicine. The majority of residency and fellowship programs are accredited by the Accreditation Council for Graduate Medical Education. After completing the residency or fellowship program and passing the respective exams, the physician will become "board certified" in that specialized field of medicine. Thus the entire process of becoming a board-certified physician may take 11 years or more: 4 years of college, 4 years of medical school, and 3 to 7 years of residency and fellowship.

Physicians are the primary providers of medical care to patients. They diagnose illnesses and prescribe and administer treatment for people suffering from injury or disease. They examine patients; obtain medical histories; and order, perform, and interpret diagnostic tests. They counsel patients on diet, hygiene, and preventive health care. Surgeons are specialized types of physicians who treat injuries and diseases through operations, although they may perform many of the same duties as other physicians. Using invasive surgical procedures, surgeons are able to correct physical deformities, repair bone and tissue after injuries, and perform preventive surgeries on patients with debilitating diseases or disorders. Additionally, some surgeons may choose to specialize in a specific area of surgery, such as orthopedic surgery or plastic or reconstructive surgery.

To maintain medical licensure and board certification, physicians must complete a specific number of **continuing medical education (CME)** credits, specified through the Federation of State Medical Boards. Thus an important role of the health services administrator will be to monitor the physician's completion of the CMEs and to ensure compliance with state and specialty boards.

An important role of the physician is to create an individualized **care plan** for the patient. In general, the patient's care plan includes an accurate and comprehensive assessment of the patient's health status, a problems list of the medical diagnoses, and the treatment plan. The purpose of the care plan is to guide all who are involved in the care of the patient—other physicians, nurses, or medical assistants—through a plan to appropriately care and treat the patient to ensure that the patient's **continuity of care** is complete. This care plan will be included in the patient's medical records for proper documentation, which will also be necessary for insurance and medical billing for services rendered.

Nurses

A **nurse** is a clinical health care professional who provides care to patients. The nurse's responsibility and duties are extensive and include performing physical exams and health histories; providing health promotion, counseling, and education; administering medications (Fig. 2.2); wound care; and numerous other medical interventions. Nurses may also coordinate care, based on the care plan created by the physician, and direct and supervise care delivered by other health care staff.

Although nurses may share similar duties to a physician, nurses, in general, do not require as much education and do not receive as extensive of a medical education or training. As a result, nurses have a more limited scope of practice, authority, and responsibility in patient care compared with physicians. However, some nurses with advanced training may be able to interpret patient information, diagnose illnesses and diseases, prescribe medication, and make critical decisions about patient care.

Today, nursing can take widely divergent paths. Nurses are divided into a variety of credentials and thus **scope of practice**, which determines the extent and limits of the types of procedures and actions a health care professional is permitted to perform based on his or her professional license. From a licensed practical nurse (LPN) or licensed

continuing medical education (CME) unit a measure of the amount of education a medical professional has acquired after a degree or credential, required to stay current in the field.

care plan the assessment of problems and plan for treatment of a patient.

continuity of care the communication and coordination of care among various health care professionals and facilities for the treatment of a patient's specific period of illness, or across a patient's lifetime.

nurse a clinical health care professional trained and licensed to provide care to patients.

TAKE AWAY ●·········

Nurses perform physical exams, take health histories, provide patient education, administer medications, and perform and coordinate care.

scope of practice the types of procedures a health care professional is permitted to perform in accordance with his or her licensure.

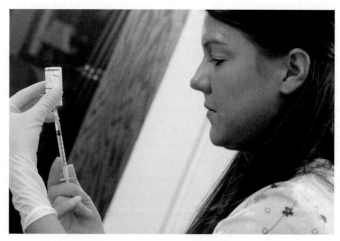

Figure 2.2 A nurse prepares to administer medication.

vocational nurse (LVN) to an advanced practice registered nurse (APRN), these types of nurses differ in the length of education, training, certification and licensing, and thus scope of practice. Additionally, each state has its own licensing board and statutes associated with the scope of practice.

Licensed practical nurses (LPNs) (or **licensed vocational nurses [LVNs]** in Texas, California, and Vermont) are nurses who work under the supervision of a registered nurse or physician. LPNs provide more basic nursing care and are responsible for the comfort of the patient, such as checking blood pressure, inserting catheters, helping patients bathe or dress, providing patient education, and reporting the patient's status to the registered nurse and doctor.

To become an LPN, the candidate must complete a year-long training program and pass the National Council Licensure Examination for Practical Nurses (NCLEX-PN) exam. LPNs are required to complete continuing education as stipulated by the state in which they practice to renew their licenses. LPNs are more often hired in nursing facilities and long-term care facilities.

Registered nurses (RNs) are able to administer medications, educate patients regarding their conditions (Fig. 2.3), and coordinate care. They interview patients about their medical history, record symptoms, and document progress. They can also supervise nursing students, practical nurses, and nursing assistants. RNs are fairly evenly distributed throughout the various health care settings.

To become an RN, there are three educational levels: Bachelor of Science in Nursing (BSN), an Associate's Degree in Nursing (ADN or ASN), or a diploma from an approved nursing program. BSNs usually take 4 years to complete, and ADN and diploma programs usually require 2 to 3 years to complete. All programs include courses in social, behavior, and physical science and clinical experiences in various health care settings. Once the program has been completed, the graduate must pass the National Council Licensure Examination for Registered Nurses (NCLEX-RN) to become a registered nurse. An RN's license is regulated by the individual state's board of nursing and, although continuing education requirements vary by state, RNs are generally required to complete 15 to 30 CMEs every 2 years to maintain their license.

RNs work under the supervision of a physician, and their scope of practice varies by state. In addition, some RNs may choose to become certified through professional associations in certain specialties, such as pediatrics, oncology, and surgical. Certification is usually voluntary, but some advanced positions require it.

An **advanced practice registered nurse (APRN)** has completed a master's degree or doctoral-level degree program and has obtained a variety of skills and knowledge

licensed practical (vocational) nurse (LPN, LVN) a nurse working under the supervision of an RN who measures vital signs and performs some interventions.

registered nurse (RN) a clinical health care professional trained and licensed to deliver interventions to promote patient well-being, including administering medications, educating patients regarding their conditions, and coordinating care.

advanced practice registered nurse (APRN) a clinical health care professional who provides patient care and who has advanced training and authority to prescribe medication and practice independently without physician oversight in some states.

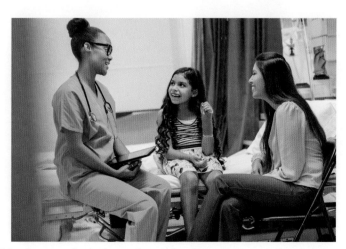

Figure 2.3 RNs educate patients about what to do after treatment, such as how to care for a cast.

required for advanced clinical practice. As a result, APRNs may work in more advanced positions and roles, including clinical nurse specialists, certified nurse practitioners, certified registered nurse anesthetists, and certified nurse-midwives. APRNs play a more active and central role in direct patient diagnosis and treatment.

Depending on individual states, some APRNs work under the supervision of a physician, whereas others may work independently and in a similar capacity to that of the physician, allowing them to develop care plans, prescribe medication, and provide primary care in a variety of health care settings. In fact, APRNs may be the lead practitioners in retail clinics that offer more basic health services in national drug store chains and grocery stores. In addition to the CME requirements for RNs, some states require a minimum number of practice hours before licensure renewal.

Physician Assistants (PAs)

Physician assistants (PAs) grew out of the need for more primary care physicians during the mid-1960s. The role of PAs was originally filled by medics in the military, specifically former US Navy Hospital Corpsmen. Now, there are now more than 222 accredited PA programs in the United States, represented by the Physician Assistant Education Association.

PAs, like APRNs, are responsible for diagnosing and treating patients, providing patient education, and documenting treatment. PAs are able to prescribe medication in the United States, although their scope of practice varies according to jurisdiction and care setting. Most PAs work independently of physician supervision but maintain an agreement with a supervising physician. They generally practice on medical teams with physicians and other health care professionals.

A PA will have earned a master's degree from an accredited school in either Physician Assistant Studies (MPAS), Health Science (MHS), or Medical Science (MMSc), and must pass the Physician Assistant National Certifying Examination (PANCE) administered by the National Commission on Certification of Physician Assistants (NCCPA). Licensure is regulated by the medical boards of the individual states. To maintain their license, PAs are required to complete 100 CMEs every 10 years.

Medical Assistants

Medical assistants (MAs) are trained to fill both clinical and administrative roles in health care settings. Although they work under the license of a physician, in some states, MAs may be supervised by a podiatrist, physician assistant, nurse practitioner, or nurse midwife. Medical assistants take vital signs (Fig. 2.4), record patient information,

physician assistant (PA) a clinical health care professional who provides primary care under the supervision of a physician.

TAKE AWAY

PAs practice medicine: they diagnose and treat patients and prescribe medication working with a physician.

medical assistant (MA) a health professional who provides both clinical and administrative support in a health care setting.

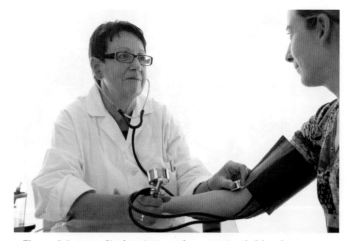

Figure 2.4 A medical assistant takes a patient's blood pressure.

take patient history, administer medications and injections, and collect and prepare specimens for laboratory testing. They instruct patients about medications and special diets, authorize drug refills as directed, telephone prescriptions to a pharmacy, draw blood, prepare patients for x-rays, take electrocardiograms, remove sutures, and change dressings. They also facilitate communication between the patient and other health care professionals. Additionally, MAs can manage medical offices, schedule patients, answer phones, and code and bill for services rendered in the medical office.

The training programs for MAs vary, although most complete formal education at postsecondary institutions, such as vocational schools, technical institutes, community or junior colleges, proprietary colleges, or online educational programs. MA training programs most commonly lead to a certificate or a diploma, which can take 9 to 12 months to complete, or an associate degree, which takes 2 years to complete.

There is no requirement for MAs to become licensed or certified, except in a few states. However, job duties in many states may be limited for those who are not certified. In addition, an increasing number of employers are looking for certified or registered MAs and often show them preference when hiring.

CURRENT TRENDS IN HEALTH CARE

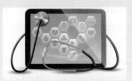

Many employers insisted their MAs be certified or registered after the 2008 passage of the Health Information Technology for Economic and Clinical Health (HITECH) Act. This legislation offered extra payments through the Centers for Medicare and Medicaid Services for using the electronic health record when eligible professionals, which includes MAs, are certified or registered.

A number of certifying agencies provide certification or registration to MAs:

- Registered Medical Assistant (RMA), through the American Medical Technologist (AMT)
- Certified Clinical Medical Assistant (CCMA) and Certified Medical Administrative Assistant (CMAA), through the National Healthcare Association (NHA)
- Certified Medical Assistant (CMA), through the American Association of Medical Assistants (AAMA)
- National Certified Medical Assistant (NCMA), through the National Center for Competency Testing (NCCT)
- Nationally Registered Certified Medical Assistant (NRCMA), through the National Association for Health Professionals (NAHP).

Depending on the certifying agency, registered or certified MAs usually must complete 12 CMEs every year.

Medical Billers and Coders

Medical billers and coders perform the important task of translating patient medical information into numeric or alphanumeric codes to submit a *claim* to insurance companies for them to determine the appropriate charge for the patient visit. Through this process of billing, the medical biller and coder ensures that the health care provider and the medical facility are paid or reimbursed for the services they provided to the patient. Additionally, the health services administrator will use this information, along with other practice costs, to manage the overall operation and finances of the clinic.

The reimbursement process begins with the medical coder translating the patient's medical report into a code using three main code sets: Current Procedural Terminology,

International Classification of Diseases, and Healthcare Common Procedure Coding System. Each of these code sets will be further discussed in Chapter 5. These code sets help medical coders document the condition of a patient and describe the medical procedure performed on the patient. Next, the medical billers take this information from the coder and, using a different code set, then code for the procedures and services. The medical biller is also responsible for preparing the invoices and claims to submit to the insurance companies and other payers. Medical billers work closely with patients and insurance companies to ensure invoices are paid on time and that health care providers are appropriately reimbursed for procedures they perform. Depending on the size and type of medical facility, one person may serve as both the medical biller and coder.

Medical billers and coders may be trained on the job, but they are more likely to receive formal training through courses offered by schools or community colleges or other accredited institutions, which may lead to a certificate, diploma, or degree. Although certification for medical billing and coding are not required for employment, most employers look for some type of certification. There are several different credentialing associations and a number of different certifications, depending on the type of practice and facility the medical biller and coder will be working at. The American Health Information Management Association (AHIMA) offers two certifications: Certified Coding Specialist (CCS) and the Certified Coding Specialist-Physician-based (CCS-P). The American Association of Professional Coders (AAPC) also has several coding credentials, the most notable being the Certified Professional Coder (CPC) and Certified Outpatient Coder (COC). Another certification for medical billers is the Certified Professional Biller (CPB) through the AAPC. To maintain certification, 20 CME credits are required every 2 years for the CCS-P, and 36 CME credits every 2 years for the CPB.

Other Health Professionals

In addition to the health care professionals discussed above, the health services administrator will interact with a wide range of other allied health professionals, listed in Table 2.2.

Allied health professionals are a part of a health care team and provide a wide range of diagnostic, technical, therapeutic, and direct patient care and support services that

TABLE 2.2

ALLIED HEALTH CARE PROFESSIONALS

Health Care Professional	Description
Acupuncturist	An alternative medical professional who inserts needles into the skin to relieve pain and other ailments.
Chiropractor	An alternative medical professional who manipulates the spine and other joints to promote the general health of the body.
Electroencephalographic (EEG) Technologist	A health care professional who records the electrical activity of the brain to help detect epilepsy, sleep disorders, cerebrovascular accidents (strokes), and other conditions.
Electrocardiograph (ECG or EKG) Technician	A health care professional who records the electrical activity of the heart to help detect myocardial infarction (heart attack) and dysrhythmias that may indicate a heart problem.
Occupational Therapist	A health care professional who helps people with physical and mental disabilities achieve their highest possible level of independence.
Pharmacist	A health care professional knowledgeable in the use and effects of medication. A *community pharmacist* is usually responsible for dispensing drugs prescribed by a physician.

TABLE 2.2

ALLIED HEALTH CARE PROFESSIONALS—cont'd

Health Care Professional	Description
Pharmacy Technician	A health care professional who performs administrative functions in the pharmacy and dispenses drugs under the supervision of the pharmacist.
Phlebotomist	A health care professional who draws blood from patients for analysis by a laboratory, blood donation, or medical research.
Physical Therapist	A health care professional who treats conditions that limit a person's mobility.
Radiographer	A health care professional who produces x-rays, CT scans, MRIs, and other types of anatomical images.
Registered Dietician	A trained nutritional professional who advises and counsels others on food and nutrition.
Respiratory Therapist	A specialized practitioner who diagnoses and treats problems associated with the pulmonary system, that is, the lungs and heart.
Sonographer	A health care professional who uses ultrasound waves to produce anatomical images.

are critical to the other health professionals they work with, particularly physicians and nurses.

They can be found in a variety of health care settings, and their training and education may vary. Some allied health professionals receive on-the-job training, whereas others must complete degrees or diplomas, be certified or licensed, and complete continuing education. Although all of these allied health professionals provide patient care, their scope of practice is specialized and limited, and they usually do not diagnose patients.

LEARNING CHECKPOINT 2.1

Health Care Professionals

1. What do the credentials DO stand for? _____

2. Which member of the health care team creates the care plan?
   _____

3. Which credential allows the nurse to deliver primary care?
   _____

4. A PA and an APRN will have earned at least a(n) _____ degree.

5. The abbreviation MA stands for which member of the health care team?
   _____

6. Medical billers and coders submit a(n) _____ to the insurance company.

7. A(n) _____ is an allied health professional who produces x-rays, computed tomography (CT) scans, magnetic resonance images (MRIs), and other types of anatomical images.

AMBULATORY CARE SETTINGS

ambulatory care outpatient health care provided to patients who arrive at the facility, receive treatment, and leave on the same day.

outpatient a patient who receives treatment during a visit on a single day.

visit an episode of service to a patient in an outpatient setting. Also called an encounter.

encounter an episode of service to a patient in an outpatient setting. Also called a visit.

acute care inpatient health care for severe illnesses or injuries requiring a hospital stay in a facility where the average stay is 30 days or less.

inpatient a patient admitted to a facility at least overnight by order of a physician.

Health care settings are generally divided into two basic types, usually depending on how severe the patient's illness or disease is and how long the treatment will take: *ambulatory care* (outpatient) and *acute care* (inpatient). When treatment occurs on the same day, it is called **ambulatory care**. The term *ambulatory* comes from the Latin root *ambulo-*, meaning to walk. You might remember this by thinking of ambulatory care patients as able to walk in and back out of the facility, such as a medical office, versus a patient who is transported by an ambulance and carried on a gurney into the hospital. Patients treated in ambulatory care settings are called **outpatients**, and the patients' interactions with health care professionals are called **visits** or **encounters**. In contrast, care for severe injuries or illnesses, such as when a patient is admitted to a hospital, is called **acute care,** and these patients are called **inpatients**. In the United States, patients in an acute care facility stay an average of 6 days or less.

Ambulatory care offers several advantages to patients, providers, and payers, including health insurers. Compared to inpatient hospital care, ambulatory settings offer a shorter length of total treatment time, more flexibility in scheduling, and other efficiencies that have led to lower costs. Some ambulatory care centers perform laboratory tests, diagnostic procedures, and treatments that would traditionally have been part of an inpatient stay, but are now able to be performed outside the hospital. This allows for shorter inpatient stays at lower costs to both the patient and insurance company.

There are two types of ambulatory care centers: hospital based and free-standing. Hospital-based ambulatory care is operated by a hospital or associated with a hospital in some way. In some cases, a hospital shares resources with an ambulatory care center, or it is overseen by the same owner or board of directors. Although located on hospital grounds, an emergency department (ED) is a type of ambulatory care setting (Fig. 2.5). Although patients in the ED are sometimes admitted to the hospital as inpatients, their treatment is intended to be a single occurrence, where the patients arrive and leave on the same day. It is common for the ED to share staffing, technology, billing, and other resources with the hospital. If additional care or treatment is needed, the ED works in conjunction with the hospital to admit a patient for additional or advanced health care services and monitoring.

Types of hospital-based ambulatory care centers are shown in Table 2.3. These offer treatments normally associated with inpatient stays, in conjunction with acute care centers, and as part of a larger treatment regimen.

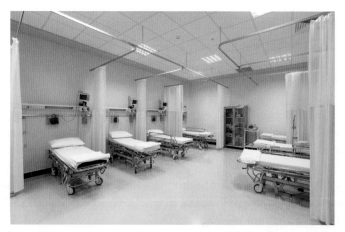

Figure 2.5 An emergency department is an ambulatory care setting.

TABLE 2.3

HOSPITAL-BASED AMBULATORY CARE SETTINGS

Setting	Services
Emergency Department (ED)	Provides medical care to patients who are critically ill or have suffered trauma and is offered on a walk-in basis.
Clinic	Provides specialty medical services such as dialysis, cancer treatment, prenatal care, and rehabilitative services, which may be offered on a scheduled or walk-in basis.
Diagnostic Facility	Provides diagnostic, radiology, and imaging centers to perform procedures such as x-rays, CT scans, MRIs, cardiac stress tests, ultrasounds, and other provider-ordered tests. These services can be offered on a scheduled or walk-in basis.
Ambulatory Surgery Center (ASC)	Provides medical services in the form of same-day surgical procedures, including patient intake, preoperative care, recovery care, and postoperative care. Services are usually scheduled by appointment.
Urgent Care Clinic	Provides medical treatment to those who cannot wait for a scheduled primary care physician appointment, do not have a designated primary care physician, or have an acute care situation that does not require emergency room treatment. Services are offered on a walk-in basis or by appointment.
Physician's Office	Physicians and other health care providers offering primary care in a group or individual office setting. Offices usually offer appointments and accept walk-ins.
Public Health Department	Preventative care, vaccinations, health screenings, and various other services offered to the public on a walk-in basis.
School Clinic	Medical services offered on a college or university campus, usually on a walk-in basis or by appointment.
Health Clinic	Offered either as part of a business, group of businesses, or in communities to offer general medical services at reduced or lower costs. Services can be delivered as an appointment or walk-in basis.

The second type of ambulatory care center is free-standing. These centers are individually owned and operated or associated with a hospital. Some outpatient surgery centers and many specialized clinics offering services, such as dialysis centers, are hospital based and some are free-standing.

Physician's Office

The foundation for much of the health care delivery system in the United States is the physician's office, where patients are served by an individual or group of providers and health care team. Most **physician offices** provide patients with **primary care**, which is the first and most basic level of treatment for injury or illness. They serve as the entry point for health care consumers into the health care delivery system (Fig. 2.6). Patients receive basic medical services from their **primary care provider (PCP)**, who may be a specialist in family medicine, internal medicine, or pediatrics. A PCP is often referred to as a *family doctor* or *physician*.

In the physician's office, patients receive routine medical care, treatment for chronic illness, limited acute care, and preventive care. In some health care systems and insurance

physician's office an ambulatory care setting served by an individual or group of primary care providers.

primary care the first and most basic level of treatment for injury or illness, serving as the entry point for health care consumers into the health care delivery system.

primary care provider (PCP) a physician or other provider designated by the patient to deliver primary care and refer the patient to other specialists as necessary.

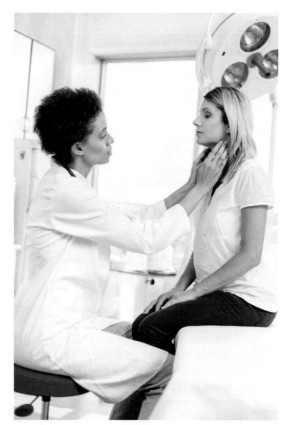

Figure 2.6 The physician's office is an ambulatory care setting where the primary provider is a physician.

CURRENT TRENDS IN HEALTH CARE

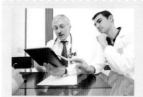

A primary care provider may be a physician, physician assistant, or nurse practitioner. Most physician assistants or nurse practitioners will work under the direction or supervision of a physician and provide care within their scope of practice or may refer the patient to see the physician, when necessary.

gatekeeper a primary care provider who sees the patient first to control access to other parts of the health care delivery system.

referral a provider's request for the services of another provider, often a specialist.

plans, PCPs may function as **gatekeepers**, where, after seeing the patient, they may order imaging or laboratory work, admit the patient to a hospital, or request a **referral** to a specialist. Oftentimes, insurance coverage may require a patient to see the PCP before seeing another health care provider, particularly a specialist. The use of PCPs as gatekeepers results in greater continuity of care for the patient and reduces the number of referrals and costs.

Organization

Physician offices are usually structured with one or more physicians overseeing medical treatment at the facility. Most physician offices have a health services administrator or medical office manager, who oversees the daily functions and operation of the office. Fig. 2.7 illustrates the organization of a typical physician's office.

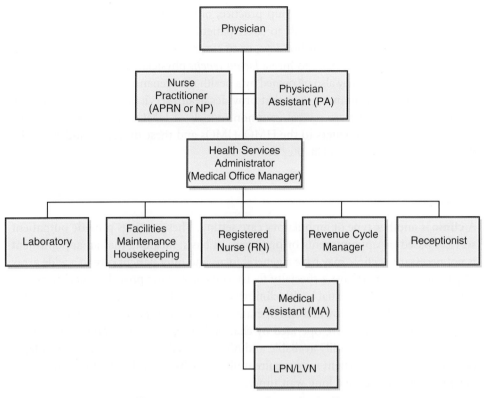

Figure 2.7 Organization of a medical office.

Ownership

Physician's offices may have several different arrangements. A sole proprietorship (also called a *solo practice* or *private practice*) is the simplest business structure available for a provider practice. The sole proprietorship is owned by one physician. All income and debts incurred by the practice are the sole responsibility of the physician. The advantage of this practice is the owner/physician makes all decisions regarding the operation of the practice and is not accountable to other owners. The disadvantage is that the owner bears the sole financial responsibility for the practice and must find another physician to fill in when the owner/physician is on vacation, ill, or for any other reasons. This physician is often referred to as *locum tenens* physician and may serve on a temporary basis for a few days or several months.

A partnership is where two providers own the practice. Oftentimes, partnerships are formed among doctors of the same specialty. For instance, two obstetricians can set up a partnership for an obstetrical practice. The advantage is that there are two providers available to offer services, and the facility, equipment, and expenses can be shared. The disadvantage is that there may be disagreements in the decision-making process.

In a group practice, multiple physicians share ownership of the practice. A group practice may be a single specialty, such as a group of pediatricians or gynecologists or composed of multiple specialties. For example, a group of internal medicine physicians may include a gerontologist (for patients who are 65 years old and older) and an endocrinologist (for patients with diabetes). These doctors are then able to offer medical care for specific groups of patients under one roof. The compensation in a group practice may be by sharing of the profits, a salary, or both. Bonuses may also be paid when the practice does financially well within a fiscal term.

TAKE AWAY ●·········

Physician practices may be a sole proprietorship, partnership, or group practice or be owned by a health maintenance organization (HMO).

In both the partnership and group practice, one great advantage is the ability to share the burden of being "on call" to cover patients during nonbusiness hours, such as nights, weekends, and major holidays, or to cover when one of the physicians is on vacation. This avoids the need to hire a *locum tenens* physician.

A physician's office may also be owned by a health maintenance organization (HMO), which is a medical insurance group that provides health services for a fixed annual fee or prepaid basis. There are several common models of HMOs, differing only in the relationships of the providers to the HMO. HMOs and these different models will be discussed in more detail in Chapter 3.

Clinic

clinic an ambulatory setting providing general or specialized care, sometimes on a walk-in basis and sometimes at a reduced cost for disadvantaged populations.

A **clinic** is another type of ambulatory care setting. These settings provide outpatient services based on appointments or on a walk-in basis, meaning that an appointment is not necessary. A clinic may have a general focus and offer patient care to a wide array of patients, or it may have a specialty focus, such as a clinic providing health care to expectant mothers or a sexual health clinic that treats and prevents sexually transmitted diseases. Some clinics are owned and operated by government entities, such as counties or cities, whereas others are operated by charitable organizations. Patients use clinics because health care is readily available and often at a reduced cost. The disadvantages of clinics are that the patient may require multiple visits to see different providers, and patients may experience a long wait time.

Diagnostic Facility

TAKE AWAY •·········

Diagnostic facilities provide imaging or lab services.

A diagnostic outpatient facility operates for the purpose of conducting medical diagnostic tests on patients, as ordered by the provider. These facilities are usually independent of a physician's office or hospital. Diagnostic tests are performed, and the results are utilized by other health care professionals at other health care facilities. Diagnostic facilities may offer various imaging studies, including radiography (x-rays), mammography, ultrasonography, electrocardiography, MRIs, and computerized axial tomography (CAT or CT scan). Other types of diagnostic facilities provide laboratory services and perform tests on blood, body fluids, and other specimens. Patients are not provided any other services other than diagnostic tests, and the facility does not provide any type of patient care.

Ambulatory Surgery Center (ASC)

ambulatory surgery center (ASC) a surgical facility that performs procedures on patients who are not admitted to a hospital for recovery.

Ambulatory surgery centers (ASCs), commonly referred to as *same-day surgery centers*, are health care facilities that provide surgical procedures to patients in a single visit without an overnight stay. Outpatient surgeries have increased dramatically over the last several years because more types of surgeries can be minimally invasive and performed in shorter periods. This has resulted in fewer complications, patients being able to go home within a few hours after surgery, and reduced costs of procedures. Some of the most common ambulatory surgical procedures performed include cataract surgery (Fig. 2.8), upper and lower gastrointestinal (GI) endoscopy, spinal injections, and knee and shoulder surgeries.

Ambulatory surgery centers may be owned by physicians, but they are usually owned by an inpatient health care facility or health care corporation, such as a hospital system. Physicians are generally employees of the outpatient surgical facility and are paid per procedure performed.

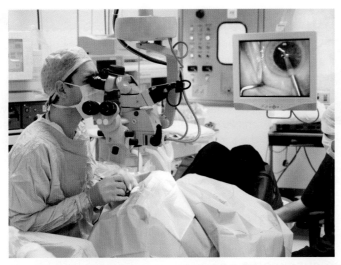

Figure 2.8 Cataract surgery is a procedure commonly performed in an ambulatory surgery center.

Urgent Care Clinic

Urgent care clinics are a type of walk-in clinic that provides services for patients who need immediate medical care but whose injuries or illnesses are not serious enough to be seen in an emergency department. Urgent care clinics operate on a walk-in basis during regular business hours, with some clinics open on weekends and evenings. These clinics provide a broad range of services, including minor medical procedures, and are staffed by a licensed provider, such as a physician, physician assistant, or nurse practitioner. Most urgent care clinics have onsite diagnostic services, such as phlebotomy and x-ray. Urgent care clinics are often owned by a health care corporation, but may also be owned by a group of physicians. It is also quite common to see urgent care clinics owned by a franchise corporation and have multiple clinics of the same name and organization throughout a region.

> **urgent care clinic** walk-in clinic that provides services for patients who need immediate medical care but whose injuries or illnesses are not serious enough to be seen in an emergency department.

Retail Health Clinic

A **retail health clinic** is a walk-in clinic that is offered onsite at a retail store, such as a large department store or pharmacy. These clinics are equipped to treat uncomplicated, minor illnesses and are often staffed by nurse practitioners or physician assistants. Most clinics operate on a walk-in basis, but some take appointments. Some patients who utilize a retail-based health clinic are unable to get an appointment with their primary care provider within a reasonable amount of time; others are traveling and unsure about where to find a physician. Other patients may not have health insurance or do not have a primary care provider. Retail health clinics also offer lower costs to patients compared with a physician's office visit and are open in the evenings and on weekends.

> **retail care clinic** a walk-in clinic offered onsite at a retail store, such as a large department store or pharmacy, equipped to treat uncomplicated, minor illnesses.

These clinics are filling a growing need by providing fast, high-quality, low-priced health care to a population of patients who need to be seen by a health care provider for minor health concerns. Common ailments treated at retail clinics are cold and flu symptoms, ear and eye infections, and skin and foot conditions. They offer physicals, vaccinations, and even pregnancy tests. Because of limited space and services, retail clinics do not treat more serious illnesses or injuries, such as fractures or lacerations.

CURRENT TRENDS IN HEALTH CARE

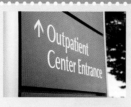

The number and types of procedures done in hospitals are on the decline, whereas those performed in outpatient settings are rising. According to the Medicare Payment Advisory Commission (MedPAC) 2016 report to Congress, payments for inpatient services decreased 7% between 2013 and 2014, whereas outpatient payments increased 11% for the same period.

Medicare Payment Advisory Commission: Report to the Congress: Medicare payment policy. Availavble at http://www.medpac.gov/docs/default-source/reports/march-2016-report-to-the-congress-medicare-payment-policy.pdf?sfvrsn=0. Accessed June 29, 2017.

LEARNING CHECKPOINT 2.2
Ambulatory Care Settings

1. What do the initials PCP stand for? _____

2. A(n) _____ facility offers imaging studies like x-rays and MRIs.

3. A(n) _____ provides services for patients who need immediate medical care but whose injuries or illnesses are not serious enough to be seen in an emergency department.

4. A(n) _____ offers care for mild ailments in a department store or drug store chain.

ACUTE CARE SETTINGS

TAKE AWAY

Acute care settings treat patients with a medical condition or trauma that requires around-the-clock care for a severe episode of illness or injury.

○ **hospital** a facility that provides medical services to the general population in the form of emergency care, critical care, intensive care, and various types of patient care requiring inpatient treatment.

Most health care provided in a hospital setting is classified as acute care. Acute care is needed when there is a medical condition or source of trauma that will require immediate or around-the-clock care for a severe episode of illness or injury. In acute care facilities, medical care is intended to take place at least overnight, and the average stay must be less than 30 days, according to state licensure standards. Most acute care facilities have an average stay of 3 to 6 days.

Hospital

Hospitals are a type of acute care facility. There are many different types of hospitals that focus on the care and treatment of a designated population and their specific medical needs. General hospitals provide medical services to the general population in the form of emergency care, critical care, intensive care, and various types of patient care requiring inpatient treatment. Other hospitals may focus on specialized populations or treatment, such as a children's hospital or a cancer treatment facility. Another type of inpatient facility is a rehabilitation hospital that specializes in the recovery process of patients who have dealt with trauma, stroke, or other issues that have caused impairment to their ability to perform activities of daily living. Behavioral health hospitals

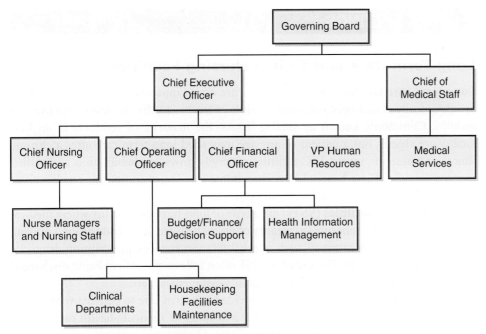

Figure 2.9 Hospital organization chart.

provide treatment in the form of psychiatric, psychological, and social services to patients with mental and emotional disorders.

Hospitals range in size and scope. Hospital size is often measured by its bed count, which is the number of beds the facility has ready to treat patients. It references the total number of patients who can be treated at any one time. Small rural hospitals can maintain 10 beds, whereas larger facilities may have 500 beds or more.

In general, the hospital organization is divided by function, which usually includes nursing, laboratory services, medical records, billing, information technology, human resources, environmental services, administrative support, security, and other ancillary departments. Fig. 2.9 shows an organizational chart for a typical hospital.

Hospital are regulated by federal, state, and local laws and regulations that ensure compliance and standards of care. Hospitals may be single hospitals or part of a multi-hospital system that is owned or managed as part of a system of two or more medical facilities. Hospitals may be organized as a corporation, government funded (such as the Veterans Administration), for profit, or not-for-profit, such as hospitals owned by religious institutions. Regardless of ownership, a board of directors oversees strategic initiatives and the overall business of providing health care. Some hospitals may have various organizational structures with a chief executive officer or a controller who is a physician in charge of operations.

Some doctors who see patients in a hospital are employees of the hospital, but many are not. Instead, hospitals may grant hospital *privileges* to physicians who are not employees of the hospital. **Privileges** allow a licensed physician to perform certain procedures or operations and to admit patients to the hospital. In order to be approved for hospital privileges, the hospital must determine if the physician is qualified by evaluating the physician's education, residency training, and references. The hospital may then grant the physician either *courtesy privileges* or *full privileges*. Courtesy hospital privileges limit the physician to admitting only a nominal number of patients to the hospital. Full hospital privileges allows physicians to admit an unlimited number of patients to the hospital, and they are usually given all the privileges needed to perform procedures based on their medical specialty.

privileges a physician's permission to use hospital facilities to treat patients.

TAKE AWAY ●·········

Hospitals grant *privileges* to physicians who are not employees of the hospital, allowing them to practice medicine there.

OTHER SETTINGS

Long-Term Care and Skilled Nursing Facilities

long-term care facility (LTC)
a health care facility that provides care on an inpatient basis to patients who are chronically ill and need extended services or treatments; commonly called a *nursing home.*

Long-term care facilities (LTCs) provide care on an inpatient basis to patients who are chronically ill and need extended services or treatments from a few weeks to a few months. Commonly known as *nursing homes,* the majority of residents in an LTC facility are elderly, but a patient of any age may need long-term care after a chronic illness or traumatic injury. LTC facilities generally provide rehabilitation and skilled nursing services after a hospital stay when home care is not an option. The length of stay in an LTC is intended to be 30 days or more.

skilled nursing facility (SNF)
a type of long-term care facility providing subacute nursing care.

Skilled nursing facilities (SNFs) are a type of long-term care facility where medical professionals provide subacute (a category of illness between acute and chronic) nursing care and administer treatments such as rehabilitation services, prescription drugs, IV therapy, and wound care. The use of an SNF often follows the patient being discharged from an acute care facility and needing additional medical care.

intermediate care facility (ICF)
a health care facility that provides long-term care most often to developmentally disabled patients who do not require the degree of medical care given at a hospital or subacute health care facility

Intermediate care facilities (ICFs) provide long-term care to patients who do not require the degree of medical care given at a hospital or subacute health care facility, but still require more than just custodial care. Oftentimes, patients in an ICF are developmentally disabled. Services often performed in this type of health care setting include the daily administration of prescription medication, occupational and physical therapy, psychological services, and assistance with basic daily activities, such as meal preparation and housekeeping. These facilities may receive licenses to operate by their state, but are federally regulated to be able to bill for Medicare and Medicaid reimbursements.

assisted living facility facilities that provide housing and support services, such as personal care, housekeeping, and coordinated recreational activities.

Assisted living facilities provide housing services to residents on a monthly basis and provide support services, such as personal care, housekeeping, and coordinated recreational activities (Fig. 2.10). This type of facility is not to be confused with an LTC (nursing home) facility, where medical care and treatment are administered. Assisted living facilities are similar to *independent living facilities* that provide health care and social support to residents who live in an apartment or condominium. Assisted living usually provides more in-depth services compared with independent living facilities, and these facilities often offer both independent and assisted living in different parts of the facility, allowing residents the option of transferring as their level of care increases.

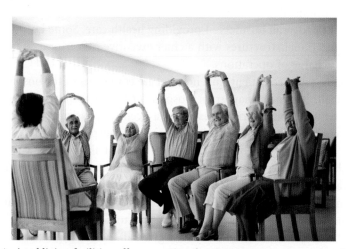

Figure 2.10 Assisted living facilities offer recreational activities to promote and maintain health.

Home Health Care

Home health care is an outpatient treatment for patients who are chronically or terminally ill. This service provides patients with the comfort and convenience of receiving necessary medical treatment in the familiar setting of their own home. Home health agencies offer medical services, such as nursing care, personal care, treatment administration, rehabilitative services, and the administration of prescribed medication. Some agencies may offer more advanced medical services and may employ nurses for medical service provisions and home health aides who can assist with basic needs, including bathing, housekeeping, and meal preparation.

> **home health care** health care services provided in the patient's home.

Hospice Care

Hospice care is medical care and service for terminally ill patients, usually with a life expectancy of fewer than 6 months. In this setting, treatment is not curative, but **palliative care,** which is to provide relief from the symptoms of the illness and to relieve or reduce pain. Although hospice care can be offered in a hospital or nursing home setting, it may be offered in the patient's home.

Hospice care not only manages pain and symptoms during the duration of its service, but also considers the emotional needs of the terminally ill patient and family. Hospice care encompasses services such as counseling for physical, emotional, and spiritual needs, as well as bereavement support for the patient's family after the end of care. Hospice care providers are skilled in dealing with end-of-life conversations and situations and help make patients and family members more comfortable during this time. Some hospice care agencies incorporate music therapists and clergy as members of their care options for patients.

> **hospice care** noncurative care delivered to patients at the end of their lives.

> **palliative care** a medical treatment to ease a patient's pain or reduce symptoms, but which is not intended to cure a disease or disorder.

CASE STUDY

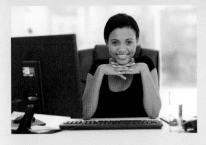

As Amala finished clearing her desk for the day, she reflected on the different employees whom she met on her tour of the office. Although she still knew that she would need to review all of the notes she took during the day, she now was able to sort out the employees and the types of duties that they performed. Mr. Saardi showed her how the staff was progressing on their required CMEs, and she had a new appreciation for how certifying and credentialing bodies ensured their members were current in their fields. Amala was also impressed with Mr. Saardi's oversight of the training and education of the office's staff. She could see how the importance of being certified and maintaining certification helps in ensuring quality patient care and reducing employee turnover and the costs of hiring and training new employees.

REVIEW QUESTIONS

1. What is the difference between certification and licensing?

2. What is a scope of practice?

3. How are physician assistants (PAs) and advanced practice registered nurses (APRNs) similar to physicians? How are they different?

4. List three clinical roles of the medical assistant (MA) in the medical office.

5. What do medical billers and coders do, and who offers their certification?

6. Besides physicians, nurses, and MAs, what other clinical health care professionals help deliver patient care? List three and briefly describe what they do.

7. What is the difference between ambulatory care and acute care?

8. List and describe three different ambulatory care settings.

9. List and describe three different inpatient care settings.

10. Describe the function of hospice care. What services does it provide?

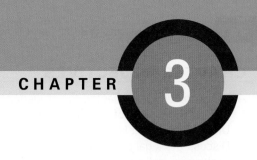

CHAPTER

3

HEALTH CARE DELIVERY[1]

Jaime Nguyen and Carol Colvin

CHAPTER OUTLINE

INTRODUCTION
HISTORY OF HEALTH CARE IN
THE UNITED STATES
Health Care Providers
Health Insurance
Federal Government Involvement
The HMO Act of 1973
*Employee Retirement Income
and Security Act (ERISA)
of 1974*
*Tax Equity and Fiscal
Responsibility Act (TEFRA)
of 1982*
*Consolidated Omnibus
Reconciliation Act (COBRA)*
*Health Insurance Portability
and Accountability Act
(HIPAA)*

*Balanced Budget Act (BBA)
of 1997*
Affordable Care Act (ACA)
LEGAL AND REGULATORY
OVERSIGHT
Federal
State
Local
Accreditation
Professional Standards
PAYING FOR HEALTH CARE
Insurance
Assumption of Risk
Types of Health Insurance
Indemnity
Managed Care
*Health Maintenance
Organizations (HMOs)*

*Preferred Provider
Organizations (PPOs)*
Point of Service (POS)
*High-Deductible Health Plans
(HDHPs)*
The Affordable Care Act (ACA)
Medicare
Medicaid
CHARACTERISTICS AND
CHALLENGES
Integrated and Fragmented Care
Rising Costs
Uninsured and Underinsured
Populations

VOCABULARY

Accountable Care Organization
(ACO)
accreditation
Affordable Care Act (ACA)
assignment
Centers for Medicare and Medicaid
Services (CMS)
claim
coinsurance
Conditions of Participation (CoP)
continuum of care
copay (copayment)
deductible
deemed status
Department of Health and Human
Services (DHHS)

Emergency Medical Treatment and
Active Labor Act (EMTALA)
entitlement program
gatekeeper
group plan
guarantor
Health Insurance Portability and
Accountability Act (HIPAA)
health maintenance organization
(HMO)
indemnity insurance
indigent
interoperability
licensure
managed care
Medicaid

Medicare
payer
Point of Service (POS)
preferred provider organization (PPO)
premium
primary care provider (PCP)
prospective payment system (PPS)
referral
reimbursement
subscriber
Tax Equity and Fiscal Responsibility
Act of 1982 (TEFRA)
The Joint Commission
underinsured
universal health care

---

[1]The editors wish to acknowledge the work of Nadinia Davis, whose writing on reimbursement in *Foundations of Health Information Management* provides the basis for much of the content of this chapter.

CHAPTER OBJECTIVES

After completing this chapter, the student should be able to do the following:

1. Outline the history of health care delivery in the United States and key US government initiatives.
2. Discuss the legal and regulatory structures that guide health care delivery.
3. Distinguish among the various ways people pay for health care.
4. Explain the characteristics and challenges of the US health care system.

INTRODUCTION

There are more than 320 million people currently living in the United States, and almost every single person will interact with the health care system. Whether it is at the time of birth in a hospital or birthing center, a trip to the emergency room after a house project gone awry, sitting at the bedside of a loved one as they battle illness, or having money taken out of each paycheck for health insurance, most people will have multiple encounters with the health care system in their lifetime. But for a society so dependent on health care, we have a limited amount of knowledge about what it is and how it operates. The purpose of this chapter is to discuss the health care delivery system—its history and evolution, current models of delivery, and how it is managed and regulated.

CASE STUDY

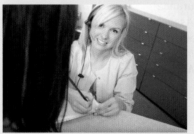

Annabelle has been a patient access specialist at a local urgent care center for 2 years. Although she enjoys her job, she is taking classes 2 days a week to earn the credits that will qualify her to sit for the Certified Medical Manager (CMM) exam.

When she started, one of the hardest parts of her job was answering patients' questions about how health services are paid and what is covered. The urgent care center sees a lot of young adults who don't know the details of their health insurance policy, sometimes because they are still getting insurance through one of their parents' employers. Other patients recently purchased insurance for the first time when "Obamacare" became the law in 2010 and are unfamiliar with how much out-of-pocket they are responsible for. Almost every day, Annabelle sees the misconceptions patients have about how health care is paid for and considers it part of her job to make sure patients understand the way their insurance policies work.

HISTORY OF HEALTH CARE IN THE UNITED STATES

Nearly everything about health care has changed in the past 100 years, from the way providers are trained to the way patients receive and pay for health care services. This section provides an overview of the development of the health care system as it exists in the United States today.

Health Care Providers

The delivery of health care in the United States has come a long way in the past century. It has evolved from a patchwork of home remedies and untrained barbers performing

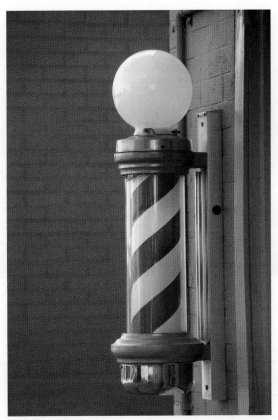

Figure 3.1 In the past, the barber pole's red and white stripes signified blood and bandages, advertising the shop as a place for health care services. The blue stripe was added later, either to represent the blue color of veins, or as a symbol of American patriotism.

unsterile surgeries to our current system of evidence-based medicine, with health care providers who are highly trained and regulated.

Before the turn of the 20th century, anyone who had the desire and resources to set up a medical practice could do so. Health care practitioners had minimal training, and what knowledge they had was not formalized but learned through internships and on-the-job training with existing physicians. For example, historically, the local clergyman or barber would serve as the town physician. Barbers erected red-and-white poles outside of their shops, which represented blood and bandages (Fig. 3.1), to signify that they performed medical procedures, such as amputations, cupping, and bloodletting.

Medical schools slowly began to organize, mostly under the direction and leadership of other physicians who sought to improve medicine and raise the medical profession in the United States. It was during the mid- to late-1700s that the United States began seeing physicians with more formal education and scientific training. The first medical school opened at the University of Pennsylvania in 1765, and, in 1781, the Massachusetts Medical Society was the first organized body to license physicians. With scientific training, physicians became more authoritative and practiced medicine as small entrepreneurs, charging a fee for their services. In 1847, the American Medical Association (AMA) was established for the purpose of protecting health care providers, although it did not have a meaningful impact until the 1900s, when it organized the membership of its physicians and set guidelines to begin standardizing medical education.

During and after the Civil War, health care drastically changed in the United States. Both the Union and Confederate militaries were devastated by battle injuries and disease and employed physicians to care for the troops. The Civil War also established

TAKE AWAY •·········

Before the 20th century, health care was virtually unregulated.

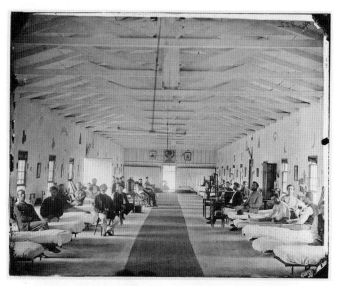

Figure 3.2 Patients in a Civil War hospital. (By USG (Library of Congress, Prints & Photographs Division) [Public domain], via Wikimedia Commons.)

nursing as a profession: more than 3000 women left home to serve in a profession that previously had been considered unsuitable for women. With no training or experience and only the willingness to serve, these military physicians and nurses learned how to treat battle wounds and cared for sick and wounded soldiers in makeshift field medical facilities and hospitals (Fig. 3.2). During the Civil War, more than 412,000 soldiers were wounded and more than 620,000 soldiers died, with two-thirds dying from diseases and not from their wounds. Hospitals and clinics were overwhelmed with patients. The massive amount of injuries presented new challenges and highlighted the broad deficiencies in the medical field.

Additionally, after the Civil War, life in the United States changed drastically as a result of industrialization, which brought new needs for health care. Despite rampant workplace injuries and deaths from diseases resulting from poor sanitation and overcrowding, there were little to no legislative or public programs to address these public health issues.

The early 20th century saw efforts to reform health care and improve social and health conditions for the working class. In 1906, an advocacy group called the American Association of Labor Legislation (AALL) led the campaign for health insurance in the United States. The AALL drafted a bill in 1915 that created the cornerstone of modern-day national health insurance: medical coverage for the working class and their dependents, sick pay, and maternity benefits. Costs were to be shared among workers, employers, and the state. However, because of heavy opposition from several physician organizations, labor parties, and insurance companies, it was not until the 1930s that there was a significant dialogue on how to finance and expand health care services because of the increased use and rising cost of medical services, especially for hospital care.

In the 1900s, as a part of this health care reform, medical education became more formalized as colleges set standards for enrollment and graduation. In 1893, Johns Hopkins University required students entering its medical program to complete a 4-year degree before enrollment. The AMA also established guidelines for medical education and drug manufacturing. It inspected 160 medical schools in the United States, rating them as acceptable, doubtful, or unacceptable. This information was first published in 1906, along with a list of licensed physicians in the United States.

The American Hospital Association (AHA) was organized in 1899. Hospitals, which were initially funded by local city governments or charitable groups to serve the poor, became both public and private institutions where physicians treated both poor and the wealthy alike.

In 1910, the *Flexner Report*, a study commissioned by the AMA, was published and provided a commentary on the lack of standardization and quality control of medical education during this time. As a result of the report, major reforms occurred in medical education in the United States, such as strengthening state regulation of medical licensure, increasing the prerequisites to enter medical school, and teaching medicine aligned with protocols of mainstream science and research. The *Flexner Report* was also instrumental in changing the governance of health care providers, with state governments beginning to regulate licensing physicians. The Federation of State Medical Boards (FSMB) was formed in 1912 to organize state medical boards and currently serves 70 medical boards in the United States. Since 1915, the FSMB issues a monthly publication and now an electronic database listing physicians who have been sanctioned and disciplined. This brought a new accountability to the medical profession.

TAKE AWAY ●·········

The findings of the *Flexner Report* spurred major reforms in medical education in the United States.

Health Insurance

After the standardization of medical education and the practice of medicine, the medical field became a reputable career, and physicians became trusted authorities in society. In the early 20th century, labor unions and employers began offering payment for medical care as incentives to membership and employment. In the 1920s, officials at Baylor University Hospital were noticing empty hospital beds night after night and recognized that patients sought care from hospitals only when they were seriously ill, often after it was too late for treatment. To offset costs and, hopefully, encourage early medical intervention, Baylor University officials offered local school teachers a deal: if they paid 50 cents each month, Baylor would pay the costs in the event of hospitalization. This system spread the expenses of costly hospital care among the teachers who paid in and supplied the hospital with the money necessary to provide care to those who needed it. The first medical insurance company, Blue Cross and Blue Shield, followed the Baylor University model. Within 10 years, several other health insurance companies entered the market, working on the same principle: if a large pool of people (the policyholders) paid a fixed amount each month (a **premium**), the cost of hospitalization for any single individual would be offset by the premiums collectively paid by the policyholders. This spreads the risk of an expensive medical bill for any single individual and is the basis for health insurance plans today.

Although medical insurance made affordable care easier to obtain, its introduction made the business of health care more complicated than a patient paying a physician directly for treatment. The health insurer is a third-party **payer**, responsible for most or all of a patient's bill to the provider. When a patient receives medical care, the physician or other provider submits a **claim** to the insurer, who then sends a payment to the provider for services rendered. This payment is called a **reimbursement**. Because the insurer is the entity who is paying for services, it reviews claims to make sure they are medically necessary and covered by the individual policy and may deny some or all of the claim for noncovered services. We will explore the way health insurance works in greater detail later in this chapter.

During World War II, health insurance became more a part of the national dialogue and landscape. To prevent inflation, the United States government instituted price and wage controls limiting the amount of money a company could pay an employee. This created a backlash from labor groups. To circumvent these restrictions, the War Labor Board ruled that certain benefits were not subject to wage controls, such as vacation time and health insurance. As a result, employers began offering health insurance packages to attract employees. In a short time, employer-sponsored coverage became widespread, and health insurers gained millions of new clients.

○ **premium** a fixed amount paid to subscribe to an insurance policy.

○ **payer** the entity responsible for most or all of a patient's bill to the provider.

○ **claim** a statement of services sent to a health insurer for payment to the provider.

○ **reimbursement** the payment to the provider for health care treatments, supplies, and services rendered.

TAKE AWAY ●·········

A health insurance company is a *third-party payer*.

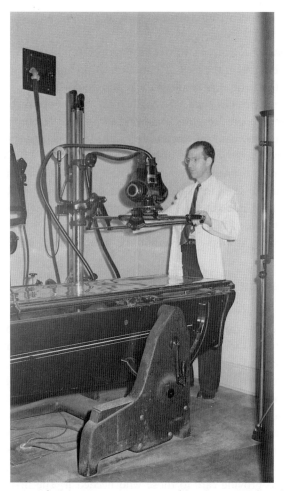

Figure 3.3 A laboratory technician uses an x-ray machine in a 1946 hospital. By Russell Lee [Public domain], via Wikimedia Commons.

After World War II, advances in technology and medicine, such as the introduction of x-rays (Fig. 3.3) and the development of inoculations for life-threatening diseases, opened the door for the beginnings of the allied health professional. The expansion of the medical field and the increasing demand for health services created the need for specialists to assist in medical practices, in positions such as respiratory therapists, x-ray technicians, lab technicians, and nutritionists and dieticians.

Federal Government Involvement

Despite employer-based health insurance becoming commonplace, efforts to implement government health insurance, wherein the state or federal government pays for some or all of an individual's medical care, gained little traction. President Harry Truman proposed a nationwide public health insurance system in 1945 but faced political opposition. Instead, labor groups supported the expansion of the current employer-based system rather than a new system of public insurance on the national level.

However, one glaring flaw with an employer-sponsored health insurance system is that those without jobs, specifically the elderly, the indigent, and the unemployed, did not have access to health insurance coverage. During the 1950s and 1960s, the United States Congress acknowledged the need for legislation to support health care for this vulnerable population, but disagreed on the best way to provide that support. The Department of Health, Education, and Welfare (HEW) was formed in 1953, a Cabinet-level

TAKE AWAY ●··········

Employer-based health insurance became widespread during the 1940s. In 1965, Medicare and Medicaid began to offer health care assistance to the elderly and indigent population.

agency that would later become the Department of Health and Human Services (DHHS). In 1965, Congress passed Title XVIII and Title XIX of the Social Security Act, which enacted **Medicare**, which focused on providing health care to the elderly, and **Medicaid**, which offered health care to those in poverty. In 1973, Medicare coverage was expanded to include the disabled and those with end-stage renal disease (ESRD), or kidney failure.

The **Centers for Medicare and Medicaid Services (CMS),** a division under HEW (now known as the DHHS), is responsible for overseeing Medicare and Medicaid. However, individual states are responsible for administering Medicaid programs based on their own state needs. Government programs like these are called **entitlement programs** because their benefits are guaranteed to people who meet certain circumstances. Currently, CMS provides health insurance coverage for more than 120 million people and is the largest payer of medical services in the United States.

Other government agencies provide health care to current and former members of the military and their families. Table 3.1 summarizes federal agencies and their roles in providing health insurance and medical care to specific populations.

The HMO Act of 1973

Besides being a provider of health insurance, the United States government created laws and regulations to hone and reform health care delivery. The 1970s introduced a new model of the way patients received services from a physician called **managed care**. Managed care focused on providing affordable, quality health care while controlling medical costs. Managed care insurers sought to control costs by limiting the providers who can be seen by the patient and, in turn, discount payments to those providers. Managed care plans typically arrange to provide medical services for members in exchange for fees paid to a managed care insurer. Members receive services from a network of approved physicians or hospitals that also have a contract with the managed care insurer. Members benefit from reduced health care costs, and the health care providers profit from a guaranteed client base. The first type of managed care insurers were **health maintenance organizations (HMOs)**, which received government funding through start-up grants and loans after passage of the HMO Act of 1973. Health care providers

Medicare a federal program paying for the health care costs of those over 65 and those with certain chronic illnesses.

Medicaid a federal program funded by each state that pays for the health care costs of those in poverty.

Centers for Medicare and Medicaid Services (CMS) a division of the Department of Health and Human Services responsible for overseeing Medicare, Medicaid, and CHIP.

entitlement program government financial support based on an individual's age, medical condition, employment status, or other circumstances.

managed care an insurance coverage and reimbursement structure that seeks to control costs by limiting the providers who can be seen by the patient and, in turn, discount payments to those providers.

health maintenance organization (HMO) a type of managed care health insurance that seeks to reduce costs by limiting the providers and facilities from which a subscriber may obtain services.

TABLE 3.1
FEDERAL PROGRAMS FOR HEALTH CARE DELIVERY

Program	Description	Coverage
Medicare	Title XVIII of the Social Security Act (1965)	Elderly, disabled, renal dialysis, and transplant patients
Medicaid	Title XIX of the Social Security Act (1965)	Low-income or indigent patients
TRICARE	Medical services for members of the armed services, their spouses, and families	Administered by the Department of Defense and applying to members of the Army, Air Force, Navy, Marine Corps, Coast Guard, Public Health Service, and the National Oceanic and Atmospheric Administration
VHA	Veterans Health Administration	Health services for veterans
CHAMPVA	Civilian Health and Medical Program of the Department of Veterans Affairs	US Department of Veterans Affairs (Health Administration Center)–administered programs for veterans and their families
IHS	Indian Health Service	Provides, or assists in providing and organizing, health care services to American Indians and Alaskan Natives

From Davis NA and LaCour M: *Foundations of Health Information Management,* ed 4, St. Louis: Elsevier, 2017.

are not independent under an HMO but work for a hospital or corporation that receives its income from prepaid health care payments, or premiums. Additionally, health care providers are not paid for services rendered, but receive an overall payment based on diagnosis. The goal of HMOs was to decrease the cost of health care delivery through these lowered payments and preventive medical services, such as wellness screenings.

Since their inception, there have been critics and proponents of the HMO managed care model. Regardless, as we will discuss later in this chapter, it remains the most prevalent insurance model in the United States today.

Employee Retirement Income and Security Act (ERISA) of 1974

The Employee Retirement Income Security Act of 1974 (ERISA) is a federal law that sets minimum standards for most voluntarily established pension and health plans in private industry to provide protection for individuals in these plans. Although the main intention of the ERISA was to regulate and protect employee pensions, the law forever changed health policy in the United States. If an employer's health plan is administered by the employer itself, known as self-insuring, ERISA took governance and regulation away from the states and placed it under federal jurisdiction. This is important because the rights of beneficiaries to sue their insurer are more limited in federal courts. If an employee is denied coverage for treatment, under state law they may sue for punitive damages, lost income, and pain and suffering; under federal law, a person can only recover the cost of the benefits for which they were denied and their own legal fees. These exclusions encouraged more large companies to switch their health plans to self-insurance.

Tax Equity and Fiscal Responsibility Act (TEFRA) of 1982

Through Medicare and employer-sponsored insurance, more people had access to health care services than ever before. The use of health care services rose accordingly, which in turn drove health care costs upward at an alarming rate. Compounding the issue was that improved access for older adults meant better care and, therefore, longer life expectancy, which further increased health care costs. Thus cost containment became a critical issue, and the federal government wanted better oversight of the care for which it paid.

One initiative was the Professional Standards Review Organizations (PSROs), established to conduct local peer reviews of Medicare and Medicaid cases for the purpose of ensuring that only medically necessary services were being provided and appropriately reimbursed. To further increase consistency and effectiveness and improve quality control, Congress later dismantled PSROs and replaced them with peer review organizations through a federal law called the **Tax Equity and Fiscal Responsibility Act of 1982 (TEFRA)**. TEFRA included a broad array of provisions, many of which had nothing to do with health care, but its effect on health care included a major modification of the Medicare reimbursement structure. Until the passage of TEFRA, Medicare payments were retrospectively adjusted: the amount paid to the provider was determined by the actual costs incurred by the patient *after* the patient was treated. However, Congress wanted more Medicare beneficiaries enrolled in HMOs to take advantage of their cost-saving measures since HMOs worked on a flat, monthly payment rather than one determined by the health services provided. This required Medicare reimbursement amounts to be determined *before* the service, or *prospectively*.

Prospective payment systems (PPS) operate on the assumption that patients with the same diagnoses will require roughly the same level of care, consuming roughly the same resources, and incurring roughly the same costs. The payment amount for any given condition is known upfront and based on the patient's diagnosis. However, if the patient requires more care, the provider receives no additional payments. This created strong incentives for the HMO or hospital to operate efficiently and at the lowest cost, sometimes at the expense of the patient.

TAKE AWAY ●‥‥‥‥

Managed care is the most prevalent insurance model in the country today.

○ **Tax Equity and Fiscal Responsibility Act of 1982 (TEFRA)** legislation that established the prospective payment system for Medicare reimbursement.

TAKE AWAY ●‥‥‥‥

Following the passage of TEFRA, Medicare and Medicaid payment amounts to doctors and hospitals were determined before the patient was treated, based on diagnosis, using a prospective payment system (PPS).

○ **prospective payment system (PPS)** a system of reimbursement in which the payment amount is determined based on the diagnosis or the treatment provided.

Consolidated Omnibus Reconciliation Act (COBRA)

In 1985, President Ronald Reagan signed the Consolidated Omnibus Reconciliation Act, referred to simply as "COBRA." Like TEFRA, COBRA included provisions unrelated to health policy, but the law is best known for its changes to the landscape of employer-sponsored health insurance. Under COBRA, companies with 20 or more employees must continue health coverage for individuals and their families who are no longer employed there for a period of 18 months. An employee and his or her family are entitled to continue receiving employee health benefits in case of resignation, layoff, strike, medical leave, and death. Further, a dependent child of the employee may receive COBRA benefits until he or she reaches a specific age set by the health plan, and a divorcee may receive benefits under his or her ex-spouse's plan for up to 36 months.

Another provision of COBRA is the **Emergency Medical Treatment and Active Labor Act (EMTALA)**, enacted by Congress in 1986. This law required hospitals to screen and treat anyone who presented to their emergency department (ED) with an "emergency medical condition." Under EMTALA, hospitals may not deny medical services and must stabilize a patient presenting with an emergency condition, and they may not inquire about insurance coverage or payment options until after the patient is stable. However, the hospital is not required to treat and cover the costs of a patient who arrives with a nonemergency condition, such as a severe cold or earache. Hospitals are also prohibited from discharging or transferring the patient to another hospital to avoid incurring further medical costs from caring for the patient.

It is also important to note that just because EMTALA legally binds a hospital to treat a patient without knowing whether or not he or she can pay, it does not mean that the patient receives care for free. The hospital can bill the patient later and the patient is still legally responsible for the amount due.

> **Emergency Medical Treatment and Active Labor Act (EMTALA)** legislation that requires health care providers to screen and treat anyone who presents to their emergency department with an "emergency medical condition."

TAKE AWAY

The provisions of EMTALA dictate that a hospital must assess and treat a patient with an emergency condition without regard for the patient's ability to pay.

Health Insurance Portability and Accountability Act (HIPAA)

The next major federal health care law was the **Health Insurance Portability and Accountability Act (HIPAA)**, passed in 1996. HIPAA has two primary purposes:

1. To protect the health insurance coverage of an employee if he or she switches employers
2. To protect the privacy of individuals' health data

Chapter 12 of this book discusses HIPAA in detail. But it is important to understand the effects of HIPAA's Privacy Rule. This part of the legislation protects information about a person's health, including diagnosis, treatment history, and patient care. Health care team members must be careful when discussing the care of patients (Fig. 3.4). Patient information must be kept strictly confidential, and there are limitations on the sharing of information from a patient's medical record with other organizations.

Balanced Budget Act (BBA) of 1997

By the 1990s, continued increases in the cost of health insurance and health care heightened the urgency of broad-based health care reform at the federal level. In 1993, President Bill Clinton appointed the First Lady, Hillary Clinton, head of the newly formed Task Force on National Health Care Reform. The Task Force's goal was to come up with a comprehensive plan to provide *universal health care* for all Americans. Although **universal health care** has many forms, in general it is defined as an organized package of benefits from the government offering access to health services and protection from financial risk. Known officially as the *Health Security Act*, the bill faced sharp criticism from the pharmaceutical and health insurance industries, conservatives, libertarians, and even some Democrats. As a result, the bill for universal health care was defeated in 1994.

Forced to give up on broad health care reform, the Clinton administration pursued a smaller plan to offer health coverage to the children of lower-income families and

> **universal health care** an organized package of benefits from the government offering access to health services and protection from financial risk.

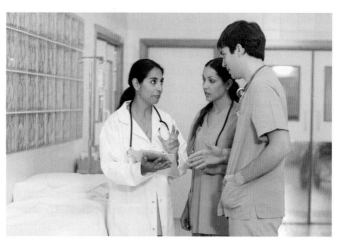

Figure 3.4 Under HIPAA, health care workers must maintain confidentiality when discussing patient care. (Copyright Wavebreakmedia/istock.com 24049244.)

those who did not qualify for Medicaid. The program, eventually titled the Children's Health Insurance Program (CHIP), was passed as part of the Balanced Budget Act (BBA) of 1997 and is administered by the states through Medicaid.

The BBA's other provisions included expanding the prospective payment approach to other health care settings, like nursing homes, home health care, hospital outpatient services, and hospice care. It also created a new Medicare program (called *Medicare Part C*) that encouraged managed care coverage for Medicare beneficiaries.

Affordable Care Act (ACA)

Through the 1990s and 2000s, the cost of medical care continued to rise, and, as a result, the cost of health insurance rose. Companies who provided insurance to their employees were paying more money every year for their health benefits, which had a negative effect on how much they could afford for employee wages and raises. Many employers began shifting their health insurance costs to the employee in the form of higher premiums or lowering the total cost of the insurance policy by eliminating certain covered services. Insurance was even more expensive for the unemployed or for individuals who were not eligible for employer-sponsored coverage, such as the self-employed, because they had no employer with whom they could share the costs of premiums. For many, health insurance was unaffordable.

Health care reform was among the largest issues of the campaign for the 2008 presidential election, and it was President Barack Obama's first major legislative effort after his inauguration. In 2010, he signed into law the Patient Protection and Affordable Care Act (PPACA), often referred to as the **Affordable Care Act (ACA),** or "Obamacare," becoming one of the most significant health care reforms since the implementation of the Medicare and Medicaid programs (Fig. 3.5). The law's provisions intended for better patient outcomes, lower health care costs, expanded health insurance availability, and increased access to health care for all. The measures of the law aimed at financial, clinical, and technical transformations in the operations of primary care providers and in hospitals. The ACA will be discussed in further detail later in this chapter, but its main reforms included:

- Health insurers may not deny coverage for individuals who have preexisting conditions, and they may not drop their coverage if the policyholder becomes ill.
- All individuals must obtain health insurance either through their employer, through public insurance (Table 3.1), or by purchasing it privately through the newly formed marketplace or state-based exchange.
- Businesses with 50 employees or more must offer health insurance to their employees.

○ **Affordable Care Act**
(ACA) legislation that set new guidelines for health insurers, mandated insurance coverage for all Americans, and reformed the way individuals who are not eligible for employer-sponsored coverage purchase insurance.

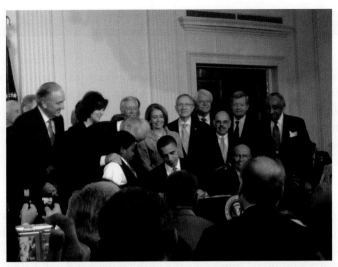

Figure 3.5 President Barak Obama signs the Patient Protection and Affordable Care Act on March 23, 2010. (By Keith Ellison [President Obama Signing The Health Care Bill] [CC BY 2.0 {http://creativecommons.org/licenses/by/2.0}], via Wikimedia Commons.)

LEARNING CHECKPOINT 3.1
History of Health Care in the United States

1. In 1910, the _____ Report critiqued the lack of standardization and quality control of medical education.

2. A _____ is a fixed amount paid each month for an insurance policy.

   a. deductible
   b. reimbursement
   c. claim
   d. premium

3. _____ is an entitlement program created in 1965 to provide health care to the poor.

4. Which legislation changed CMS reimbursement to a prospective payment system?

   a. Consolidated Omnibus Reconciliation Act (COBRA)
   b. Emergency Medical Treatment and Active Labor Act (EMTALA)
   c. Tax Equity and Fiscal Responsibility Act of 1982 (TEFRA)
   d. Employee Retirement Income and Security Act (ERISA) of 1974

5. In what year did the Affordable Care Act (ACA) become law?

   a. 1910
   b. 1965
   c. 1973
   d. 2010

LEGAL AND REGULATORY OVERSIGHT

As we have discussed, the federal government's involvement in health care delivery expanded greatly through the last century, especially in regard to how it is paid for and how it is delivered. Various health care facilities have different ways of operating, but the way in which activities are performed often arises from legislation, regulation, and accreditation requirements. Federal, state, and local governments monitor health care institutions and regulate the way they deliver health services.

Federal

In regard to regulating health care services in the United States, the primary regulatory agency was the *Department of Health, Education, and Welfare (DHEW)*, and, in 1979, DHEW was renamed the **Department of Health and Human Services (DHHS)** or HHS. The agency's motto is "Improving the health, safety, and well-being of America." HHS is responsible for administering and overseeing programs that enhance and protect the well-being of all Americans by providing effective health and social services and public health.

The HHS is responsible for almost one-fourth of all federal government expenditures and administers more grant dollars than all other federal agencies combined. The HHS administers more than 115 programs across its 11 operating divisions. Those most important to our discussion are listed in Table 3.2.

Earlier in this chapter, we discussed the development of federal programs, such as Medicare, Medicaid, and CHIP, administered by the CMS. More than $950 billion are spent on these CMS programs each year[2] to cover the care of more than 129 million adults and children in the United States.[3]

To ensure individuals in these programs are receiving quality care, providers must meet specific standards to receive reimbursements for treating patients participating in CMS programs, such as Medicare and Medicaid. The standards with which a health care facility must comply are called Medicare's **Conditions of Participation (CoP)**.

---

[2]http://www.hhs.gov/about/budget/budget-in-brief/cms/
[3]http://kff.org/health-reform/state-indicator/total-monthly-medicaid-and-chip-enrollment/

Department of Health and Human Services (DHHS) the agency of the US government with oversight of health care.

TAKE AWAY

CMS is the largest third-party payer in the United States.

Conditions of Participation (CoP) the terms that a facility or provider must follow to receive reimbursement from the Centers for Medicare and Medicaid Services.

TABLE 3.2
HHS AGENCIES AND OFFICES

Agency/Office	Function
Agency for Healthcare Research and Quality (AHRQ)	Supports ways to improve the quality, safety, and accessibility of health care.
Centers for Disease Control and Prevention (CDC)	Studies and fights disease and other threats to public health.
Centers for Medicare and Medicaid Services (CMS)	Administers Medicare, Medicaid, and CHIP.
Food and Drug Administration (FDA)	Assures the safety of drugs, medical devices, and food.
National Institutes of Health (NIH)	Fosters research to improve health and longevity and reduce illness and disability.
Office of Inspector General (OIG)	Promotes efficiency and fights fraud in health entitlement programs.
Substance Abuse and Mental Health Services Administration (SAMHSA)	Provides policy and resources to reduce the effects of substance abuse and mental illness.

CoP standards address the quality of providers, dictate certain policies and procedures for patient care and safety, and set requirements for facility administration and governance. For instance, the CoPs set rules for infection control, require certain information to be recorded in a patient's medical record, and specify which types of health care professionals can perform what levels of care.

State

Every health care facility needs a license from its state government to operate, and the process of **licensure** varies among states. In most states, the state's legislature passes a licensing act or a similar law that requires facilities to be licensed and delegates the authority to regulate that process to a state agency, often the state's department of health. The state agency then develops and administers the detailed regulations, which are part of the state's administrative code. Some states' regulations are very detailed and specific as to the organization and structure of a facility, including services that can be provided, medical staff requirements, nursing requirements, committees, and sanitation. Licensure is specific to the type of health care facility being operated. In addition to facilities, states license the practice of physicians, nurses, and other health care providers in their state.

States also track and monitor the well-being of their populations. In the interest of public health, health care facilities are required to report certain patient data to their state agencies. For example, hospitals, clinics, physicians, and laboratories must report certain diseases and conditions, such as cancer, trauma, birth defects, and infectious disease (Box 3.1). In addition, health care professionals have an obligation to report certain types of suspected abuses to the authorities. Most state laws require health care professionals who find evidence of inappropriate activities, such as child abuse, to notify local law enforcement. Laws in most states also require providers to report:
- A physician practicing medicine while impaired
- Conditions that would impair a person's ability to operate a motor vehicle, such as failing vision, seizures, or dementia
- Stillbirths and fetal deaths
- Injuries caused by weapons, such as gunshot and knife wounds

Local

Local government may also be involved in overseeing health care organizations, for example, in zoning regulations and tax exemption. Local governments dictate zoning regulations that require businesses, including health care organizations, to be located only in certain areas of the city. If a health care organization is not for profit, it is likely exempt from property and income taxes, but it is required to report community benefits offered by the organization. Therefore health care organizations often play an active role in the local governments and in the communities they are located.

Accreditation

Another issue that has an effect on the operation of a health care facility is accreditation. Whereas licensure is mandatory to operate a health care facility within a given state, accreditation is voluntary.

Accreditation begins with voluntary compliance with a set of standards that are developed by an independent, not-for-profit organization. That organization then audits and evaluates the facility to ensure compliance based on its accreditation standards, which may include enforcement of policies and procedures regarding activities of medical

licensure official permission to practice or operate.

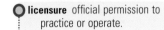
TAKE AWAY

Every health care facility needs a license from its state government to operate.

accreditation voluntary compliance with a set of standards for operation developed by an independent, not-for-profit organization.

BOX 3.1   REPORTABLE CONDITIONS

DISEASES REPORTABLE TO THE CENTERS FOR DISEASE CONTROL

Regulatory bodies at the local, county, state, and federal levels require that certain diseases be reported when diagnosed. These agencies use the information to track occurrences and establish policy to control outbreaks.

- Anthrax
- Arboviral diseases, neuroinvasive and non-neuroinvasive
  - California serogroup virus diseases
  - Chikungunya virus disease
  - Eastern equine encephalitis virus disease
  - Powassan virus disease
  - St. Louis encephalitis virus disease
  - West Nile virus disease
  - Western equine encephalitis virus disease
- Babesiosis
- Botulism
  - Botulism, foodborne
  - Botulism, infant
  - Botulism, wound
  - Botulism, other
- Brucellosis
- Campylobacteriosis
- Cancer
- Carbon monoxide poisoning
- Chancroid
- *Chlamydia trachomatis* infection
- Cholera
- Coccidioidomycosis
- Congenital syphilis
  - Syphilitic stillbirth
- Cryptosporidiosis
- Cyclosporiasis
- Dengue virus infections
  - Dengue
  - Dengue-like illness
  - Severe dengue
- Diphtheria
- Ehrlichiosis and anaplasmosis
  - *Anaplasma phagocytophilum* infection
  - *Ehrlichia chaffeensis* infection
  - *Ehrlichia ewingii* infection
  - Undetermined human ehrlichiosis/anaplasmosis
- Foodborne Disease Outbreak
- Giardiasis
- Gonorrhea
- *Haemophilus influenzae*, invasive disease
- Hansen's disease
- Hantavirus infection, non-Hantavirus pulmonary syndrome
- Hantavirus pulmonary syndrome
- Hemolytic uremic syndrome, post-diarrheal
- Hepatitis A, acute
- Hepatitis B, acute
- Hepatitis B, chronic
- Hepatitis B, perinatal virus infection
- Hepatitis C, acute
- Hepatitis C, chronic
- HIV infection (AIDS has been reclassified as HIV Stage III)
- Influenza-associated pediatric mortality
- Invasive pneumococcal disease
- Lead, elevated blood levels
  - Lead, elevated blood levels, children (<16 Years)
  - Lead, elevated blood levels, adult (≥16 Years)
- Legionellosis
- Leptospirosis
- Listeriosis
- Lyme disease
- Malaria
- Measles
- Meningococcal disease
- Mumps
- Novel influenza A virus infections
- Pertussis
- Pesticide-related illness and injury, acute
- Plague
- Poliomyelitis, paralytic
- Poliovirus infection, nonparalytic
- Psittacosis
- Q fever
  - Q fever, acute
  - Q fever, chronic

- Rabies, animal
- Rabies, human
- Rubella
- Rubella, congenital syndrome
- Salmonellosis
- Severe acute respiratory syndrome-associated coronavirus disease (SARS)
- Shiga toxin-producing *Escherichia coli*
- Shigellosis
- Silicosis
- Smallpox
- Spotted fever rickettsiosis
- Streptococcal toxic shock syndrome
- Syphilis
  - Syphilis, primary
  - Syphilis, secondary
  - Syphilis, early latent
  - Syphilis, late latent
  - Syphilis, late with clinical manifestations (including late benign syphilis and cardiovascular syphilis)
- Tetanus
- Toxic shock syndrome (other than streptococcal)
- Trichinellosis
- Tuberculosis
- Tularemia
- Typhoid fever
- Vancomycin-intermediate *Staphylococcus aureus* and Vancomycin-resistant *Staphylococcus aureus*
- Varicella
- Varicella deaths
- Vibriosis
- Viral hemorrhagic fever
  - Crimean-Congo hemorrhagic fever virus
  - Ebola virus
  - Lassa virus
  - Lujo virus
  - Marburg virus
  - New World arenavirus—Guanarito virus
  - New World arenavirus—Junin virus
  - New World arenavirus—Machupo virus
  - New World arenavirus—Sabia virus
- Waterborne Disease Outbreak
- Yellow fever
- Zika virus disease and Zika virus infection
  - Zika virus disease, congenital
  - Zika virus disease, non-congenital
  - Zika virus infection, congenital
  - Zika virus infection, non-congenital

OTHER REPORTABLE CONDITIONS AND DISEASES

In addition, states may require notification of any unusual cluster of isolates, or the following diagnoses:

AIDS (Acquired Immune Deficiency Syndrome)
Amebiasis
Animal bite
Cat scratch disease (infection caused by Bartonella species)
Congenital adrenal hyperplasia (CAH) (<5 y/old)
Creutzfeldt-Jakob Disease
Encephalitis
Galactosemia (<5 y/old)
Granuloma inguinale
Guillain-Barre syndrome
Histoplasmosis
Influenza (laboratory-confirmed only)
Kawasaki disease
Leprosy (Hansen's Disease)
Lymphogranuloma venereum
Maple syrup urine disease (MSUD) (<5 y/old)
Meningitis
Neonatal sepsis
Phenylketonuria (PKU) (<5 y/old)
Primary congenital hypothyroidism (<5 y/old)
Respiratory syncytial virus
Shingles (via zoster disease)
Toxoplasmosis

staff, environment of care, information management, and provision of care. Numerous accrediting bodies exist for different industries. Table 3.3 lists some health care accrediting bodies and the scope of their activities and oversight.

The oldest and largest accrediting agency for health care organizations in the United States is **The Joint Commission**. The Joint Commission is an independent, not-for-profit organization that sets standards for acute care facilities, ambulatory care networks, long-term care facilities, and rehabilitation facilities, as well as certain specialty facilities, such as hospice and home care agencies. The standards set by The Joint Commission reflect best practices and, in many ways, define how health care facilities should operate in terms of patient care and safety measures, clinical data flow, documentation standards, and performance measurements. It currently accredits and certifies more than 21,000 health care organizations and programs in the United States.

Before The Joint Commission's formation, hospitals followed accreditation standards and were approved through the American College of Surgeons (ACS). In 1951, the ACS, along with the AHA, the AMA, and the Canadian Medical Association, formed the Joint Commission on Accreditation of Hospitals, which took over that accrediting function. In 1987, the organization changed its name to the Joint Commission on Accreditation of Healthcare Organizations (JCAHO) to better reflect the variety of organizations that were seeking accreditation. In 2007, JCAHO simplified its name to The Joint Commission.

To maintain accreditation, The Joint Commission conducts onsite audits or surveys of accredited health care organizations a minimum of once every 39 months and every 24 months for laboratories to ensure the facilities are adhering to its standards for operation. During the site survey, The Joint Commission surveyors will look at the organization and management of the facility, examine medical records, review infection control protocols, check emergency plans, and even observe medical procedures. Because accreditation standards may change annually, facilities are required to stay abreast of these changes and implement procedures to comply.

Although accreditation is not mandatory, being accredited by The Joint Commission provides multiple benefits to health care organizations, such as strengthening patient safety, reducing liability insurance, and improving business operations and marketing. Moreover, when a health care organization is accredited or certified, it is eligible to submit claims for reimbursement from insurance companies and for Medicare and Medicaid. As previously discussed, CMS allows reimbursement from Medicare to those health care organizations that comply with Medicare's CoPs, which ordinarily entails a survey to ensure that the facility complies with the CoPs. However, in lieu of the CoP review, the health care organization can choose to seek accreditation through The Joint Commission or a number of different accrediting agencies. This is called **deemed status** because the facility is deemed to have complied with the CoPs through its accreditation, thus reducing the number of required surveys the facility must undergo. In some areas, accreditation is also a prerequisite for eligibility to participate in health and managed care plans.

Professional Standards

In addition to licensure and accreditation requirements, professional standards serve to regulate health care delivery. Licensing and accrediting agencies take a general overview of the facility and its operation but tend not to specifically address the day-to-day activities of individual health care providers and staff members. However, professional standards are developed by professional organizations that grant the credentials and licenses to health care professionals themselves.

Professional standards play an important role in determining the activities of health care professionals. For those directly involved in patient care, the professional standards

The Joint Commission an independent, not-for-profit organization that sets standards for acute care facilities, ambulatory care networks, long-term care facilities, and rehabilitation facilities, as well as certain specialty facilities, such as hospice and home care agencies.

TAKE AWAY •·········

A health care facility that achieves accreditation is one that has met standards for quality patient care.

deemed status the compliance of a health care entity with federal regulations through a survey by an accreditation agency.

TABLE 3.3
ACCREDITING ORGANIZATIONS IN HEALTH CARE

Accrediting Organization	Facilities/Organizations Accredited
Health Care Facilities	
Accreditation Association for Ambulatory Health Care (AAAHC)	• Ambulatory health care clinics • Ambulatory surgery centers • Birthing centers • College and university health centers • Community health centers • Dental group practices • Diagnostic imaging centers • Managed care organizations • Pain management centers • Podiatry practices • Radiation oncology centers • Single specialty group practices • Surgical recovery centers • Immediate/urgent care centers • Women's health centers
Accreditation Commission for Health Care (ACHC)	• Home health services • Hospice • Durable medical equipment (DME) suppliers • Pharmacy services • Private duty care • Sleep centers • Behavioral health facilities
The Joint Commission	• Critical access hospitals • Physician practices • Immediate/urgent care centers • Behavioral health facilities • Home health services • Hospitals • Laboratories • Nursing care centers
National Integrated Accreditation for Healthcare Organizations (NIAHO)	• Hospitals • Critical access hospitals
Commission on Accreditation of Rehabilitation Facilities (CARF)	• Rehabilitation facilities
National Committee for Quality Assurance (NCQA)	• Managed care organizations
Healthcare Facilities Accreditation Program (HFAP)	• Hospitals • Critical access hospitals • Ambulatory surgery centers • Laboratories • Behavioral health facilities • Ambulatory care/office-based surgery
Community Health Accreditation Partner (CHAP)	• Home health services • Pharmacy services • Private duty care • DME suppliers • Hospice • Infusion therapy nursing • Public health
The Compliance Team (TCT)	• Critical access hospitals • Rural health clinic • Physician practices • Immediate/urgent care clinics • Pharmacy services • DME suppliers

BOX 3.2   PAHCOM CODE OF ETHICAL STANDARDS

1. PAHCOM members shall be dedicated to providing the highest standard of managerial services to employers, employees, and patients, showing compassion and respect for human dignity.
2. PAHCOM members shall maintain the highest standard of professional conduct.
3. PAHCOM members shall respect the rights of patients, employers, and employees, and within the constraints of the law, maintain the confidentiality of all privileged information.
4. PAHCOM members shall use only legal and ethical means in all professional dealings, and shall refuse to cooperate with, or condone by silence, the actions of those who engage in fraudulent, deceptive, or illegal acts.
5. PAHCOM members shall respect the laws and regulations of the land, and the bylaws of the Association, and recognize a responsibility to seek to change those laws which are contrary to the best interest of patients, employers, employees, and other Association members.

6. PAHCOM members shall pursue excellence through continuing education in all areas applicable to the management of the medical office.
7. PAHCOM members shall strive to maintain and enhance the dignity, status, competence, and standards of medical office management and its practitioners.
8. PAHCOM members shall use every opportunity, including participation in local health care associations, to promote and improve public understanding and enhancement of the status of the profession.
9. PAHCOM members shall respect the integrity and protect the welfare of employers, employees, and patients.
10. PAHCOM members do not exploit professional relationships with patients, employees, or employers for personal gain. Nor do they condone or engage in sexual harassment or discriminatory hiring and supervisory practices.

of the individual provider dictate the level of care and the extent of documentation required while treating or evaluating patients. In addition, each professional organization has a code of ethics that governs the conduct of its members. For example, the Professional Association of Health Care Office Management (PAHCOM) is a national organization that promotes professionalism in physician office practice by providing professional development opportunities, continuing education in health care office management principles and practice, and certification for health care office managers. Box 3.2 lists the Code of Ethical Standards for members of PAHCOM.

▪ LEARNING CHECKPOINT 3.2
Legal and Regulatory Oversight

1. The Centers for Medicare and Medicaid Services (CMS) is an agency under:

    a. Department of Health and Human Services (HHS)
    b. Department of Health, Education, and Welfare (HEW)
    c. The Joint Commission
    d. The Professional Association of Health Care Office Management (PAHCOM)

2. Whereas licensure is mandatory, _____ is voluntary.

3. Which organization accredits hospice care organizations?

    a. Commission on Accreditation of Rehabilitation Facilities (CARF)
    b. Community Health Accreditation Partner (CHAP)
    c. The Compliance Team (TCT)
    d. The Joint Commission

PAYING FOR HEALTH CARE[4]

Patients and providers were, historically, the only parties involved in a health care relationship. Patients were free to seek whatever services they were able to afford, and providers could charge whatever the market would bear. This one-on-one relationship has evolved into a multiparty, complex system. The following section explores this system.

Reimbursement takes many different forms. In the past, it was not uncommon for a physician to be "paid in kind." For example, a physician makes a house call to treat a patient and receives chickens as the form of compensation. These types of bartering arrangements were mutually acceptable to both physician and patient and still exist in many parts of the world and the United States. However, reimbursement today is generally monetary, especially for hospitalization services.

In the past, the amount paid for medical services was not dependent on what the physician charged, but what the patient thought the physician's services were worth. This changed in the early 1900s with physicians setting prices for specific medical services rendered. More recently, the amount of reimbursement is decided not by the patient or physician, but by the third-party payer, namely, an insurance company or government program. These third-party payers have assumed the risk that a particular group of patients will require health care services and incur the cost of paying for the services.

Insurance

Insurance is a contract between two parties in which one party assumes the risk of loss on behalf of the other party in return for some monetary compensation. The insurer receives a premium payment, often on a monthly basis, and in return it pays for some or all of the contracted amount for health services rendered.

Ultimately, the patient is financially responsible for services that he or she has received. If the patient is a dependent, a person other than the patient, such as a parent, is responsible for the bill. The person who is ultimately responsible for paying the bill is called the **guarantor**. For example, if a child goes to the physician's office for treatment, the child, as a dependent, cannot usually be held responsible for the invoice. The parent or legal guardian is responsible for payment and is the guarantor.

guarantor the person who is ultimately responsible for paying for health care services.

Assumption of Risk

Health care providers render services for which they expect to be fairly compensated. Patients need these services, but the high cost of medical services is largely unaffordable. Thus insurance companies are willing to assume the risk of having to pay for these expensive medical services, but they cannot spend more than they collect in premiums. To avoid this, insurance companies try to balance their risk by insuring a large number of patients, or **subscribers**, many of whom will likely need limited health care services. **Group plans**, such as those negotiated through employers, consist of pools of potential patients—in this case, employees—whose risk can be averaged by the health insurer. This assumption of risk is the foundation of the concept of insurance.

subscriber the primary enrollee of an insurance policy.

group plan a type of insurance policy that averages risk over a group of covered individuals.

Insurance companies serve the public by assuming the risk of financial loss. Let us look at auto insurance as a simple example. Car owners pay periodic premiums to the auto insurance company, which in turn covers all or part of the costs incurred in an accident. The auto insurance company, although assuming the risk of financial loss in the event of an accident, is gambling that its customers will not have an accident. In fact, it goes to great lengths to predict the likelihood of accidents in certain populations,

[4]The editors wish to acknowledge Nadinia Davis and Melissa LaCour, whose writing in *Fundamentals of Health Information Management* provides the basis for this section of the chapter.

geographical areas, and types of vehicles. If you pay $1000 per year in auto insurance premiums for 40 years and never have an accident, the insurance company keeps the $40,000 (plus interest) accumulated over the life of the policy. If the auto insurance company insures a very large number of drivers, in theory and under normal circumstances, only a small percentage of drivers will ever have a costly accident, so the insurance company makes a profit. In some states, auto insurance companies are permitted to choose which drivers they wish to insure. Obviously, they would prefer to choose drivers with good driving records and no history of accidents. However, in some states, insurers may not pick and choose and must offer insurance to anyone who applies for it. This requirement raises the risk that the insurer will be required to pay for the costs of accidents and resulting settlements. This in turn raises the cost of auto insurance for all, unless the premiums of the high-risk drivers are increased significantly.

Health insurance works in a similar way. If employers provide a majority of their employees' private insurance plans, health insurers have fewer ways to limit their exposure to "high-risk" patients. Nevertheless, this model remains attractive to health insurers: insuring large numbers of individuals so that the risk that someone will require expensive medical care is offset by the large numbers of individuals who require less expensive care (Fig. 3.6).

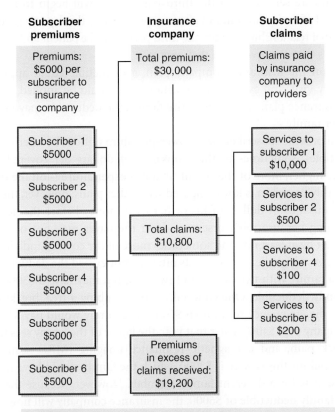

This is not the insurance company's PROFIT, since it does not take into consideration administrative and other costs. However, as long as the insurance company keeps those under control, it will make money. Theoretically, the larger and more diverse the pool of subscribers, the less risk the insurance company has of receiving claims in excess of premiums.

Figure 3.6 Insurance companies spread risk by collecting monies from a larger pool of subscribers and assuming only a small number of them will make claims. (From Davis NA, LaCour M: *Foundations of Health Information Management*, ed 4, St. Louis, 2017, Elsevier.)

Originally, the focus of insurance was on the coverage of services of the health care provider's fee. If the provider raised the fee, the insurance company raised its premiums to cover these fees. As health care costs increased, premiums also increased dramatically, becoming too expensive for many employers to pay in full. As a result, many employers pay only a part of the premiums, with employees bearing the rest.

Premiums can be lowered by limiting the types of covered services. When the employer pays the cost (premium) of the health insurance, it is the employer who negotiates what services will be covered. For example, monthly premiums will be lower if the employer chooses not to cover infertility services, such as in vitro fertilization. Although there are some federal and state mandates regarding what must be covered and under what circumstances, it is usually the employer's decision, which is generally based on what the employer can afford to pay in premiums for the group.

copay (copayment) a fixed amount the insured owes to the provider at the time of service.

Depending on the type of insurance, the patient may have responsibilities, such as *copays, coinsurance,* or *deductibles.* A copayment, commonly called a **copay**, is a fixed amount that a patient pays at the time of service. Copays vary according to the service rendered. For example, a copay may be $20 for a physician visit and $100 for an ED visit. **Coinsurance** is the percentage of the payment for which the patient is responsible. The payer may have 80% responsibility for the payment, and the patient has 20%. A **deductible** is a fixed amount the patient is responsible for before the payer provides any payment. For example, if the patient has a $500 deductible, the patient must spend $500 for health care services, and the third-party payer will begin to reimburse for services rendered after that amount. In all cases, payment by third-party payers depends on the contractual relationship between the third party and the patient and will reimburse only for services that are covered in that contract.

coinsurance a percentage of the amount owed to a provider for which the subscriber is responsible.

deductible the amount of money a subscriber must pay for medical services before an insurer will pay claims.

Depending on the insurance company plan, a deductible could apply for every encounter, every visit, and every hospitalization, or it could be applied on an annual basis. If the insurance plan covers the entire family, the deductible may be per family member or per family.

Insurers can provide subscribers with lower-premium options by offering plans with higher deductibles, sometimes in the thousands of dollars per covered life. When deductibles are higher, more of the risk of financial expenditure is on the patient. The insured's monthly premium is low compared with other plans; however, the individual must spend thousands of dollars of his or her own money before the health insurer pays for anything because reimbursement from the payer may not occur until the deductible is met by at least one and sometimes more of the covered individuals. When deductibles are very high, health care costs often do not exceed the deductible amount. For instance, a family with two adults and two children may have a $3000 individual and $6000 family deductible. One child falls while climbing a tree, breaking his arm. The bills from the emergency room total $7000. The family would pay $3000 and the insurance company pays $4000. Later that year, the father of the family sees his provider for severe back pain, and a magnetic resonance imaging (MRI) scan is ordered (Fig. 3.7). The bill for this service is $3000, which the family would have to pay out of pocket because it is for a different family member. However, because the family has now paid the family deductible of $6000, the insurance company will now pay for any services received by any family members for the remainder of the year.

TAKE AWAY

Copays, coinsurance, and deductibles are cost-sharing devices designed to help lower monthly premiums.

Federal law allows the purchase of "catastrophic" health insurance plans, which have the highest deductibles, to individuals under the age of 30 or those who can claim certain hardships. The premiums for these plans are very low. But, in the cases of very high deductibles, the insurance company ultimately covers and pays for only unusual or extraordinary expenses, such as serious illnesses and accidents.

Between deductibles, copays, and coinsurance, the amount for which an individual or family is responsible can be complicated—and expensive. Most plans specify an

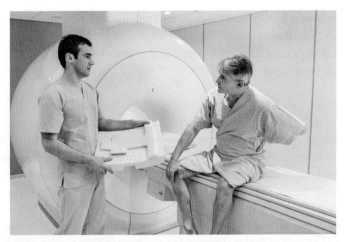

Figure 3.7 A magnetic resonance imaging (MRI) machine uses magnetic and radio waves to view the structures inside the body.

out-of-pocket maximum for the year, after which the health insurer will pay all the costs of care for the remainder of the year.

Types of Health Insurance

There are many different insurance plans, with an almost endless variety of benefits and reimbursement rules. Nevertheless, the majority of plans fall into one of two basic categories: *indemnity* and *managed care*. Managed care plans are further divided into two major types: preferred provider organizations (PPOs) and health maintenance organizations (HMOs). These managed care plans differ in their relationships among the health care provider, patient, and insurer, as well as the way patients access care.

Indemnity

In a typical **indemnity insurance** arrangement, the patient can see any provider they choose. After receiving services, the patient pays the physician or other health care providers and then submits the bill to the insurance company for reimbursement. Under the terms of the insurance contract is a list of services for which the insurance company agrees to pay, called the *covered services*. As long as the service is covered, the insurance company must reimburse the patient. Some insurance companies may pay 100% of the cost of certain covered services but a lower percentage of the cost of other covered services. Indemnity contracts often specify limits for certain covered services. If the benefit limit is $3000 for physician office visits and the patient's care is $4000 after the deductible, then the patient is responsible for the additional $1000.

Indemnity insurance plans led to an increase in the amount of money spent on health care. In a simple physician–patient relationship, the patient bears the cost of the care, but has some control on the amount spent on health care. For example, individuals may choose not to go to the physician in the first place because they feel the fee is too high and they cannot afford it, or they might be able to afford only select services. But because indemnity insurance plans reduce the out-of-pocket expense to the patient, with or without the deductible, they increase the likelihood that the services of the provider will be used regardless of the fees. Consequently, the number of people using health care services increases. In addition, if the insurance company reimburses for services without reviewing the need for those services, the physicians have no incentive to be conservative in their diagnostic and treatment plans.

○ **indemnity insurance** a type of health insurance policy that pays all or part of covered services after deductibles and within the limits of the policy.

With rising costs, health insurance companies had to find ways to control their expenses, such as imposing higher deductibles and limiting the number and types of covered services. As a result, insurance became less attractive under these circumstances, paving the way for managed care plans.

Managed Care

In general, the term *managed care* refers to the control that an insurance company or other payer exerts over the reimbursement process and over the patient's choices in selecting a health care provider. Managed care insurance plans have all the same features of indemnity plans, including copays, deductibles, premiums, and coinsurance. But, unlike indemnity plans, managed care health plans limit which providers a subscriber may use.

In a simple physician–patient relationship, the patient makes an appointment with the physician of his or her choice. The patient arrives at the office with a medical concern, and the physician determines a diagnosis and develops a treatment plan. The patient agrees (or declines) to undergo the treatment plan, the physician bills the patient, and the patient pays the physician. However, under managed care, the health care provider has a contractual arrangement with the insurer (payer) and must provide medical services to the insurer's patients. Depending on the insurer, managed care patients are called members, enrollees, or covered lives. The primary insured member is the subscriber, and those covered under the subscriber's policy are referred to as dependents or additional insured. The insurer's patients must choose their providers from those participating in the managed care plan. The scope of services paid for is determined by the insurer's contract with the subscriber, the subscriber's employer, or group manager.

Managed care organizations seek to reduce costs by controlling as much of the health care delivery system as possible. The underlying rationale for managed care is to reduce overall costs by eliminating unnecessary tests, procedures, visits, and hospitalizations through financial incentives, if the plan is followed, and financial penalties or sanctions if the plan is not followed. For example, a physician may write an order for a blood test to determine whether the patient has a vitamin D deficiency. But the managed care organization may only pay for the vitamin D blood test if the patient is known or suspected to have a bone loss condition, such as osteopenia or osteoporosis.

A major controversy in this strategy lies in the definition of what constitutes necessary health care and who makes this determination. Traditionally, physicians have determined the care that they provide to patients, whereas managed care has shifted that determination somewhat to the insurer. The managed care organization does not dictate what care will be rendered; it dictates what care it will pay for. Although this may control costs, it may drive patients to deny or neglect their own medical care and choose only that care that the third-party payer will approve.

An incentive to the provider is that managed care insurers direct their large pool of patients to specific providers, thereby offering the provider a relatively stable group of patients. Providers apply to be included on the insurers' lists of in-plan providers. In return, the insurer negotiates lower rates for the provider's services. The insurer determines the services that apply to that provider, how much the insurer will pay for those services, and under what circumstances the provider may render those services. This is a cost-saving measure for the insurer, allowing them to offer lower premiums to their policy-holders, and it helps guarantee a steady stream of patients and business for the provider. However, if insurers reduce payments and restrict services, providers may decide to avoid these payer relationships all together.

In a managed care scenario, the patient goes to the **primary care provider (PCP)**, whom the patient has chosen from a list of participating providers. The PCP diagnoses and treats the patient according to the guidelines from the managed care plan. The

---

TAKE AWAY ●········

Managed care plans lower costs by limiting the providers from which a subscriber may receive care from those providers.

◯ **primary care provider (PCP)** a physician or other provider designated by the patient to deliver primary care and refer the patient to other specialists as necessary.

patient pays the PCP a small copay. The PCP directly bills the managed care insurer for the visit. The managed care insurer may refuse to pay the PCP if the PCP does not obtain preapproval or authorization from the insurer for specific procedures or treatments, such as hospitalization. If a patient sees a PCP or any other type of physician outside the plan, the patient may not be covered at all and may be responsible for paying the entire cost of that visit, including any associated treatment or procedures. In most instances under a managed care plan, the patient is required to go to a PCP before going to see a specialist. After examination and discussion with the patient, the PCP must justify the necessity for referring the patient to a specialist also participating in the plan.

It should be noted that managed care plans do employ physicians who assist in making these medical decisions and rationales about what services to cover and what not to cover, which are based on evidence-based medicine and standards of care. For example, in the past, many managed care insurers did not consider preventive care to be necessary and, thus, would not pay for it. However, based on years of research and studies, it was concluded that preventive care was one of the best ways to reduce health care costs. Consider obstetrical care, for example. The costs of treating a pregnant woman through prenatal testing, education, and regular examinations and delivering a healthy newborn are significantly less costly than treating a newborn or new mother with complications that could have been prevented or treated with early medical intervention.

CURRENT TRENDS IN HEALTH CARE

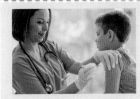

Today, federal law requires insurers to pay the full cost of certain preventive services, including immunizations, developmental assessments for children, and screening for depression, diabetes, cholesterol, obesity, various cancers, and sexually transmitted infections.

Managed care organizations focus heavily on statistical analysis of treatment outcomes and may regulate physicians whose practices appear to vary significantly from what they consider the "standard." As a result, some providers are critical of managed care because they feel a loss of control in the treatment process. They are sometimes frustrated by the medical practice standards imposed on them by the managed care organization, what some call *cookbook medicine,* and not being able to provide individualized care to their patient.

Despite controversy and criticism, managed care has become an important presence in the health care arena. In fact, most of the exchange plans available under the ACA are managed care plans. Managed care takes a number of different forms, and there are many variations in the relationship among managed care organizations and physicians and other health care providers. But at the core of managed care is the idea that the insurer has more control over cost of health care by actively engaging with the provider in determining the services to be provided.

Health Maintenance Organizations (HMOs)

An HMO is a type of managed care organization that has ownership or employer control over the health care provider. Essentially, the HMO is both the insurer (payer) and the provider. Members must use the HMO for all services, and the HMO will generally not pay for out-of-plan (also called *out-of-network*) services without prior approval. In some plans, approval to obtain health care services outside the plan is granted only in emergency situations.

TAKE AWAY

A health maintenance organization (HMO) is a type of managed care organization.

There are several types of HMOs, differing in the relationship between the providers and the HMO. The most common types are the *staff model, group practice model,* and *independent practice association (IPA) model.* In the staff model HMO, the organization owns the facilities, employs the physicians, and provides essentially all health care services. In a group practice model HMO, the organization contracts with a group or a network of physicians and facilities to provide health care services. Finally, in an IPA HMO, sometimes referred to as *individual practice association,* the HMO contracts with individual physicians, whose practices are partly devoted to the HMO. Regardless of the HMO model, an HMO generally does not reimburse for services provided by providers who are not in the HMO's network.

Preferred Provider Organizations (PPOs)

preferred provider organization (PPO) a type of managed care health insurance in which a patient may see certain providers in-network and pay a higher cost to see providers out of network; some plans allow patients to self-refer to specialists.

A **preferred provider organization (PPO)** is another type of managed care where the organization contracts with a network of health care providers who agree to certain reimbursement rates. It is from this network that patients are encouraged to choose their primary care physician and any specialists. If a patient chooses a provider who is not in the network, the PPO reimburses in the same manner as an indemnity insurer: after the deductible amount is paid for by the insured, the insurer pays for the specified services based on a specific dollar amount or percentage limit. In essence, the PPO allows patients to see the provider of their choice, but with a higher cost for those out of network.

A PPO is a hybrid plan that gives patients the option of choosing physicians outside the plan without totally forfeiting benefits. In addition, PPOs may offer patients a certain degree of freedom to self-refer to specialists. For example, some plans allow patients to visit gynecologists and vision specialists directly, without referral from the PCP.

Point of Service (POS)

Point of Service (POS) a type of managed care health insurance in which a patient may see certain providers in-network and pay a higher cost to see providers out of network; patients must have a referral to see a specialist.

A **Point of Service (POS)** plan is similar to a PPO, but the patient may see an out-of-network provider if they choose to pay more. However, POS plans require a referral from a PCP to see a specialist.

High-Deductible Health Plans (HDHPs)

Some health insurance plans allow subscribers to take advantage of income tax breaks when they choose a plan with low monthly premiums but high deductibles. For 2016, the Internal Revenue Service defines a high-deductible health plan (HDHP) as any plan with a deductible of $1300 or more for an individual or $2600 for a family. Although the individual pays more health care costs out-of-pocket, he or she can set aside money to pay for those costs in a special account called a *health savings account (HSA).* Any money contributed to this account is not subject to federal income taxes, reducing the subscriber's overall tax burden for the year. Additionally, funds in an HSA will roll over year after year and may even be invested.

CURRENT TRENDS IN HEALTH CARE

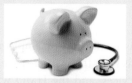

A flexible spending account (FSA) is another type of tax-advantaged account. FSAs are offered through employers and allow the employee to set aside money from each paycheck into the account to use toward medical expenses. Similar to HSAs, money contributed to an FSA account is tax free. FSAs are usually paired with traditional health plans, not HDHPs. FSA holders may roll over up to $500 of savings into the following year. However, anything over $500 in the account will be forfeited to the employer at the end of the year.

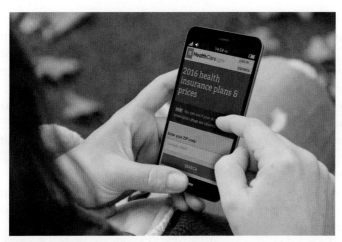

Figure 3.8 Affordable Care Act (ACA) legislation created an online exchange where individuals could compare and purchase plans.

The Affordable Care Act (ACA)

The passage of the ACA in 2010 brought about broad and sweeping changes to the health insurance industry. The law introduced provisions aimed at consumer protection, improving the quality of care, lowering costs, and increasing access to health care.

Perhaps ACA's most dramatic innovation was the implementation of the health insurance marketplace, sometimes referred to as the *health insurance "exchange"* or *"Obamacare exchange,"* named after President Barack Obama. The health insurance marketplace allowed individuals who do not have insurance through an employer, Medicare, Medicaid, CHIP, or other similar sources to purchase health insurance on the government website, Healthcare.gov (Fig. 3.8). At Healthcare.gov, individuals are able to compare all health insurance policies available to them based on the cost of each plan's monthly premium, deductibles or coinsurance for certain services, and maximum out-of-pocket costs. After a comparison, they may enroll in the policy through the marketplace or state exchange website. Employers can use the same website to find and choose plans to offer their employees.

Prices for health insurance policies on the marketplace are dependent on the individual's geographic location and income level. People with lower incomes can qualify for tax subsidies that reduce the cost of their monthly premiums, making health insurance more affordable to them. For example, Alex is a 30-year-old nonsmoker who makes $30,000 per year. He is looking for health insurance policies with low deductibles and costs of around $265 per month for premiums. Based on Alex's income, he qualifies for $65 per month in subsidies from the federal government. If he chooses to apply the subsidies, the cost of his monthly premiums would be reduced to $200, not $265, with an overall savings of $780 per year ($65 × 12 months).

Another provision of the ACA allowed states to expand their Medicaid programs to grant access to those who had previously made too much money to be eligible for Medicaid assistance but made too little to purchase insurance from the marketplace. This expansion was not mandatory, and, despite temporarily being funded by the federal government, some states declined to participate in the expansion partly because the entire cost of the expansion would be shifted back to the states after 3 years. In addition, the ACA requires insurers to offer eligibility for adults under the age of 26 who are insured or able to be insured under their parent's health plan. Both of these provisions increased the number of people with health coverage, increasing access to health care.

Outside of the exchanges, the ACA enacted multiple restrictions and standards for health care coverage to protect consumers. Earlier in this chapter, we mentioned that under the ACA, health insurers may not deny coverage for individuals who have preexisting conditions and they may not drop coverage if the policyholder becomes ill. Other consumer protections included:

- Ended the possibility of health care insurance being withdrawn or terminated because of mistakes on the insurance application
- Gave consumers the right to appeal denial decisions made by the health care insurance provider
- No lifetime limit on payments for care made by insurance companies
- No increases in rates on health care coverage plans unless publicly justified
- Premiums paid by the insured must be spent primarily on health care, not on administrative costs

The ACA also sought to improve the quality of health care. Before the ACA, consumers might have been restricted by their health care coverage plans to certain health care providers, even in emergency situations. The ACA provided the following regulations for health care insurance companies to follow:

- Preventive care must be covered under health coverage plans at no cost to the consumer.
- Consumers are free to choose their doctor from their plan's network.
- Emergency services can be sought from providers outside of the plan's network.[5]

The ACA encourages preventive care as a means to control costs, for example, allowing employers to discount an employee's share of premium costs when they participate in a wellness program. Employers can also offer their employees weight loss or smoking cessation programs, discounts for gym memberships, and education on nutrition and healthy living. These programs are developed to assist consumers in maintaining a healthy lifestyle and take measures to prevent future medical issues. As a result, the insurer is able to offer its policyholders a lower rate because their lifestyle reduces their risk for chronic illnesses.

Consider one of the most common diseases in the country: diabetes. More than 22 million people are diagnosed with diabetes in the United States, incurring more than $306 billion in direct medical costs and accounting for more than 1 of 5 dollars spent on medical care. The cost to provide annual screenings and education on diet and exercise that would prevent diabetes is far lower than the amount spent on insulin therapy, dialysis, amputation, and other treatments for diabetes and its complications. Clearly, it is cheaper and easier to prevent people from becoming ill than it is to treat a patient after they have developed the illness.

Another way that the ACA is attempting to control costs is through the development of the **Accountable Care Organizations (ACO)**, a network of diverse health care providers who are jointly responsible for the care and outcome of their Medicare patients. The ACA offers incentives to the ACO when they coordinate health care services more efficiently and with better patient outcomes.

Accountable Care Organization (ACO) a network of diverse health care providers who are jointly responsible for the care and outcome of their Medicare patients.

Medicare

Medicare helps pay for the health care for adults over the age of 65, individuals with certain disabilities, or those with ESRD requiring dialysis or kidney transplantation (Fig. 3.9). Over 55 million Americans are Medicare beneficiaries, and the program pays for more than 50% of the reimbursements received by some health care providers.

TAKE AWAY

Many insurance companies follow Medicare's guidelines when adopting reimbursement strategies.

[5]US Department of Health & Human Services. "About the law." http://www.hhs.gov/healthcare/about-the-law/index.html

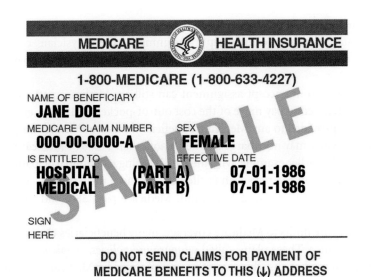

Figure 3.9 Medicare beneficiaries are issued a card with a unique identification number.

Its status as the largest payer in the country means that it drives health care policy decisions for a large number of Americans. In fact, many insurance companies follow Medicare's guidelines when adopting reimbursement strategies. For example, if Medicare decides that a particular surgical procedure will be reimbursed only if is it performed in the inpatient setting, other insurance companies often choose to enforce the same rule.

Medicare has four categories:

- **Medicare Part A** covers hospital services, nursing home stays, home health visits, and hospice care. There is no monthly premium for Part A (individuals pay into Medicare throughout their working lives from payroll taxes), but there is an annual deductible. Beneficiaries begin to pay a daily coinsurance after a 60-day hospital stay or after 20 days in a nursing home.

- **Medicare Part B** pays for visits to the physician's office and other outpatient services. Individuals must pay a monthly premium depending on their yearly income. There is a 20% coinsurance for most services and an annual deductible.

- **Medicare Part C**, also called *Medicare Advantage,* is a voluntary managed care option. It allows individuals to buy private insurance that pays for similar services covered under Parts A, B, and D. Part C also offers additional benefits, such as vision, dental, and hearing, and many include prescription drug coverage. These plans often have networks, which means the insured may have to see certain doctors and go to certain hospitals in the plan's network to receive care.

- **Medicare Part D**, implemented in 2006, is a prescription drug program purchased through Medicare-approved private insurers. The monthly premium varies depending on the enrollee's income, and there is usually some cost sharing. For example, an individual may pay 5% of the cost of a prescription, and the Part D plan pays the rest. Many Part D plans feature catastrophic coverage that pays for very expensive drugs after a threshold is met.

Medicare decides how much it will pay for each treatment, procedure, or service. Providers who participate in Medicare must accept **assignment**, meaning that they agree to accept the Medicare-approved amount as payment in full. For example, a patient on Medicare goes to the physician for a bad cough. The physician examines the patient and prescribes medicine and respiratory therapy. The physician's usual

assignment the amount of money Medicare will pay for medical services.

charge for the visit is $150; however, Medicare has only agreed to pay $100 for this service. Because the physician accepts assignment, the physician can only bill $100 to Medicare. However, CMS will pay $80, and the patient pays the $20 coinsurance.

Providers who do not accept assignment can still see Medicare patients as long as the patient is prepared to pay more of the cost out-of-pocket. CMS does enforce a price cap on services provided to any Medicare beneficiary, called a *limiting charge.* The rule states that a provider may not charge a patient more than 115% of Medicare's approved amount. Using the earlier example, with the patient going to a nonparticipating provider, the maximum amount the physician is allowed to charge the patient is $115, which is 115% of the Medicare-approved $100 limit. Medicare pays $80, and the cost to the patient is $35.

Because there are limits to Medicare coverage, many beneficiaries choose to purchase additional insurance. These plans, called *wraparound policies, supplemental policies,* or *"Medigap,"* are aimed at absorbing costs not reimbursed by Medicare. These help pay for deductibles and copays and any care an individual might need if they were traveling outside the United States. However, these plans do not pay for prescription drugs. Medigap plans are sold by private insurers but regulated by CMS. It is also important to note that Medicare may be the secondary payer for individuals who are still employed or retired and still covered primarily by the employer's insurance plan. In these cases, the private insurer is billed first and then Medicare. The patient pays any costs not covered by the primary insurance and Medicare.

Medicaid

TAKE AWAY

Medicaid is partially funded by the federal government and administered by the states to help pay for the health care of those in poverty.

Also administered by CMS, Medicaid is a shared federal and state program. The federal government allocates funds to states through the Federal Medical Assistance Program according to the average income of the residents of the state. Unlike Medicare, which reimburses through fiscal intermediaries, Medicaid reimbursement is handled directly by each individual state. Medicaid coverage and reimbursement guidelines vary from state to state, with some states contracting with insurers to offer HMO plans to Medicaid beneficiaries.

The federal government specifies minimum requirements for Medicaid programs, with states having the option to expand coverage. Eligibility for Medicaid is determined by the individual states on the basis of the state's income criteria. The federal government mandates that the following services be included in each state's program:

- Inpatient hospital services
- Outpatient hospital services
- Early and Periodic Screening, Diagnostic, and Treatment (EPSDT) Services
- Nursing facility services
- Home health services
- Physician services
- Rural health clinic services
- Federally qualified health center services
- Laboratory and x-ray services
- Family planning services
- Nurse midwife services
- Certified pediatric and family nurse practitioner services
- Freestanding birth center services (when licensed or otherwise recognized by the state)
- Transportation to medical care
- Tobacco cessation counseling for pregnant women

● CASE STUDY

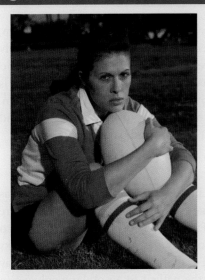

Just a few weeks ago, one of Annabelle's colleagues checked in a patient named Skyler who presented with a sore index finger. Her passion is playing rugby with a local club, and she jammed her finger catching a pass. Her insurance policy specified a $50 copay. During the visit, she got x-rays, a temporary splint, and a referral to an orthopedic specialist. Today, Skyler called the clinic, furious about the bill she received.

"This bill says I owe you $176 for diagnostic x-rays!" Skyler says. "I don't understand. I pay $267 every month for premiums, and I paid you a $50 copay before the visit. Why isn't this covered by my insurance?"

"I'm truly sorry for the confusion," Annabelle said, "but it looks to me like you haven't met your yearly deductible yet, which is $1000. That means you have to spend $1000 of your own money before the insurer will pay for certain services, like x-rays."

"That's just too much money," Skyler said. "I guess when it's time to choose a new plan this November, I'll look for one with a lower deductible."

"Unfortunately, it's always a trade-off," Annabelle cautioned. "Health insurance policies with lower deductibles usually require higher monthly premiums. So you have to decide what's best for you."

▪ LEARNING CHECKPOINT 3.3
Paying for Health Care

1. Regarding the insurance of a minor, the parent or legal guardian is responsible for payment and is the _____.

2. Anita's hospital bill was $7199.00, and she owed $720.00 after insurance. Her insurance policy stipulates that she pay a 10% _____ for hospitalization services.

3. A preferred provider organization is a type of _____ care.

4. Under the Affordable Care Act (ACA), children could remain on their parent's insurance policies until the age of _____.

5. Which component of Medicare helps pay for outpatient services?

   a. Part A
   b. Part B
   c. Part C
   d. Part D

CHARACTERISTICS AND CHALLENGES

Currently, more than 32 countries have some type of a universal health care system, some since the 1940s. Not all countries with universal health care have government-only health care. Many of these countries with universal health care systems continue to have both public and private insurance and medical providers. The United States is one of the few developed countries that does not have a universal health care system. As we have already seen in this chapter, the United States health care system is instead a mixture of government, private, and nonprofit services and payers.

Integrated and Fragmented Care

Whether the patient has a type of managed care plan, is a Medicare beneficiary, or has some other third-party payer, most individuals have a relationship with a primary care provider (PCP), also called a *family physician* (Fig. 3.10). This physician is trained to identify and treat a wide variety of conditions. However, the family physician also seeks guidance from other specialists when necessary. For example, the family physician may identify a lump in the patient's neck and send the patient to an otolaryngologist (a physician specializing in the ear, nose, and throat) for further evaluation. In most cases, the PCP serves as the access point for health care. However, there are times when the PCP will need to send the the patient to a specialist. The process of sending a patient to another physician, usually a specialist, is called a **referral**, and most health insurance plans require a referral from the PCP for the patient to see a specialist. Similarly, patients cannot access diagnostic or other allied health services without an order from a physician. The system where a PCP controls access to other parts of the health care delivery system is called a **gatekeeper** model. The gatekeeper model helps control health care cost by reducing the number of patients' self-referral to specialists.

Some conditions or diseases require the services of multiple health care providers. A woman fighting metastatic breast cancer, for example, would access health care from many different health care providers at many different settings. She would see her PCP for routine complaints, but her oncologist would coordinate care related to the cancer. She might visit a radiation oncologist for radiation therapy, a chemotherapy center for infusions, a lab for blood tests, and an acupuncturist for pain and nausea treatment. She may be admitted to the hospital for blood and platelet transfusions.

Being able to track and guide health services, either during an individual illness or over the course of one's life, is called the **continuum of care** (Fig. 3.11). The continuum

referral a provider's request for the services of another provider, often a specialist.

gatekeeper a primary care provider who sees the patient first to control access to other parts of the health care delivery system.

continuum of care the tracking and guiding of health services, either during an individual illness or over the course of one's life.

Figure 3.10 Most individuals have a relationship with a family physician, also called a primary care provider (PCP).

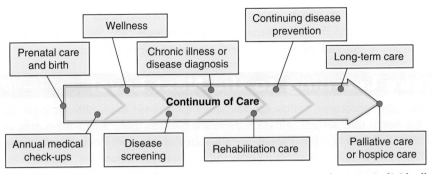

Figure 3.11 The continuum of care can refer to the health care accessed over an individual's life or to the care received in the treatment of a particular illness.

of care tracks and guides the health care services that are provided to a patient at all levels and stages of care. For this to work, communication is required among the various health care professionals and providers who treat the patient. For example, if the above patient presents at the ED late one night because of dizziness and shortness of breath, the staff at the hospital would be able to provide more accurate and appropriate care if they knew the patient's cancer diagnosis, treatment history, medications, and recent blood work. Without such communication, the providers at the hospital may order unnecessary tests or even pursue an incorrect diagnosis. In an *integrated* delivery system, all the various health care providers are connected to provide the best patient care, to produce the optimal patient outcome, and in the most efficient way.

However, health care delivery in the United States is a complex mixture of many different people and organizations, and achieving an integrated system has proven difficult, often leading to a fragmented health care system. In a *fragmented* health care system, one health care provider is responsible for one part of care and another health care provider is responsible for another part. It would be more efficient and beneficial to the patient for there to be a single decision maker or to have coordinated care between health care providers in order to reduce the potential for multiple treatments and tests.

The Institute of Medicine reported that fragmented care is a common obstacle to controlling cost and wastes in the usage of government health care programs. The average Medicare beneficiary sees two physicians and five specialists each year. However, it is more common for patients or their family members to communicate and coordinate the patient's care than the physicians. This ineffective management of patient care decreases the likelihood that patients will receive timely care and increases the likelihood of poor patient outcomes and higher rates of morbidity and mortality.

Consider the case of Elizabeth Young, a 75-year-old Medicare beneficiary who was recently hospitalized for a routine surgery to correct an issue with her carpal tunnel syndrome. Due to her age, Elizabeth was kept in the hospital for 2 nights, during which time she contracted pneumonia, which extended her hospital stay. Her attending physician treated the pneumonia with powerful antibiotics that caused extreme diarrhea. She then developed a bacterial infection that later caused colitis. The sequence of events caused Elizabeth to become very frail, necessitating her move to a rehabilitation facility upon her release from the hospital. Once discharged to the rehabilitation facility, her primary care physician resumed overseeing her care. During one of her examinations, the physician heard her coughing and ordered a chest x-ray. He noticed on the x-ray an abnormality and ordered a strong round of antibiotics to treat the finding. As a result, Elizabeth's diarrhea and bacterial infection returned. Had the primary care physician been made aware of Elizabeth's pneumonia during her hospital stay, he would have recognized the abnormality in the chest x-ray as a result of that illness.

TAKE AWAY ●·········

The fragmented health care system in the United States presents challenges to providing continuity of care.

This example is an unfortunate result of a fragmented health care system where health care providers do not communicate to coordinate care. Situations such as this result in inefficient and ineffective patient care and poor health outcomes.[6]

Take Learning to the Next Level····················

Patient care advocates and patient navigators are used in many different capacities in the health care system. Although there are overlaps, patient care advocates and patient navigators do differ. Patient care advocates usually work independently outside of the medical center to assist patients in their health care decision making. Patient navigators, on the other hand, usually work within the medical center and are employed by the organization. They assist patients in locating services and making appointments at the medical center and may even help patients understand their diagnoses and treatment plans. They may be nurses, therapists, or social workers or have other types of medical training and education.

Considering the fragmented health care system in the United States and the reports of the high number of preventable deaths that occur in the health care system each year, what are some suggested roles that patient care advocates could serve to improve patient outcomes? Do you think that there should be government incentives for health care providers to use patient care advocates? What do you think cost savings would look like if patient care advocates were routinely used?

Various efforts have attempted to reduce fragmentation in health care delivery. As mentioned earlier in this chapter, parts of the ACA encouraged health care providers to voluntarily share responsibility in patient care, coordinating treatment efforts through the establishment of ACOs. But those unfamiliar with medical records may wonder why it is so difficult for different providers to share patient information, especially in our digital age. Isn't it all computerized? Can't patient data be sent electronically?

Although the technology needed to collect and transmit patient care data electronically is not new (Fig. 3.12), some providers have struggled to implement electronic health records (EHRs) capable of collecting and sharing patient data. The shift from paper-based charting to computerized systems has been in progress for decades. But a fully electronic system is expensive, and transmitting patient data is complicated by concerns for privacy. Furthermore, such a system needs standardized data formats so that computers using

---

[6]Institute of Medicine: To err is human: building a safer health system. Washington, DC, 2000, The National Academies Press. https://doi.org/10.17226/9728.

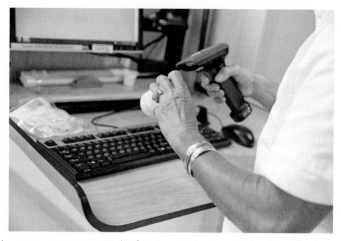

Figure 3.12 A nurse uses a computerized system to access a patient's medical record and track the administration of medication.

different software at different clinics can process the information. This is known as **interoperability,** or the ability of different information technology systems to exchange data and communicate.

> **interoperability** the ability of different information technology systems to exchange data and communicate.

Health information professionals have long recognized how fully interoperable EHRs can reduce inefficiencies and improve patient safety. As part of the American Recovery and Reinvestment Act legislation, passed in 2009 and commonly known as the *Recovery Act*, the federal government funded a stimulus bill that provided incentives for health care providers to embrace EHR technology. The program, commonly called *meaningful use,* increased Medicare reimbursements to providers who purchased and used EHRs capable of collecting and sharing certain kinds of patient data electronically and, in the later stages, penalized those providers that did not implement an EHR system by reducing payments. CMS announced the end of the program in 2016 but has not yet announced a replacement.

Rising Costs

Health care makes up a huge portion of the US economy. It will account for almost 20% of the gross domestic product (GDP) by 2021. In 2015, the United States' spending on health care rose to the equivalent of 17% of the GDP, totaling more than $3 trillion. Spending significantly increased with the implementation of the ACA, which produced a nearly 12% increase in Medicare spending.

Additionally, several factors contributed to these rising costs:

- **Lack of competition and inability to compare prices**. Prices are lower when businesses compete. However, the ability to compare prices for health care is problematic because care is almost always paid for by a third party, such as employers or the state or federal government. This means that many people may not care to make cost-saving decisions or find the task too laborious. Some patients may also look at the price of services and assume that higher cost means higher quality—they would purposely avoid the lowest-priced care. Additionally, even though insurers negotiate prices of health care services directly with individual providers, patients often do not have access to these negotiated prices. Thus it is difficult for a patient to make an informed decision about cost when prices are not transparent. These factors work together to eliminate the downward pressure on prices that would normally arise from comparing prices and choosing the lowest-cost service.
- **Overtreatment**. Health care is generally billed by the service provided. According to the Congressional Business Office, up to 30% of health care provided in the United States is unnecessary. The Institute of Medicine estimates that the industry driven by fee-for-service payments for treatment has led to excessive costs of $210 billion a year for services, resulting in unnecessary tests and procedures and poorer patient outcomes.[7] This may be caused by more health care providers practicing *defensive medicine,* where the provider recommends or performs treatments and procedures not because he or she believes the patient requires it, but to safeguard against malpractice and litigation.
- **Lack of patient care coordination**. Many patients, especially the elderly, have multiple health issues that require them to see multiple health care providers. As discussed earlier, the lack of coordination of care between providers may result in test duplication, medication mismanagement, and unnecessary treatments. Poor continuum of care may also result in complications for the patient and more hospital stays, resulting in even more cost.
- **Technology**. Advances in medicine and technology have saved millions of lives, but they come at a higher cost. A computer tomography (CT) scanner provides images

---

[7]Parker-Pope, T. (Aug. 2012). Overtreatment is taking a harmful toll. *The New York Times.*

of the body, but the machine can cost anywhere from $50,000 to $150,000, with a cost to the patient of $350 to $1000 for the procedure. Sometimes, new technology may provide little or no additional value compared with current treatments. For example, if a patient presented with chest pain, a physician used to perform an exercise stress test to determine if there is coronary artery disease. But now, with the development of the coronary CT angiogram (CTA), the exercise stress test has lost favor. The CTA is 10 times more expensive than the exercise stress test but has not been shown to improve patient outcomes.[8]

- **Prescription drugs**. New drug treatments represent some of the biggest advances in health care and improved patient outcomes. However, prescription drug innovation is also one of the major contributors to the increase in health care spending. Pharmaceutical companies will invest in specialty medicines and injectable drugs that are expensive to develop and costly to patients when they reach the market.

- **Fraud and abuse**. Health care fraud is a national problem occurring in federal and state-funded health programs, as well as in private insurance programs. Health care fraud is when a company, health care provider, or a patient submits false or misleading information or a claim to receive a profit. For example, a physician may bill Medicaid for a medical procedure that was either not performed or billed at a higher rate than the actual procedure. Although it is difficult to determine what the actual financial impact is, health care fraud has been estimated to cost more than $272 billion in health care spending in the United States, which squanders tax dollars and drives up health care costs.[9]

The cost of health care deductibles and premiums is growing from year to year at a rate matching the increase in the cost of health care. Employers are facing an increase of more than 20% in premium costs, which they try to offset by offering higher-deductible plans to their employees. Over the past 5 years, average deductibles have almost doubled. With both deductibles and health care insurance premiums rising, the out-of-pocket costs paid by consumers increased by more than 11% from 2014 to 2015. Unfortunately, the growth in income from year to year has not kept up with health care costs, with income increasing from only 1% to 2% annually.

Shifting demographics in the United States have also resulted in increases in health care costs, especially in regard to its aging population. People require more care as they age. As a result, older people will need to see PCPs and specialists for a myriad of different health conditions: muscle and joint aches, failing hearing and eyesight, dementia, incontinence, and heart conditions. Currently, the population consists of approximately 14.5% senior citizens, or an estimated 45 million people. In the next few decades, however, the number of older adults will swell as the generation called the *baby boomers* (the 76 million babies born in the two decades after World War II, from 1945–1964) advance in age (Fig. 3.13). By 2060, the population over the age of 65 is expected to reach 21.7% of the total population, an increase to 98 million people.

Uninsured and Underinsured Populations

Even though the United States spends more than most other industrialized countries on health care, there are disparities in accessing health care. Lack of insurance is the largest barrier to the United States health care delivery system, and the increasing cost of insurance premiums and deductibles of those covered has made many people reluctant to even use health services and preventive care. The medically **indigent**, or those without

indigent the condition of being unable to afford care.

---

[8]Patel et al. (March 11, 2010). Low diagnostic yield of elective coronary angiography. *N Engl J Med* 2010;362: 886–895.
[9]Berwick DM, Hackbarth AD. (April 11, 2012). Eliminating waste in US health care. *JAMA* 307(14):1513–1516.

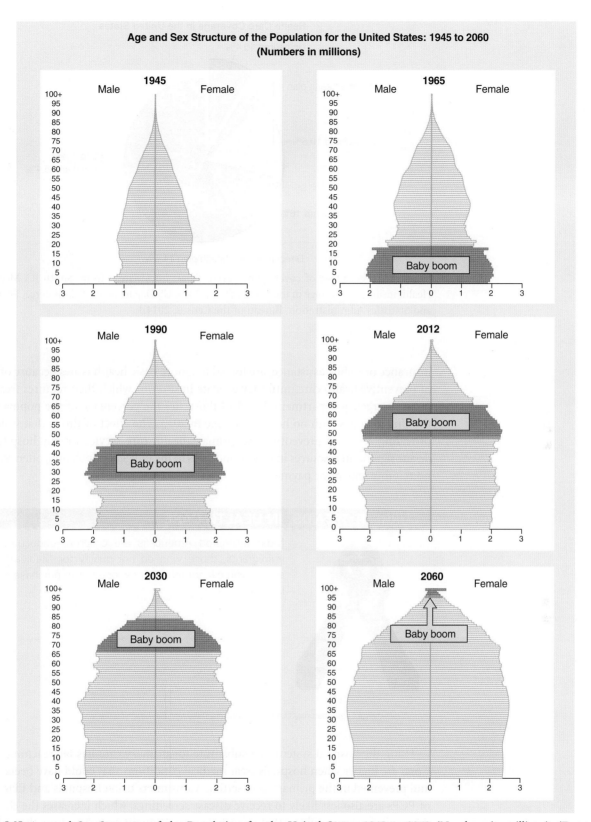

Figure 3.13 Age and Sex Structure of the Population for the United States: 1945 to 2060 (Numbers in millions). (From Colby SL, Ortman JM. The baby boom cohort in the United States: 2012 to 2060: Population estimates and projections. US Census Bureau, May 2014.)

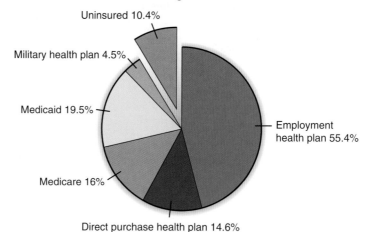

Figure 3.14 Percentage of coverage by payer. (Chart information from: Smith JC, Medalia C. Health insurance coverage in the United States: 2013. US Department of Commerce, Economics and Statistics Administration, Bureau of the Census, 2014.)

insurance or public assistance, are forced to ignore basic health issues because of a lack of preventive health care until they escalate in severity, which then requires treatment in an emergency department. Fig. 3.14 illustrates the percentage of the population in the United States with no health coverage in 2013. The effect of this is that instead of providing access to preventive and primary health care services, many hospital EDs devote significant resources in service and costs to the indigent population, often receiving no reimbursement or payment.

CURRENT TRENDS IN HEALTH CARE

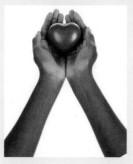

Most uninsured Americans are children, undocumented immigrants, those who do not qualify for Medicaid, and adults who cannot afford or choose not to purchase health insurance.

http://fivethirtyeight.com/features/33.million-americans-still-dont-have-health-insurance/

Using the hospital system as a substitute for primary care has far-reaching effects. Costs are higher when hospitals treat medical conditions that could have been treated and prevented in the primary care setting. Consumers using hospitals and EDs in lieu of PCPs are also less likely to receive disease screenings, which increases the chance of developing a chronic illness that is costly to treat. Without early detection, these chronic illnesses have lower positive outcome rates than illnesses detected early in the disease process.

Beyond the uninsured population, there are more than 31 million **underinsured** people in the United States. The underinsured are covered by a health care plan but have high deductibles or out-of-pocket expenses that are not in relationship to their

underinsured a term describing individuals who are covered by a health care plan but have high deductibles or out-of-pocket expenses that are not in relationship to their income level.

income level. The numbers of lower income Americans seeking care has increased, but the out-of-pocket costs has risen for those covered under private or group plans, which has led to missing regular medical visits, requesting minimal services, putting off medical procedures, avoiding filling prescriptions, and the rationing of medicines—all practices once characteristic of the uninsured population.

REVIEW QUESTIONS

1. How is the HMO model different from other types of insurance? What are the benefits to patients and insurers?

2. What is the function of the Medicare Conditions of Participation (CoP)?

3. What is the difference between Medicare and Medicaid?

4. List and explain three reasons for rising health care costs.

ADMINISTRATIVE MANAGEMENT

4 HEALTH CARE PROCESSES AND WORKFLOW

5 DOCUMENTATION

6 TECHNOLOGY

7 MANAGING SUPPLIES AND INVENTORY

8 BASIC FINANCE AND HEALTH CARE ACCOUNTING

9 THE REVENUE CYCLE

10 QUALITY, PERFORMANCE IMPROVEMENT, AND RISK MANAGEMENT

CHAPTER 4

HEALTH CARE PROCESSES AND WORKFLOW

Betsy Shiland

CHAPTER OUTLINE

INTRODUCTION
WORKFLOW
   Scheduling
      Triage
      Scheduling Methods

Check-in
Clinical Assessment
Checkout
Revenue Cycle

THE FACILITY
   Housekeeping
   Facility Layout

VOCABULARY

buffer time
chief complaint
cluster scheduling
double booking
fixed appointment scheduling
modified wave scheduling

open access scheduling
patient portal
progress note
revenue cycle
scheduling matrix
staggered schedule

stream scheduling
triage
walk-in
wave scheduling
workflow
workflow map

CHAPTER OBJECTIVES

After completing this chapter, the student should be able to do the following:

1. Summarize the workflow in an ambulatory care setting.

2. Describe the ambulatory care facility and the physical layout of various medical offices.

INTRODUCTION

Now that you have reviewed the role of the health services administrator, the array of professionals and settings, and the landscape of health care delivery, the remaining chapters of this book speak to the day-to-day activities of the health services administrator. This chapter provides an overview of the processes that occur in most ambulatory care settings, from the way patients are scheduled in the medical office to the payment for services rendered. It also discusses the design of a medical office and offers best practices for time management.

WORKFLOW

Although each ambulatory care facility has its own distinct methods and processes, the activities of providing patient care are usually similar and include scheduling of the patient, the clinical assessment, and the e-prescribing of the patient's medication. All of these activities comprise health care processes, with the sequences of these processes called the **workflow**. A visual tool that a health services administrator uses to understand the workflow process is called a **workflow map**, which, similar to a flowchart, shows the steps in any given process (Fig. 4.1).

It is critical for the medical office to have an efficient and effective workflow to optimize productivity and ensure high patient satisfaction and health outcomes. For example, improving a medical practice's workflow may lead to better patient access and a greater understanding of patient demand, strengthen prevention efforts, increase disease detection, and help manage chronic conditions.

Oftentimes, the health services administrator is responsible for developing and reevaluating the medical office's workflow. The evaluation of the office's workflow and processes should occur routinely to allow for changes in regulations and laws, staffing, patient care, and equipment and technology. For example, identifying problems and areas of improvements in the medical office's workflow will make the check-in process more efficient, decrease the wait times for patients, improve patient flow from intake to discharge, and help in the transition from paper medical charts to an electronic medical system.

○ **workflow** the sequence of processes in a medical office.

○ **workflow map** a graphic display of the steps in a process.

TAKE AWAY ●·········

The health services administrator must evaluate the office's workflow regularly.

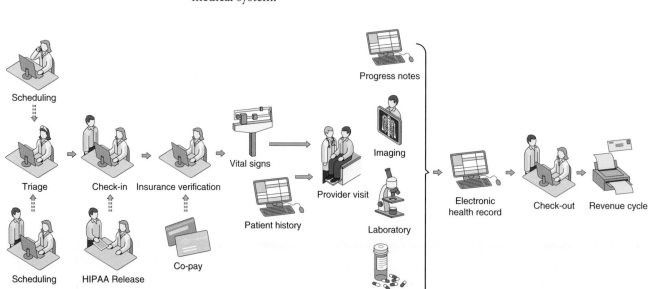

Figure 4.1 Health care processes in an ambulatory care workflow map.

CASE STUDY

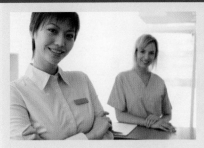

Julie, a student in an online health services administration program, was asked to review the scheduling process and workflow at her clinical site to see if there were any changes in the past year. The clinic administrator introduced her to the staff in the registration area where she was to sit with Ashley, the patient registration technician, for the morning. Julie reviewed the clinic's workflow map, made notes, and then began her interview to determine the process. Ashley, who has been working in patient registration for 4 years, immediately pointed out that the process is not as straightforward as it had been previously. Although many of the appointments for established patients were made by a telephone call, some of the patients were now using the *patient portal* to make their appointments, which is something they were not able to do in previous years.

"You mean they can log on to a website and request an appointment online?" Julie asked.

"Exactly," Ashley said. "They can search for appointment times and select the one they want, and even fill out an intake form electronically."

"That sounds convenient for the patients," Julie said, "but I can see how it takes some getting used to. What happens next?"

Scheduling

Workflow in the medical office begins with a patient arriving at the facility. Scheduled appointments remain the norm in many ambulatory settings, and patients make appointments through a variety of means. They could call the office on the telephone, set a time after their last visit, or request an appointment through a consultation or referral. They may also set up an appointment through a **patient portal**, which is a secure, web-based tool that allows the medical office and its patients to communicate (Fig. 4.2).

Using the patient portal, patients are able to make their own appointments by logging in and viewing the medical office's schedule for available appointments. Patients are also able to see their upcoming appointments, confirm or cancel appointments, and even choose their reminder call preferences. Once the patient selects an appointment time, the system automatically sends a notification to the patient registration staff. A staff member monitors the appointments that are made through the patient portal and for each appointment made determines if the time allotment is correct. This staff member may verify the appointment with the patient and may also maneuver the time slot if the appointment doesn't allow the amount of time needed based on the reason for the visit. A clinical staff member—usually a nurse or medical assistant—also monitors the portal for patient information of a clinical concern. *Does the patient need a laboratory test before being seen? Does this patient need to be seen right away?* By monitoring appointment requests on the portal, the clinical staff member helps keep the workflow of the office running smoothly.

Using the patient portal, the medical office can save time and money by minimizing calls and missed appointments. Additionally, the patient portal allows patients to view their health information and records, such as recent physician visits, discharge summaries, medications, and laboratory test results. Patients are also able to communicate directly with the provider through secure messaging and ask questions in between visits.

An increasing number of ambulatory care settings see patients on a **walk-in** basis, where no appointment is required. At retail care clinics, urgent care clinics, diagnostic facilities, dialysis centers, and other such facilities, patients can generally arrive during normal business hours and be seen in a reasonable amount of time.

TAKE AWAY

The patient may schedule appointments in person, by telephone, through referral, or by using the patient portal.

patient portal a web-based tool that allows the medical office and its patients to communicate securely.

walk-in a type of encounter for which no appointment is required.

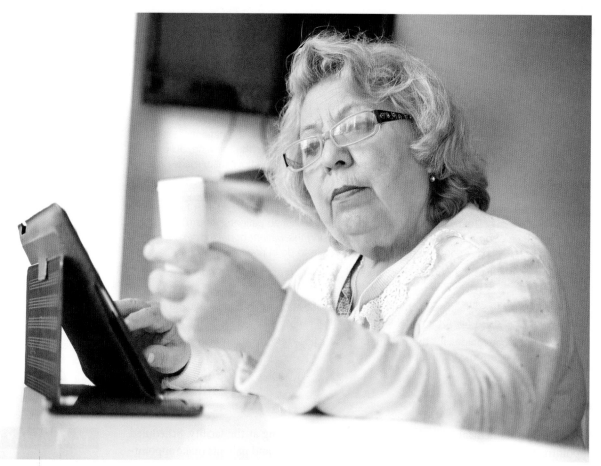

Figure 4.2 Patients can set up an appointment with the provider using a patient portal.

When scheduling appointments, patients are categorized as either *new* or *established* patients. The difference is important because of the amount of time and work involved in getting information from a new patient compared with one who has already been seen by the physician. This is true for both administrative and clinical processes: when a new patient requests an appointment, office staff must collect detailed demographic information, such as the patient's medical history and current conditions and insurance information. Patients may be sent the new patient forms ahead of time, asked to arrive early so they may complete these forms before being seen by the physician, or asked to submit their patient information on an electronic intake form using a patient portal. Established patients will also be asked to update their information either through the patient portal or upon their arrival at the medical office.

Take Learning to the Next Level

Another important reason why a patient needs to be differentiated between a new and an established patient is due to the coding process and how to bill for the services rendered. As defined by the coding system CPT-4, an established patient is one who has previously received care within the last 3 years by the particular physician or the same physician specialty group.

staggered schedule the placement of providers in a variety of days and times that best meet the needs of the organization.

Not all providers work in an ambulatory setting on a standard 9 AM to 5 PM schedule. Some providers have hours at other practices and/or in other locations, and some will work early mornings or into the evening. A **staggered schedule** has physicians in a variety of days and times that best meet the practice's needs. To make appointments, the patient registration technician needs to know when the providers are available, making sure to exclude each provider during their vacation, travel, and personal time. This information helps create a **scheduling matrix**, which is a tabular map of the times each provider is available (Fig. 4.3).

    Time allotments for appointment duration will vary. The appointment may be quick and short if the patient only needs simple laboratory work, a blood pressure check, or a wound check by a nurse. Others may need more of the provider's time, such as for a physical exam, a consultation, a new patient visit, or a sick visit. Each of these will have a predetermined amount of time set by the medical office that is helpful when scheduling patients (Fig. 4.4). In addition, the length of appointment times may vary by provider preference. Some physicians choose to see their established patients for 20-minute appointments, whereas others use 10- or 15-minute appointment times. The length of the appointment may also depend on the physician's specialty. For example, a cardiologist may require more time with a patient than a family physician.

scheduling matrix a tabular map of the times each provider is available.

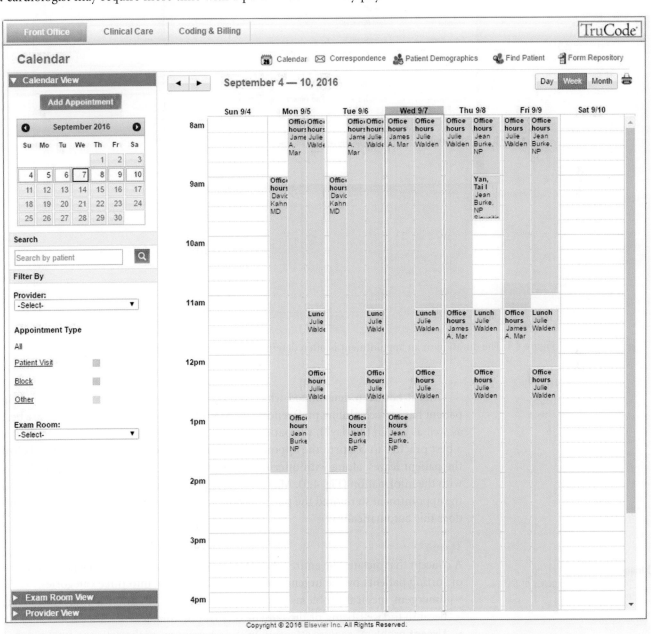

Figure 4.3 The scheduling matrix shows the times when each provider is available in this staggered schedule.

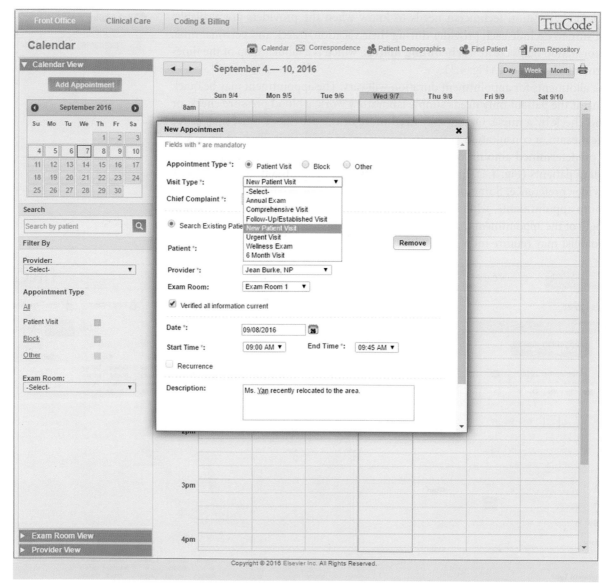

Figure 4.4 The duration of an appointment is often determined by the type of appointment.

Once it has been determined what type of time slot is necessary and whether the patient has any scheduling preferences (for example: "Wednesdays and Fridays are best, as well as late in the day"), the patient is offered an appointment date and time. It is a best practice to confirm the appointment date, time, location, and physician before the patient leaves, along with offering a "reminder" card or sticker for their calendar with the information (Fig. 4.5). Many offices routinely call a set number of days before the appointment to remind the patient again, and scheduling software is available that does this automatically.

Triage

A concept that dictates the entire scheduling process is that of *triage*. **Triage** is a method of sorting patients by the urgency of their needs, usually into three categories:
- **Emergent** medical problems require the immediate attention of the clinical staff because the well-being of the patient is currently threatened.
- **Urgent** problems require attention in the near future, or the patient's condition will worsen, threatening their well-being.

triage a method of sorting patients by the urgency of their needs.

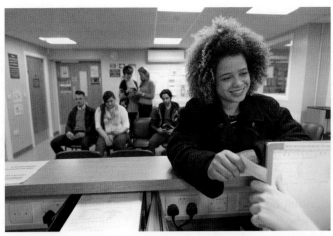

Figure 4.5 The patient receives a reminder card for her next appointment.

- **Nonurgent** problems do not require immediate attention because they do not pose a threat to the well-being of the patient.

Certainly, a patient with an emergency medical condition would need to be seen much sooner than a patient with a nonurgent condition. For example, if one patient calls with a cold (a nonurgent problem) and another calls with a suspected broken wrist (an urgent problem), the triage process would give the patient with the suspected broken wrist an earlier appointment.

Scheduling Methods

Scheduling appointments efficiently is crucial to the successful operation of a medical office. Scheduling will affect resource and staff utilization; profitability; and the general satisfaction of patients, physicians, and staff. Some appointments take longer than usual, whereas others may be shorter; sometimes patients are late, and sometimes they do not show up at all. Traffic problems, forgetfulness, family matters, and other problems can and do cause patients to miss or appear late for appointments. Each medical office must have a policy for those patients who are chronically late or miss schedule appointments because they will negatively affect scheduling and waste the providers' time and profitability.

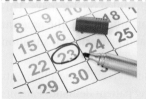

CURRENT TRENDS IN HEALTH CARE

In 2007 the Centers for Medicare and Medicaid Services began allowing providers to charge patients a fee for missed appointments to help provide an incentive for patients to show up when scheduled.

https://www.cms.gov/Regulations-and-Guidance/Guidance/Manuals/Downloads/clm104c01.pdf

When scheduling, staff should allow for *lead time,* which is a short amount of time before the physician actually sees the patient. Using lead time, the patient's appointment time might be 8:15 AM, but the physician may see the patient at 8:30 AM. The 15-minute difference allows for patients to be slightly late and gives the staff time for the check-in, collection of vitals, and taking of the patient history and reason for the visit.

As mentioned earlier, many ambulatory care settings see patients on a walk-in basis, including laboratories, imaging centers, chemotherapy centers, dialysis centers, and clinics. **Open access scheduling** is a method that has no appointments at all and allows for patients to be seen as they arrive at the facility, usually on a first-come-first-serve (FCFS) basis. Open access scheduling is often effective in these settings because the

open access scheduling a method that has no appointments at all and allows for patients to be seen as they arrive at the facility, usually on an FCFS basis.

buffer time a section of the schedule that is open for walk-ins or patients who need to see the physician urgently.

stream scheduling a method of assigning a set appointment time to each individual patient. Also called *fixed appointment scheduling*.

wave scheduling a method of appointment scheduling in which a group of patients are placed at the top of the hour and seen in the order in which they arrive.

modified wave scheduling a method of appointment scheduling in which a small group of patients is scheduled at the top of an hour, with single patients also scheduled within the hour.

double booking the scheduling of two patients to see the same provider at the same time.

cluster scheduling a method of scheduling that assigns similar patients or medical care on the same days.

duration of the encounter is roughly the same for all patients, and the facility can generally count on a consistent level of traffic each day. Although this is convenient from a patient's point of view, it may be inefficient for a conventional family physician to wait for patients to appear. As a result, a hybrid scheduling method provides a **buffer time**, a section of the schedule that is open for walk-ins or patients who need to see the physician urgently, to satisfy both patients and physicians.

Stream scheduling or **fixed appointment scheduling** is a traditional method of assigning a set appointment time to each individual patient. For example, one patient is scheduled for 8:15 AM, the next for 8:30 AM, and the third for 8:45 AM. This scheduling method works well in theory but does not account for normal variability of patients' arrival times and patients whose problems require more of the provider's time than was scheduled, resulting in the provider falling behind and patients having to wait despite having a scheduled appointment. Other scheduling methods are available that help add some flexibility to the scheduling process without turning away late patients and losing revenue.

Wave scheduling places a group of patients at the top of an hour: 9 AM, 10 AM, or 11 AM. The patients are then seen in the order that they arrive. For example, three established patients—Ms. Abbot, Mr. Brown, and Ms. Clark—are scheduled for an 11 AM appointment, with the physician seeing patients in 15-minute intervals. Mr. Brown shows up first, Ms. Clark second, and Ms. Abbot last. Mr. Brown is the first person seen, and, when he leaves, Ms. Clark is next, and followed by Ms. Abbot. The advantage to this type of scheduling is a reduced chance of the provider waiting for late patients and having them alter the schedule for the remainder of the day.

Modified wave scheduling allows a small group of patients to be scheduled at the top of an hour, with single patients also scheduled at 10- to 15-minute intervals within the hour. The more complicated patients are scheduled and treated first. This type of scheduling allows for the same advantage as wave scheduling with the additional advantage of mixing shorter and longer appointments.

Double booking is when two patients are scheduled for the same time slot with the same provider. If this occurs, patients should be seen in the order in which they arrive or the order in which they are triaged. Some medical offices may double book patients when one needs to be sent for diagnostic testing, allowing time for the provider to see both patients without keeping either one waiting.

Cluster scheduling is used to assign similar patients or medical care on the same days. For example, all well-baby visits or new patients are scheduled on Tuesdays. This type of scheduling helps maximize efficiency in the office by minimizing the amount of equipment being used and providing similar information about a particular situation to many patients.

Each practice should routinely evaluate their scheduling methods and time allotments to see if its current system is effective and efficient and meeting patient demand. Patients may request appointment times outside the currently available schedule. As the health services administrator, you may want to continually evaluate and survey patients and their requests and consider a change in the schedule method.

Check-In

Upon arriving for the visit, the first component of the medical office workflow is the patient check-in. The patient will provide the patient registration staff his or her name and which provider the appointment is with. The patient registration technician will access the patient's record and verify the patient's date of birth, gender, address, contact information, insurance information, and any other required information specified by the clinic's protocol. If the patient is new or his or her insurance company has changed,

TAKE AWAY ●·········

Registration staff verify the patient's information at check-in.

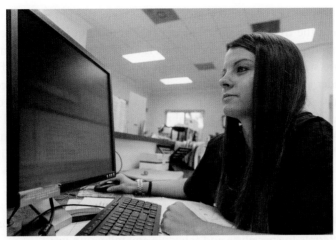

Figure 4.6 A patient registration technician checks the insurance card to ensure the practice has the patient's most current insurance information.

the staff member will make a photocopy of the patient's insurance card to be placed in the patient's record or scan an image of the card and upload it to the patient's electronic health record (EHR) (Fig. 4.6). Having the current insurance policy numbers and the contact numbers listed on the card is essential for determining if certain services or prescription drugs are covered and which specialists are in-network, should the patient need a referral. The insurance card also lists the amount of the copay required for the visit, if any.

The claim submitted to the patient's third-party payer for the reimbursement of services contains sensitive information about the patient's health. Thus the patient must sign a Health Insurance Portability and Accountability Act (HIPAA) release or privacy notice, granting the facility permission to share information regarding the visit. A copay, if required by the patient's policy, may be collected at this time, and a receipt is then provided either electronically or as a hard copy. The patient registration technician may then ask the patient to return to the reception area to wait to be called by a medical assistant or nurse. Once the patient registration technician has inputted the patient's information in the EHR and insurance eligibility has been confirmed, the medical assistant or nurse will see an alert on the EHR screen that the patient is ready to be roomed.

Clinical Assessment

After retrieving the patient from the reception area, the patient's weight, height, and vital signs (blood pressure, pulse, respiratory rate, and temperature) are measured and recorded. The patient is asked about the **chief complaint** (the primary reason for the visit), any changes in health status, and the names and dosages of any current medications. This information is documented in the patient's medical record or EHR. The patient is then asked to wait for the provider, which may be a physician, a physician's assistant, or nurse practitioner.

Upon entering the examination room, the provider should greet the patient and review the documentation of the medical assistant or nurse. The provider confirms the patient information and will continue questioning the patient in regard to the duration, severity, and location of the presenting problem.

A common method of documenting the medical evaluation and treatment plan is by using SOAP notes. The four components of a SOAP note are Subjective, Objective, Assessment, and Plan. It consists of collecting data in four specific categories: the

chief complaint the primary reason for the visit.

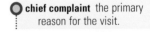

Clinical findings are documented in the patient's medical record.

patient's *subjective* view, the physician's *objective* view, the physician's evaluation or *assessment*, and the treatment *plan*. The patient's complaint is the subjective portion ("I have a sore throat"), and the objective part is the physician's physical findings—that is, temperature, strep test, physical examination. Assessment is a judgment of the findings by the provider as to support the diagnosis, and the plan is the proposed treatment and follow-up. Although providers may not always follow this format exactly, they record patient information in this general manner. If the visit is brief and specific and does not require an extensive SOAP note, each patient visit will result in a **progress note** from the provider with documentation to support the resulting diagnosis and treatment.

Once the provider is finished examining the patient, laboratory tests, procedures, or medications may need to be ordered. Some EHR systems have automatic standardized order sets based on the provider's specialty or on specific diseases. The provider may also make referrals to specialists and schedule any follow-up visits.

progress note the documentation of a patient's care and response to treatment.

Checkout

The last step in the patient visit is the patient checking out with the patient registration technician (Fig. 4.7). Often, the same patient registration technician may perform both check-in and check-out functions, depending on the volume of patients. At this time, the patient will be scheduled for any needed follow-up appointments, will receive any discharge instructions or any educational material, and pays for any services.

The patient registration technician will use the scheduling software to find an acceptable follow-up appointment for the patient in the provider's schedule. The software will not only enter the appointment for the patient and the provider, but, in many cases, place the appointment in a "reminder" file that automatically contacts the patient before the appointment. Once the patient leaves, the medical assistant or nurse will clean the patient room and prepare it for the next patient.

Revenue Cycle

revenue cycle the series of processes related to billing for medical services performed and other resources consumed.

The term **revenue cycle** refers to the series of processes related to billing for medical services performed and other resources consumed, such as medical supplies. It is a critical component of the office workflow. The revenue cycle and its management will be discussed in further detail in Chapter 9.

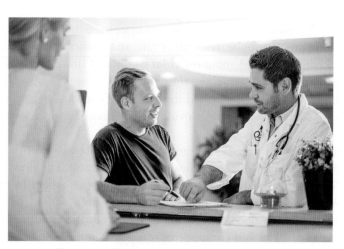

Figure 4.7 The patient checks out after a visit.

The documentation of the patient visit, which includes the provider's assessment and treatment plan, serves as the basis for billing. In fact, only the services recorded in the patient's EHR are billable. First, a medical coder examines the provider's documentation and assigns codes to the patient's diagnosis and any procedure or services performed by the provider. The medical coder will create electronic claims and transmits them to the patient's third-party payers for reimbursement. The third-party payer reviews the claim to ensure it is complete and accurate and that the received services are covered benefits. Payers also check whether the service provided was appropriate for the patient's condition and whether the test or treatment was necessary. For example, if a patient presents with dysuria (pain with urination), it would be reasonable for the provider to request a urinalysis to be performed, and the payer would cover the cost of the service. However, if an x-ray was ordered, the payer would deny the claim because there is not a clear relationship between the symptom (dysuria) and the test ordered (an x-ray).

The patient's third-party payer may cover all, some, or none of the costs of a patient's visit. The patient is responsible for any amount not paid for by the payer, with the medical biller sending the patient a separate invoice. Once the full balance is paid, the patient's file is updated. If the patient fails to pay a bill on time, the medical office is responsible for following up with the patient and handling any billing issues. If the balance remains unpaid for a certain amount of time as specified by office policy, a collections process is initiated to receive reimbursement for the overdue bill. The patient's unpaid bills may be sent to an outside collection agency.

TAKE AWAY

Only the services documented in the patient's record are billable.

LEARNING CHECKPOINT 4.1
Workflow

1. Which type of scheduling allows walk-ins?

   a. wave scheduling
   b. modified wave scheduling
   c. open access scheduling
   d. cluster scheduling

2. The _____ is the primary reason for the patient's visit.

   a. workflow
   b. triage
   c. chief complaint
   d. SOAP note

3. Which happens first?

   a. staff make a copy of the patient's insurance card
   b. staff take the patient's vital signs
   c. the provider establishes a diagnosis
   d. the patient schedules a follow-up appointment

4. Submitting a claim to the patient's payer is part of the _____ process.

   a. check-in
   b. clinical assessment
   c. check-out
   d. revenue cycle

THE FACILITY

A well-maintained facility is not only required for an efficient workflow, but also provides a professional and compliant space for patient care. In terms of the facility itself—whether the office is a free-standing building, a floor in a high-rise, or a section of a department store—all aspects of the physical environment must be monitored by the health services administrator. This includes testing fire alarms, extinguishers, and sprinklers and having all medical and nonmedical equipment regularly serviced. The facility will employ a service for the regular inspection of the heating and cooling system, which will include cleaning the ducts to maintain healthy ventilation. Burned-out light bulbs should be replaced as soon as possible, and painting should be done every 7 years or as needed. On the exterior of the medical office, maintenance of the entrance and exit, the parking lot, and any landscaping also needs to be addressed and maintained.

Housekeeping

Aside from the daily business of treating patients, the practice needs regular custodial maintenance. Vacuuming; trash and recycling collection; cleaning of offices, exam rooms, bathrooms, and waiting rooms; and other housekeeping activities may be performed by the office's own cleaning staff or a contracted vendor. Usually, this type of housecleaning takes place at night when the office is closed. The health services administrator must develop a schedule to determine which tasks are done and how often.

The Occupational Health and Safety Administration (OSHA), discussed in more detail in Chapter 11, imposes specific regulations and guidelines regarding medical waste. In order to maintain a sanitary workplace, biohazard materials and sharps, such as used needles, must be collected and disposed of separately (Fig. 4.8). The clinical staff is responsible for properly disposing of these items, and an outside vendor will collect the waste. Potentially infectious bodily fluids must be properly and immediately cleaned. For example, if a patient with a nosebleed drips blood in the reception area, the area must be cleaned with an approved disinfectant, with the staff member wearing the proper equipment, such as gloves.

Facility Layout

The most efficient workflow also depends on the layout of the office. Of course, the physical layout varies greatly location to location, as well as by the type of ambulatory care services offered. For example, some urgent care clinics and physician's offices have a laboratory or x-ray unit on site (Fig. 4.9). A retail clinic's layout may be as simple as an exam room adjacent to the pharmacy (Fig. 4.10). The floor plan of a dialysis center may reflect a different workflow, with several chairs in an open area and close to the nurses' station (Fig. 4.11).

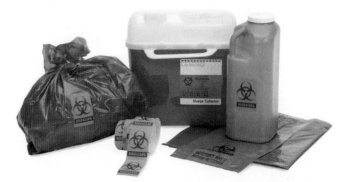

Figure 4.8 Biowaste is collected in specially designed containers.

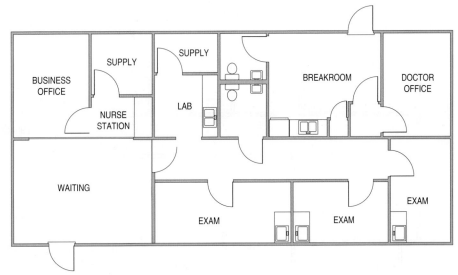

Figure 4.9 The floor plan of a small physician's office or clinic with a laboratory.

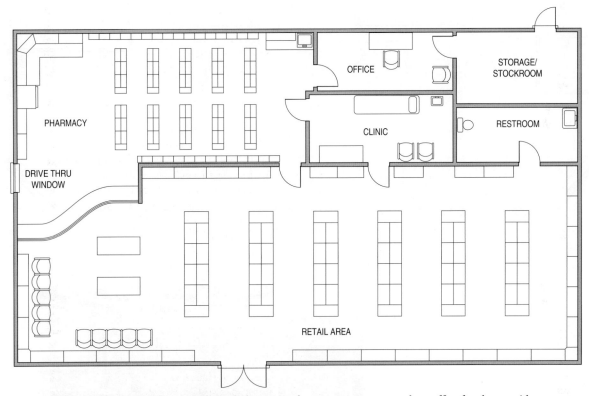

Figure 4.10 A retail clinic usually only has space for one exam room and an office for the provider.

Virtually all medical facilities and offices will have a reception area, where patients wait following check-in. In the reception area, offices usually keep on hand an array of magazines and medical pamphlets, and some may even have a television and children's play area in the room. Chairs should be comfortable and commercial grade, with some extra-wide bariatric chairs available for obese clients (Fig. 4.12). Space in the reception area, as well as the rest of the office, should be open enough to accommodate a wheelchair. Patient check-in desks should be conveniently accessible but should offer a level of privacy so conversations with patients cannot be easily heard by others in the waiting area. Because the reception area is the patients' first impression of the practice, extra care should be taken to ensure it is clean, orderly, and comfortable.

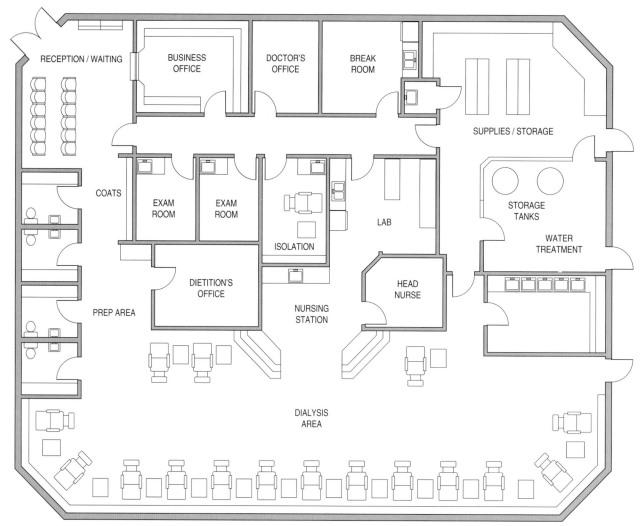

Figure 4.11 The floor plan of a dialysis center reflects its unique workflow.

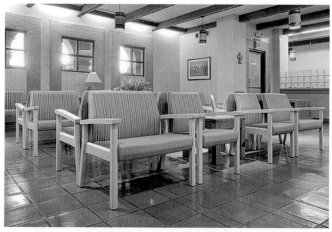

Figure 4.12 The reception area should have chairs to accommodate patients of all sizes. (Courtesy Stance Healthcare, Inc., Kitchener, Ontario.)

● CASE STUDY

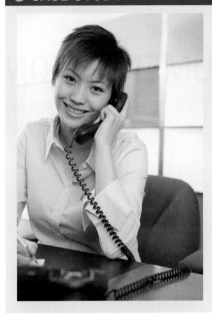

After sitting with Ashley for most of the morning, Julie got the chance to see how patient registration and scheduling begin the workflow at the clinic. She included three main notes about recent changes:

- Although still not common practice, a growing number of patients were using the patient portal to schedule appointments.
- The office had begun using a scanner to store an image of the patient's insurance card, which can then automatically be uploaded into the EHR, rather than simply making a photocopy.
- Several patients were unaware of how much their copay was and expected a lower amount.

▪ LEARNING CHECKPOINT 4.2
▪ The Facility

Circle the correct answer.

T or F   1. The maintenance of the medical office is usually monitored by the property owner.

T or F   2. Vacuuming usually takes place at night when the office is closed.

T or F   3. Used needles are referred to as sharps.

T or F   4. The reception area, as well as the rest of the office, should be open enough to accommodate a wheelchair.

REVIEW QUESTIONS

Match the term with its definition.

_____ 1. stream scheduling

_____ 2. buffer time

_____ 3. scheduling matrix

_____ 4. workflow map

_____ 5. open access scheduling

_____ 6. patient portal

_____ 7. triage

a. a tabular map of the times each provider is available

b. a graphic display of the steps in a process

c. a web-based tool that allows the medical office and its patients to communicate securely

d. a method of assigning a set appointment time to each individual patient

e. a method that has no appointments at all and allows for patients to be seen as they arrive at the facility

f. a section of the schedule that is open for walk-ins or patients who need to see the physician urgently

g. a method of sorting patients by the urgency of their needs

8. Which parts of the facility must be regularly inspected or serviced?

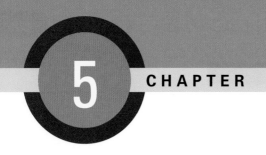

5 CHAPTER

DOCUMENTATION

Betsy Shiland

CHAPTER OUTLINE

INTRODUCTION
THE MEDICAL RECORD
  Types of Health Data
    Demographic Data
    Legal Data
    Financial Data
    Clinical Data
      Signatures
      Imaging and Laboratory
        Documentation
      Operative Reports
      Discharge Summary

  Ownership
    Retention
OTHER TYPES OF
  DOCUMENTATION
USES OF DOCUMENTATION
  Patient Care
  Support of Litigation
  Reimbursement
  Licensure, Accreditation, and
    Certification
  Administrative Functions
  Research

CODING
  International Classification of
    Disease, 10th Revision, Clinical
    Modification
  Healthcare Common Procedure
    Coding System (HCPCS)
    CPT's Evaluation and
      Management Codes

VOCABULARY

advance beneficiary notice (ABN)
advance directive
authentication
continuum of care
countersignature
Current Procedural Terminology
  (CPT)
discharge summary

do not resuscitate (DNR) order
evaluation and management (E/M)
  codes
incidence
informed consent
International Classification of
  Disease, 10th edition, Clinical
  Modification (ICD-10-CM)

litigation
master patient index
medical necessity
medical proxy
medical record
medical record number (MRN)
morbidity
mortality

CHAPTER OBJECTIVES

After completing this chapter, the student should be able to do the following:

1. Discuss the types of information kept in medical documentation.
2. Explain the ownership and retention of the medical record.
3. List other types of documentation in ambulatory settings.
4. Describe the uses of medical documentation.
5. Define medical coding and explain its purpose and uses.

INTRODUCTION

Documentation is the process of collecting different pieces of data that are critical to many functions and processes in a health care organization. The different types of documentation include demographic data about the patients, clinical and medical records, and legal and financial documents. There are many purposes to the documentation in a health care facility—from providing quality medical care to patients to ensuring accurate coding and claims being submitted for reimbursements.

This chapter explores the types of documentation and data collected in a health care setting along with the reasons for their collection. It also introduces the importance of accurate documentation for coding and reimbursement purposes and for the delivery of patient care.

CASE STUDY

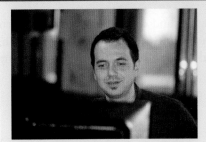

Abel, a second-year student in the health services administration program, is assigned to complete an externship at the Community Health Services Practice. One of his assignments is to follow the trail of documentation from the previous day's patients, record the level of E/M codes by the physicians, and understand the process of how documentation in the patient's record affects the level of E/M codes generated. Additionally, he is tasked with reporting on the staff's licensing status and, if he has time, to sample the patient index to check for duplicates. While at the clinic, the health services administrator reminds him of the maxim "If it's not documented, it wasn't done" to help emphasize the importance of documentation.

THE MEDICAL RECORD

The last time you visited the medical office, did you see the physician dictating or the medical assistant or nurse taking notes? What types of information were you asked to provide? Both the administrative and clinical staff asked questions and recorded the information to establish a patient record and determine the best way to provide quality care. Along with your name, contact information, age, ethnicity, marital status, financial data, and other information, the details of each encounter are documented in your patient medical record, sometimes referred to as a *health record* or *patient chart*. **Medical records** are a chronologic assemblage of all the medical data about an individual patient. Your health history, vital signs, diagnoses, procedures, medications, and treatments are recorded so that medical and legal professionals can refer to the information later, if needed. These records also include demographic information, legal consents, financial data, the history and physical examination, imaging and laboratory results, physician orders, nursing notes, and any referrals. In short, it is a report of the care a patient received and a record of relevant facts, findings, and observations about the patient's health history. Medical record documentation helps physicians and other health care providers evaluate and plan the patient's treatment and monitor the patient's health care over time. This information is crucial to providing quality care in both the short and longer term.

medical record an assemblage of all the medical data about an individual patient.

TAKE AWAY ●·········

Documentation helps ensure quality health care that is safe and legal.

Additionally, health insurance payers, including those for Medicaid and Medicare, may require accurate and sufficient documentation to ensure that a medical service is covered under the patient's insurance policy and to validate the medical necessity and appropriateness of the diagnostic and/or treatment services provided.

For example, a patient goes to sees his physician because of symptoms of a severe cold. The medical staff measures the patient's height, weight, and vital signs. The physician examines the patient, diagnoses a sinus infection, and prescribes an antibiotic. All this information is recorded in the patient's medical record. Several weeks later, the patient finishes his prescribed course of antibiotics but is still feeling ill. He returns to the medical office where his vital signs are taken again. The physician reviews the patient's medical record, including the information from his last visit. Because the details of the patient's previous visit were carefully documented, the physician can see the previous diagnosis and the specific antibiotic prescribed. The physician can also see that the patient's body temperature was normal 2 weeks ago, but is now measured at 103.1° F! Based on this patient history, the physician can confirm that the patient has not improved and may provide a different antibiotic, request additional tests, or pursue a different diagnosis and treatment plan.

Medical information has been kept in paper files and charts for most of modern medicine. Today, however, the electronic health record (EHR) is far more common. An EHR stores medical information digitally, and as we will see in Chapter 6, has many more features besides simple storage.

Types of Health Data

The types of information found in the medical record can be divided into four general categories: demographic, legal, financial, and clinical aspects. Table 5.1 summarizes each type of patient information collected in the health care setting.

Demographic Data

medical record number (MRN)
a unique number assigned to each patient's medical record.

A patient's medical record will include the patient's name, address, date of birth, gender, and contact information as part of its demographic information. In addition, each record is assigned a unique number called the **medical record number (MRN)**. The MRN represents the patient, and all information regarding the patient is filed or submitted

TABLE 5.1			
TYPES OF HEALTH DATA			
Data Type	**Examples**	**Data Type**	**Examples**
Demographic	Name	Financial	Patient's employer
	Address		Primary payer
	Date of birth (DOB)		Guarantor
	Gender		Group number
	Telephone number(s)	Clinical	Patient history
	Social Security number (SSN)		Physical exam
	Race/ethnicity		Laboratory report
	Medical record number		Imaging report
Legal	Advance directives		Nursing notes
	Medical proxy		Physician notes
	Consent to treatment		Physician orders
	Notice of Privacy Practices		Operative report
			Anesthesiology report

under that number in the practice's EHR system. The MRN number is an efficient way to connect patients to their medical data. The patient's MRN is unique to the practice, but may also be linked to other medical records the patient has in an enterprise-wide facility. The advantages of using MRNs to identify patient medical records are that they facilitate information sharing among physicians, may prevent against medical errors, and may protect health records by separating clinical data from financial data, such as Social Security numbers.

The recording and format of each piece of demographic information need to be carefully defined and standardized to ensure complete and accurate data collection. The health care organization should include instructions for the patients and staff as to how each field should be recorded. For example, the patient's address should be documented as a billing address or a mailing address if different from the patient's physical street address. Patient telephone numbers should include both landlines and any mobile phone numbers, and the area code should be recorded in a consistent format (Box 5.1).

A patient's name must be recorded in exactly the same way to prevent duplicate records and confusion between patients. For example, a patient's name could be stated as Beth B. Smith on one visit and as Elizabeth Beryl Jones on another visit. Although this is the same patient, in the second visit the patient used her full first and middle names and her married last name. What could appear to be two patients is really just one. However, the information of both visits should be kept together in the patient's medical record.

The traditional category for "sex" is distinct from the concept of gender. A patient's sex is the biological difference between male and female, such as the genitalia and genetic differences. Gender is different in that it refers to the role of a male or female in society (gender role) or an individual's concept of himself or herself (gender identity). Sometimes, a patient's biological sex does not align with his or her gender identity. These patients may refer to themselves as transgender, nonbinary, or gender-nonconforming. In the health care setting, the "sex" of the patient is recorded as to the patient's wishes, which may be based on the gender. In fact, it is becoming more common for new patient intake forms to include the option of both sex and gender. For example, some patient intake forms might include the question, "What sex was

> **TAKE AWAY** ●··········
>
> All data must be carefully recorded to ensure complete and accurate data collection.

BOX 5.1   DATA CONSISTENCY
··

How many ways can you think of to record a patient's telephone number? The format of telephone numbers themselves must be recorded the same way every time. For instance, a patient's number might be written in the following ways:

(123) 456-7890
123-456-7890
123 456 7890
456-7890
1234567890
1-123-456-7890

Data consistency means ensuring that data are standardized and recorded the same way every time. It is essential to maintaining accurate, useful records and reducing the risk of errors. The health care organization's policy should provide clear guidelines on how to record the patient's phone number and all other information. Fortunately, computerized records have greatly improved the standardization of recorded data and will either autocorrect or will only allow the inputting of information in a specific format.

recorded on your birth certificate?" It is important to accurately document this information because it may significantly affect the patient's health and health delivery. Race and ethnicity are also recorded, and, similar to gender, are based on how the patient wishes to be identified.

Legal Data

Several pieces of documentation are collected to legally protect the patient, the provider, and the health care organization. First, to receive treatment, a patient must consent, or agree, to be treated by the providers at the health care organization. A current **informed consent** form must be signed by the patient and appear in his or her medical record before any services can be provided. Chapter 11 discusses informed consent in detail.

Second, because payment for the treatment is often contingent on third-party payers, such as a health insurance company, the information regarding the specifics of the diagnoses and treatments is required for payment to occur. In other words, the patient must authorize the health care organization to release the patient's medical information to the payer so that the payer can reimburse the provider for any services. Patients routinely sign a release of information regarding their visit for the purposes of billing their health insurance companies for the cost of the care. This is called a *"Notice of Privacy Practices" (NPP)*, which will be further discussed in Chapter 12. The NPP details how a health care organization may disclose or use a patient's protected health information, what the patient's rights are, and what the organization's duties are with regard to that information. This authorization to release patient information is necessary for sharing information regarding the patient's diagnosis and treatment with the health insurance company. Releasing or sharing such information without the patient's consent is a breach of confidentiality and a Health Insurance Portability and Accountability Act (HIPAA) violation. Fig. 5.1 is an example of a consent form used in a physician's office.

Another legal document that may need patient authorization is a **do not resuscitate (DNR) order.** A DNR order is a document signed by the patient specifying that, if the patient has no heartbeat or is not breathing, no lifesaving measures should be performed, such as cardiopulmonary resuscitation. Similarly, an **advance directive** details the types and limits of care in the event that a patient is unable to communicate his or her wishes. For example, using an advance directive, patients may elect in advance to forego feeding or breathing tubes when, for example, patients are in an irreversible coma or a condition that requires life support. A **medical proxy**, also called a *health care proxy or agent,* is another legal document that specifies who will make medical decisions for the patient and under what types of circumstances. Each of these legal documents may be subject to state law, and the health services administrator should be familiar with the state laws that apply.

Financial Data

The financial data for a health care organization is composed largely of the information that captures the details of the patient's payment method and health insurance policy. Although a few patients will be "self-pay," meaning that they are responsible for the bill without the benefit of health insurance, most will use either public or private insurance to help finance the payment.

The patient's health insurance information should be collected during the patient registration. The information that needs to be recorded includes the specifics of the patient's payer, which are found on the patient's insurance card, and the company's name, address, and individual identification and group numbers (Fig. 5.2). The member's identification number identifies the individual who is covered by the insurance policy,

○ **informed consent** Voluntary agreement, usually written, for treatment after being informed of its purpose, methods, procedures, benefits, and risks.

○ **do not resuscitate (DNR) order** a document specifying the lifesaving measures that should or should not be performed if a patient ceases cardiac or pulmonary function.

○ **advance directive** documentation that details the types and limits of care in the event that a patient is unable to communicate his or her wishes.

○ **medical proxy** a document that specifies who will make medical decisions for the patient and under what circumstances.

TAKE AWAY ●·········

Each time a patient comes in for a medical visit, the demographic and financial information should be updated for any changes.

Kennedy Family Practice
414 Jacksonia St., Armandale, VA. 26004

Patient Consent for Use and Disclosure
of Protected Health Information

I hereby give my consent for Kennedy Family Practice to use and disclose protected health information (PHI) about me to carry out treatment, payment and health care operations (TPO).

I have the right to review the Notice of Privacy Practices prior to signing this consent. Kennedy Family Practice reserves the right to revise its Notice of Privacy Practices at any time. A revised Notice of Privacy Practices may be obtained by forwarding a written request to Sophia Viero, 414 Jacksonia St., Armandale, VA. 26004.

With this consent, a representative of Kennedy Family Practice may call my home or other alternative location and leave a message on voice mail or in person; may e-mail me on my approved email site; and/or may mail to my home or other alternative location any items that assists the practice in carrying out TPO such as appointment reminders, insurance items and any calls pertaining to my clinical care, including laboratory test results.

I have the right to request that Kennedy Family Practice restrict how it uses or discloses my PHI to carry out TPO. By signing this form, I am consenting to allow Kennedy Family Practice to use and disclose my PHI to carry out TPO.

I may revoke my consent in writing however previous disclosures are considered valid based on my prior consent.

_____

Signature of Patient or Legal Guardian

_____

Print Patient's Name   Date

_____

Patient Approved Telephone number   Patient Approved Email address

1

Figure 5.1 Patient consent form. (From Proctor, et al: Kinn's the administrative medical assistant, ed 13, St. Louis, Elsevier, 2017.)

whereas the group number is the identifier for the type of insurance plan. The group number identifies the type of policy for the plan and details the specifics of the benefits allowed, including the copayment required. Copayments are the amount that the individual is responsible for each visit outside of the larger amount covered by the plan. The health services administrator or the medical biller should also verify billing information and note any outstanding balances.

As we will see in Chapter 9, the successful submission of a claim for reimbursement is contingent on correctly collecting the right patient information and submitting the proper documentation to the health insurance payer. The primary payer is the health insurance company that will be billed first for services. If the patient has a secondary payer, it pays when the first one does not or will not pay any of the remaining payment. For example, if the patient is being seen for a workers' compensation claim or an automobile accident, those specific insurances will be the primary payer and will pay before the patient's primary insurance.

Another financial document related to health insurance is an **advance beneficiary notice (ABN)**, which signifies the patient is aware of an amount, service, or procedure that may not be covered by the health insurance company or that the physician believes may not be medically necessary (Fig. 5.3). In this case, the patient will be personally responsible for the charges.

advance beneficiary notice (ABN) notice to the patient of an amount, service, or procedure that may not be covered by the health insurance company or that the physician believes may not be medically necessary.

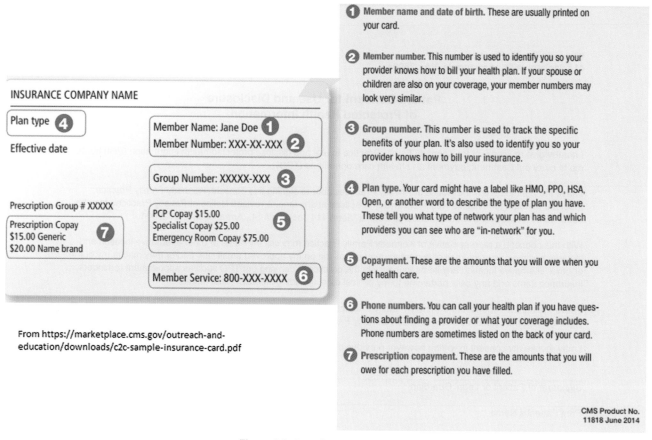

Figure 5.2 Sample insurance card.

Clinical Data

The clinical data in the medical record consist of the information gathered by the health care provider and the clinical staff. The clinical data include the patient's chief complaint, vital signs, medical history, family history, physical findings, diagnoses, and treatments. The provider conducts a patient assessment by performing and documenting the review of systems (ROS) and focusing the physical exam on the patient's chief complaint. Aside from the assessment that supports the patient's diagnosis, the health care provider must document the need for treatment, referred to as **medical necessity**. For example, ordering a chest x-ray for a patient who presents with a sore throat would not be justified unless there are other signs or symptoms to warrant the procedure, such as accompanying abnormal lung sounds, pain in the chest, or difficulty in breathing.

One method of documentation in the medical record is the "SOAP" method introduced in Chapter 4. "SOAP" stands for subjective, objective, assessment, and plan. The *subjective* section includes the symptoms that the patient is experiencing, such as nausea, pain, and confusion, that cannot be objectively measured. *Objective* signs are the other piece of the complaint—those that can be measured or observed, such as fever, weight gain, or a rash. The *assessment* piece is the compilation of signs and symptoms and evaluation to determine a diagnosis. The *plan* is the action plan or treatment regimen to the given diagnosis. As part of the treatment, documentation for any medications prescribed will be made in the medical record, along with e-prescribing the order to the pharmacy of the patient's choice and any consultations or referrals.

medical necessity regarding insurance, the need for treatment.

A. Notifier:

B. Patient Name: **C. Identification Number:**

Advance Beneficiary Notice of Noncoverage (ABN)

<u>NOTE:</u> If Medicare doesn't pay for **D.** _____ below, you may have to pay.

Medicare does not pay for everything, even some care that you or your health care provider have good reason to think you need. We expect Medicare may not pay for the **D.** _____ below.

D.	E. Reason Medicare May Not Pay:	F. Estimated Cost

WHAT YOU NEED TO DO NOW:
- Read this notice, so you can make an informed decision about your care.
- Ask us any questions that you may have after you finish reading.
- Choose an option below about whether to receive the **D.** _____ listed above.
  Note: If you choose Option 1 or 2, we may help you to use any other insurance that you might have, but Medicare cannot require us to do this.

G. OPTIONS: Check only one box. We cannot choose a box for you.

☐ **OPTION 1.** I want the **D.** _____ listed above. You may ask to be paid now, but I also want Medicare billed for an official decision on payment, which is sent to me on a Medicare Summary Notice (MSN). I understand that if Medicare doesn't pay, I am responsible for payment, but **I can appeal to Medicare** by following the directions on the MSN. If Medicare does pay, you will refund any payments I made to you, less co-pays or deductibles.

☐ **OPTION 2.** I want the **D.** _____ listed above, but do not bill Medicare. You may ask to be paid now as I am responsible for payment. **I cannot appeal if Medicare is not billed**.

☐ **OPTION 3.** I don't want the **D.** _____ listed above. I understand with this choice I am **not** responsible for payment, and **I cannot appeal to see if Medicare would pay.**

H. Additional Information:

This notice gives our opinion, not an official Medicare decision. If you have other questions on this notice or Medicare billing, call **1-800-MEDICARE** (1-800-633-4227/**TTY:** 1-877-486-2048).

Signing below means that you have received and understand this notice. You also receive a copy.

I. Signature:	J. Date:

According to the Paperwork Reduction Act of 1995, no persons are required to respond to a collection of information unless it displays a valid OMB control number. The valid OMB control number for this information collection is 0938-0566. The time required to complete this information collection is estimated to average 7 minutes per response, including the time to review instructions, search existing data resources, gather the data needed, and complete and review the information collection. If you have comments concerning the accuracy of the time estimate or suggestions for improving this form, please write to: CMS, 7500 Security Boulevard, Attn: PRA Reports Clearance Officer, Baltimore, Maryland 21244-1850.

Form CMS-R-131 (03/11)   Form Approved OMB No. 0938-0566

Figure 5.3 Medicare advance beneficiary notice.

Signatures

Upon documenting in the patient's medical record, specific sections must be *authenticated* by the provider or clinical staff. The term **authentication** means that the provider's or staff member's name and title are present and legible for each entry or notation in the patient's medical record, signifying responsibility. A **countersignature** is an additional signature on a document that may be required in some states, such as for physician assistants and nurse practitioners who practice under a physician.

authentication the assumption of responsibility for the data collected.

countersignature evidence of supervision of a subordinate's documentation.

Imaging and Laboratory Documentation

As part of the diagnostic process, the physician may write an order for additional testing that includes imaging or laboratory work. The results of these tests must be entered into the medical record, as they are integral to the substantiation of the diagnosis and the patient's treatment plan. Laboratory results, whether they are completed onsite or offsite, are directly entered into the patient's medical record and should include the normal ranges for each laboratory test. For imaging studies, such as x-ray, computed tomography (CT) scan, and magnetic resonance imaging (MRI) they will be incorporated in the medical record using a software application, such as a Picture Archiving and Communication System (PACS), that digitizes images and allows for their electronic storage and transmission (Fig. 5.4). Because of this technology, images can be taken in one facility and sent and interpreted by physicians hundreds (and sometimes thousands) of miles away.

Operative Reports

If the health care organization offers ambulatory surgeries, a report will be generated that includes the preoperative assessment and postoperative management or instructions. Any findings during the surgical procedure, such as images from a colonoscopy or biopsy results, will be included, and the entire report will be reviewed and signed by the physician responsible for the procedure. Anesthesia reports may be documented separately and are often found in hospital medical records.

Discharge Summary

○ **discharge summary** documentation of a visit given to the patient at checkout.

The discharge summary, also called a *discharge report,* is provided to the patient when he or she is discharged, or checks out, after the medical visit. The **discharge summary** includes the patient's diagnoses; any procedures that were performed; the patient's diagnostic studies, including laboratory and imaging; progress notes; physician's orders; consultation reports; and any discharge instructions.

Ownership

Ownership of the medical record is an interesting topic and the cause of some confusion among patients and even among those within the health care industry. There is no consensus on who owns medical records, and both federal and state laws are unclear or inconsistent. However, the common thinking is that the *patient* owns the information in the record

TAKE AWAY ●·········

The patient owns the information in the record but not the medium on which the information is kept.

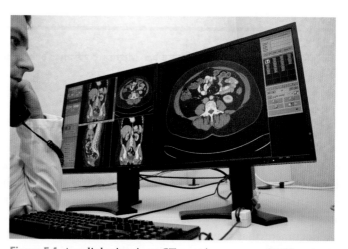

Figure 5.4 A radiologist views CT scan images on a PACS system.

but not the medium on which the information is kept. For example, in the case of paper records, the paper belongs to the *health care organization,* whereas the information belongs to the patient. This means that the patient may request certain changes be made to the information in the medical record, such as change of address and name, and how this information is used and shared outside of the health care organization. However, the organization owns the paper that the patient's information is on. Thus the patient may have to pay a processing fee to obtain copies of his or her own medical record or to have copies sent to another provider. Further, the health care organization is responsible for maintaining those medical records and protecting them against data breaches.

Retention

The data in the medical record are owned by the patient; however, the storage and maintenance of these data are the responsibility of the health care organization that collected the data. All documentation must be safely stored for a number of years based on the *statute of limitations,* which is a specific amount of time that is determined by each state (Table 5.2). The statute of limitations is extended for minors to begin at the age of consent, usually 18 in most states. Thus a child who has medical treatment in

Text continued on p. 106

TABLE 5.2

STATE MEDICAL RECORD LAWS: MINIMUM MEDICAL RECORD RETENTION PERIODS FOR RECORDS HELD BY MEDICAL DOCTORS AND HOSPITALS

State	Medical Doctors	Hospitals
Alabama	As long as may be necessary to treat the patient and for medical/legal purposes. Ala. Admin. Code r. 545-X-4-.08 (2007).[1]	5 yr Ala. Admin. Code § 420-5-7.10 (adopting 42 C.F.R. § 482.24).
Alaska	N/A	**Adult patients** 7 yr after the discharge of the patient. **Minor patients (under 19)** 7 yr after discharge or until patient reaches the age of 21, whichever is longer. Alaska Stat. § 18.20.085(a) (2008).
Arizona	**Adult patients** 6 yr after the last date of services from the provider. **Minor patients** 6 yr after the last date of services from the provider, or until patient reaches the age of 21, whichever is longer. Ariz. Rev. Stat. § 12-2297 (2008).	**Adult patients** 6 yr after the last date of services from the provider. **Minor patients** 6 yr after the last date of services from the provider, or until patient reaches the age of 21, whichever is longer. Ariz. Rev. Stat. § 12-2297 (2008).
Arkansas	N/A	**Adult patients** 10 yr after the last discharge, but master patient index data must be kept permanently. **Minor patients** Complete medical records must be retained 2 yr after the age of majority (i.e., until patient turns 20). 016 24 Code Ark. Rules and Regs. 007 § 14(19) (2008).
California	N/A[1]	**Adult patients** 7 yr after discharge of the patient. **Minor patients** 7 yr after discharge or 1 yr after the patient reaches the age of 18 (i.e., until patient turns 19), whichever is longer. Cal. Code Regs. tit. 22, § 70751(c) (2008).

Continued

TABLE 5.2

STATE MEDICAL RECORD LAWS: MINIMUM MEDICAL RECORD RETENTION PERIODS FOR RECORDS HELD BY MEDICAL DOCTORS AND HOSPITALS—cont'd

State	Medical Doctors	Hospitals
Colorado	N/A[1]	**Adult patients** 10 yr after the most recent patient care usage. **Minor patients** 10 yr after the patient reaches the age of majority (i.e., until patient turns 28). 6 Colo. Code Regs. § 1011-1, chap. IV, 8.102 (2008).
Connecticut	7 yr from the last date of treatment, or, upon the death of the patient, for 3 yr. Conn. Agencies Regs. § 19a-14-42 (2008).	10 yr after the patient has been discharged. Conn. Agencies Regs. §§ 19-13-D3(d)(6) (2008).
Delaware	7 yr from the last entry date on the patient's record. Del. Code Ann. tit. 24, §§ 1761 and 1702 (2008).	N/A
District of Columbia	**Adult patients** 3 yr after last seeing the patient. **Minor patients** 3 yr after last seeing the patient or 3 yr after patient reaches the age of 18 (i.e., until patient turns 21). D.C. Mun. Regs. tit. 17, § 4612.1 (2008).	10 yr after the date of discharge of the patient. D.C. Mun. Regs. tit. 22, § 2216 (2008).
Florida	5 yr from the last patient contact. Fla. Admin. Code Ann. 64B8- 10.002(3) (2008).	Public hospitals: 7 yr after the last entry. Florida Department of State, General Records Schedule GS4 for Public Hospitals, Health Care Facilities and Medical Providers, (2007), http://dlis.dos.state.fl.us/barm/genschedules/GS04.pdf (accessed September 12, 2008).
Georgia	10 yr from the date the record item was created. See Ga. Code Ann. § 31-33- 2(a)(1)(A) and (B)(i) (2008).	**Adult patients** 5 yr after the date of discharge. **Minor patients** 5 yr past the age of majority (i.e., until patient turns 23). See Ga. Code Ann. §§ 31-33-2(a)(1)(B)(ii) (2008); 31-7-2 (2008) (granting the department regulatory authority over hospitals) and Ga. Comp. R. & Regs. 290- 9-7-.18 (2008).
Guam	N/A	N/A
Hawaii	**Adult patients** Full medical records: 7 yr after last data entry. Basic information (i.e., patient's name, birthdate, diagnoses, drugs prescribed, x-ray interpretations): 25 yr after the last record entry. **Minor patients** Full medical records: 7 yr after the patient reaches the age of majority (i.e., until patient turns 25). Basic information: 25 yr after the minor reaches the age of majority (i.e., until patient turns 43). Haw. Rev. Stat. § 622-58 (2008).	**Adult patients** Full medical records: 7 yr after last data entry. Basic information (i.e., patient's name, birth date, diagnoses, drugs prescribed, x-ray interpretations): 25 yr after the last record entry. **Minor patients** Full medical records: 7 yr after the minor reaches the age of majority (i.e., until patient turns 25). Basic information: 25 yr after the minor reaches the age of majority (i.e., until patient turns 43). Haw. Rev. Stat. § 622-58 (2008).
Idaho	N/A	Clinical laboratory test records and reports: 5 yr after the date of the test. Idaho Code Ann. § 39-1394 (2008).

TABLE 5.2

STATE MEDICAL RECORD LAWS: MINIMUM MEDICAL RECORD RETENTION PERIODS FOR RECORDS HELD BY MEDICAL DOCTORS AND HOSPITALS—cont'd

State	Medical Doctors	Hospitals
Illinois	N/A	10 yr. See 210 Ill. Comp. Stat. 85/6.17(c) (2008).
Indiana	7 yr. Burns Ind. Code Ann. § 16-39-7-1 (2008).	7 yr. Burns Ind. Code Ann. § 16-39-7-1 (2008).
Iowa	**Adult patients** 7 yr from the last date of service. **Minor patients** 1 yr after the minor attains the age of majority (i.e., until patient turns 19). See Iowa Admin. Code r. 653- 13.7(8) (2008); Iowa Code § 614.8 (2008).	N/A
Kansas	10 yr from when professional service was provided. Kan. Admin. Regs. § 100-24-2 (a) (2008).	**Adult patients** Full records: 10 yr after the last discharge of the patient. **Minor patients** Full records: 10 yr or 1 yr beyond the date that the patient reaches the age of majority (i.e., until patient turns 19), whichever is longer. Summary of destroyed records for both adults and minors—25 yr. Kan. Admin. Regs. § 28-34-9a (d)(1) (2008).
Kentucky	N/A	**Adult patients** 5 yr from date of discharge. **Minor patients** 5 yr from date of discharge or 3 yr after the patient reaches the age of majority (i.e., until patient turns 21), whichever is longer. 902 Ky. Admin. Regs. 20:016 (2007).
Louisiana	6 yr from the date a patient is last treated. La. Rev. Stat. Ann. § 40:1299.96(A)(3)(a) (2008).	10 yr from the date a patient is discharged. La. Rev. Stat. Ann. § 40:2144(F)(1) (2008).
Maine	N/A	**Adult patients** 7 yr. **Minor patients** 6 yr past the age of majority (i.e., until patient turns 24). See 10-144 Me. Code R. Ch. 112, § XII.B.1 (2008). Patient logs and written x-ray reports— permanently. 10-144 Me. Code R. Ch. 112, § XV.C.5 (2008).
Maryland	**Adult patients** 5 yr after the record or report was made. **Minor patients** 5 yr after the report or record was made or until the patient reaches the age of majority plus 3 yr (i.e., until patient turns 21), whichever date is later. MD. Code Ann., Health–Gen. §§ 4-403(a)–(c) (2008).	**Adult patients** 5 yr after the record or report was made. **Minor patients** 5 yr after the report or record was made or until the patient reaches the age of majority plus 3 yr (i.e., until patient turns 21), whichever date is later. MD. Code Ann., Health–Gen. §§ 4-403(a)–(c) (2008).
Massachusetts	**Adult patients** 7 yr from the date of the last patient encounter. **Minor patients** 7 yr from date of last patient encounter or until the patient reaches the age of 9, whichever is longer. 243 Mass. Code Regs. 2.07(13)(a) (2008).	30 yr after the discharge or the final treatment of the patient. Mass. Gen. Laws ch. 111, § 70 (2008).

Continued

TABLE 5.2

STATE MEDICAL RECORD LAWS: MINIMUM MEDICAL RECORD RETENTION PERIODS FOR RECORDS HELD BY MEDICAL DOCTORS AND HOSPITALS—cont'd

State	Medical Doctors	Hospitals
Michigan	7 yr from the date of service. Mich. Comp. Laws § 333.16213 (2008).	7 yr from the date of service Mich. Comp. Laws § 333.20175 (2008).
Minnesota	N/A	Most medical records: Permanently (in microfilm). Miscellaneous documents: **Adult patients** 7 yr. **Minor patients** 7 yr after the age of majority (i.e., until the patient turns 25). Minn. Stat. § 145.32 (2007) and Minn. R. 4642.1000 (2007).
Mississippi	N/A	**Adult patients** Discharged in sound mind: 10 yr. Discharged at death: 7 yr.[2] **Minor patients** For the period of minority plus 7 yr.[3] Miss. Code Ann. § 41-9-69(1) (2008).
Missouri	7 yr from the date the last professional service was provided. Mo. Rev. Stat. § 334.097(2) (2008).	**Adult patients** 10 yr. **Minor patients** 10 yr or until patient's 23rd birthday, whichever occurs later. Mo. Code Reg. tit. 19, § 30-094(15) (2008).
Montana	N/A[1]	**Adult patients** Entire medical record—10 yr after the date of a patient's discharge or death. **Minor patients** Entire medical record—10 yr after the date the patient either attains the age of majority (i.e., until patient is 28) or dies, whichever is earlier. Core medical record must be maintained at least an additional 10 yr beyond the periods provided earlier. Mont. Admin. R. 37.106.402(1) and (4) (2007).
Nebraska	N/A	**Adult patients** 10 yr after a patient's discharge. **Minor patients (under 19)** 10 yr or until 3 yr after the patient reaches age of majority (i.e., until patient turns 22), whichever is longer. Neb. Admin. Code 175 § 9-006.07A5 (2008).
Nevada	5 yr after receipt or production of health care record. Nev. Rev. Stat. § 629.051 (2007).	5 yr after receipt or production of health care record. Nev. Rev. Stat. § 629.051 (2007).
New Hampshire	7 yr from the date of the patient's last contact with the physician, unless the patient has requested that the records be transferred to another health care provider. N.H. Code Admin. R. Ann. Med 501.02(f)(8) (2008).	**Adult patients** 7 yr after a patient's discharge. **Minor patients** 7 yr or until the minor reaches age 19, whichever is longer. N.H. Code Admin. R. Ann. He-P 802.06(h) (1994).[4]
New Jersey	7 yr from the date of the most recent entry. N.J. Admin. Code § 13:35-6.5(b) (2008).	**Adult patients** 10 yr after the most recent discharge. **Minor patients** 10 yr after the most recent discharge or until the patient is 23 yr of age, whichever is longer. **Discharge summary sheets (all)** 20 yr after discharge. N.J. Stat. Ann. § 26:8-5 (2008).

TABLE 5.2

STATE MEDICAL RECORD LAWS: MINIMUM MEDICAL RECORD RETENTION PERIODS FOR RECORDS HELD BY MEDICAL DOCTORS AND HOSPITALS—cont'd

State	Medical Doctors	Hospitals
New Mexico	**Adult patients** 2 yr beyond what is required by state insurance laws and by Medicare and Medicaid requirements. **Minor patients** 2 yr beyond the date the patient is 18 (i.e., until the patient turns 20). N.M. Code R. § 16.10.17.10 (C) (2008).	**Adult patients** 10 yr after the last treatment date of the patient. **Minor patients** Age of majority plus 1 yr (i.e., until the patient turns 19). N.M. Stat. Ann. § 14-6-2 (2008); N.M. Code R. § 7.7.2.30 (2008).
New York	**Adult patients** 6 yr. **Minor patients** 6 yr and until 1 yr after the minor reaches the age of 18 (i.e., until the patient turns 19). N.Y. Education § 6530 (2008) (providing retention requirements in the definitions for professional misconduct of physicians).	**Adult patients** 6 yr from the date of discharge. **Minor patients** 6 yr from the date of discharge or 3 yr after the patient reaches 18 yr (i.e., until patient turns 21), whichever is longer. **Deceased patients** At least 6 yr after death. N.Y. Comp. Codes R. & Regs. tit. 10, § 405.10(a)(4) (2008).
North Carolina	N/A	**Adult patients** 11 yr after discharge. **Minor patients** Until the patient's 30th birthday. 10 A N.C. Admin. Code 13B.3903(a), (b) (2008).
North Dakota	N/A	**Adult patients** 10 yr after the last treatment date. **Minor patients** 10 yr after the last treatment date or until the patient's 21st birthday, whichever is later. N.D. Admin. Code 33-07-01.1-20(1)(b) (2007).
Ohio	N/A	N/A
Oklahoma	N/A	**Adult patients** 5 yr beyond the date the patient was last seen. **Minor patients** 3 yr past the age of majority (i.e., until the patient turns 21). **Deceased patients** 3 yr beyond the date of death. Okla. Admin. Code § 310:667-19-14 (2008).
Oregon	N/A[1]	10 yr after the date of last discharge. Master patient index—permanently. Or. Admin. R. 333-505-0050(9) and (15) (2008).
Pennsylvania	**Adult patients** At least 7 yr after the date of the last medical service. **Minor patients** 7 yr after the date of the last medical service or 1 yr after the patient reaches age 21 (i.e., until patient turns 22), whichever is the longer period. 49 Pa. Code § 16.95(e) (2008).	**Adult patients** 7 yr after discharge. **Minor patients** 7 yr after the patient attains majority[5] or as long as adult records would be maintained. 28 Pa. Code § 115.23 (2008).

Continued

TABLE 5.2

STATE MEDICAL RECORD LAWS: MINIMUM MEDICAL RECORD RETENTION PERIODS FOR RECORDS HELD BY MEDICAL DOCTORS AND HOSPITALS—cont'd

State	Medical Doctors	Hospitals
Puerto Rico	N/A	N/A[6]
Rhode Island	5 yr unless otherwise required by law or regulation. R.I. Code R.14-140-031, § 11.3 (2008).	**Adult patients** 5 yr after discharge of the patient. R.I. Code R. 14 090 007 § 27.10 (2008). **Minor patients** 5 yr after patient reaches the age of 18 yr (i.e., until patient turns 23). R.I. Code R. 14 090 007 § 27.10.1 (2008).
South Carolina	**Adult patients** 10 yr from the date of last treatment. **Minor patients** 13 yr from the date of last treatment. S.C. Code Ann. § 44-115-120 (2007).	**Adult patients** 10 yr. **Minor patients** Until the minor reaches age 18 and the "period of election" expires, which is usually 1 yr after the minor reaches the age of majority (i.e., usually until patient turns 19). S.C. Code Ann. Regs. 61-16 § 601.7(A) (2007). See S.C. Code Ann. § 15-3-545 (2007).[7]
South Dakota	When records have become inactive or for which the whereabouts of the patient are unknown to the physician. S.D. Codified Laws § 36-4-38 (2008).	**Adult patients** 10 yr from the actual visit date of service or resident care. **Minor patients** 10 yr from the actual visit date of service or resident care or until the minor reaches age of majority plus 2 yr (i.e., until patient turns 20), whichever is later. See S.D. Admin. R. 44:04:09:08 (2008).
Tennessee	**Adult patients** 10 yr from the provider's last professional contact with the patient. **Minor patients** 10 yr from the provider's last professional contact with the patient or 1 yr after the minor reaches the age of majority (i.e., until patient turns 19), whichever is longer. Tenn. Comp. R. & Regs. 0880-2-.15 (2008).	**Adult patients** 10 yr after the discharge of the patient or the patient's death during the patient's period of treatment within the hospital. Tenn. Code Ann. § 68-11-305(a)(1) (2008). **Minor patients** 10 yr after discharge or for the period of minority plus at least 1 yr (i.e., until patient turns 19), whichever is longer. Tenn. Code Ann. § 68-11-305(a)(2) (2008).
Texas	**Adult patients** 7 yr from the date of the last treatment. **Minor patients** 7 yr after the date of the last treatment or until the patient reaches age 21, whichever date is later. 22 Tex. Admin. Code § 165.1(b) (2008).[8]	**Adult patients** 10 yr after the patient was last treated in the hospital. **Minor patients** 10 yr after the patient was last treated in the hospital or until the patient reaches age 20, whichever date is later. Tex. Health & Safety Code Ann. § 241.103 (2007); 25 Tex. Admin. Code § 133.41(j)(8) (2008).[8]
Utah	N/A	**Adult patients** 7 yr. **Minor patients** 7 yr or until the minor reaches the age of 18 plus 4 yr (i.e., patient turns 22), whichever is longer. Utah Admin. Code r. 432-100-33(4)(c) (2008).
Vermont	N/A[1]	10 yr. Vt. Stat. Ann. tit. 18, § 1905(8) (2007).

TABLE 5.2

STATE MEDICAL RECORD LAWS: MINIMUM MEDICAL RECORD RETENTION PERIODS FOR RECORDS HELD BY MEDICAL DOCTORS AND HOSPITALS—cont'd

State	Medical Doctors	Hospitals
Virginia	**Adult patients** 6 yr after the last patient contact. **Minor patients** 6 yr after the last patient contact or until the patient reaches age 18 (or becomes emancipated), whichever time period is longer. 18 Va. Admin. Code § 85-20-26(D) (2008).	**Adult patients** 5 yr after patient's discharge. **Minor patients** 5 yr after patient has reached the age of 18 (i.e., until the patient reaches age 23). 12 Va. Admin. Code § 5-410-370 (2008).
Washington	N/A	**Adult patients** 10 yr after the patient's most recent hospital discharge. **Minor patients** 10 yr after the patient's most recent hospital discharge or 3 yr after the patient reaches the age of 18 (i.e., until the patient turns 21), whichever is longer. Wash. Rev. Code § 70.41.190 (2008).[9]
West Virginia	N/A	N/A
Wisconsin	5 yr from the date of the last entry in the record. Wis. Admin. Code Med. § 21.03 (2008).	5 yr. Wis. Admin. Code Health & Family Services §§ 124.14(2)(c), 124.18(1)(e) (2008).
Wyoming	N/A	N/A[9]

All years are minimum periods (e.g., "at least" 7 years). Chart does not address retention of original x-rays or tracings, which may be subject to other requirements.

Minor = Person under 18 years old unless otherwise noted. N/A = No statute or regulation found.

Notes: [1] No statutory or regulatory requirement but state medical board or medical association recommends as follows:

Alabama: At least 10 years. See "Medical Records," available on the website of the Medical Association of the State of Alabama (MASA) at: http://www.masalink.org/uploadedFiles/Practice_Management/policy_Medicalrecords.pdf (accessed September 15, 2008).

California: Indefinitely, if possible. See CMA ON-CALL: The California Medical Association's Information-On-Demand Service, available at http://www.thedocuteam.com/docs/retention_medicalrecords.pdf (accessed August 14, 2008).

Colorado: Adult patients 7 years after the last date of treatment and the records of minor patients 7 years after the last date of treatment or 7 years after the patient reaches the age of 18, whichever is later. See Colorado Board of Medical Examiners, Policy 40-7: "Guidelines Pertaining to the Release and Retention of Medical Records." Available at: http://www.dora.state.co.us/Medical/policies/40- 07.pdf (accessed September 16, 2008).

Montana: Seven years from the date of last contact with the patient. Birth and immunization records: Until the patient's 25th birthday. See Montana Board of Medical Examiners, Statement on Physician Obligation to Retain Medical Records (2004), available at http://www.mt.gov/dli/bsd/license/bsd_boards/med_board/pdf/patient_medrec.pdf (accessed July 17, 2008).

Oregon: In accordance with Oregon's statute of limitations, at least 10 years after the patient's last contact with the physician. If space permits, indefinitely for all living patients. See Oregon Medical Board, available at http://www.oregon.gov/OMB (accessed August 8, 2008).

Vermont: Patient's lifetime if possible. Minors' records: at least until the child reaches age 21 and decedent's records at least 3 years after the patient's death. See Vermont Guide to Health Care Law, available at http://www.vtmd.org/ (accessed September 16, 2008).

[2] If a patient dies in the hospital or within 30 days of discharge and is survived by one or more minors who are or claim to be entitled to damages for the patient's wrongful death, the hospital must retain the patient's hospital record until the youngest minor reaches age 28. Miss. Code Ann. § 41-9-69(1) (2008).

[3] A person under the age of 21 is generally considered a "minor" in Mississippi. However, for purposes of consenting to health care, an "adult" is a person age 18 or older. See Miss. Code Ann. §§ 1-3-27 and 41-41-203(a) (2008).

[4] Hospital licensure rules have expired, but, as of June 2008, they were still in current use by the state Bureau of Licensing & Certification, which licenses health care facilities.

[5] The age of majority in Pennsylvania is 21. See 1 Pa. Cons. Stat. § 1991 (2008). However, minors over 18 may consent to health services in their own right. See 35 Pa. Cons. Stat. § 10101 (2008).

[6] Based only on statutes, not on regulations, which currently are published only in Spanish.

[7] The period of election is the time during which a person may elect to bring a lawsuit for malpractice that occurred while the patient was a minor, generally a maximum of 1 year after the minor reaches the age of majority. See S.C. Code Ann. § 15-3-545 (2007).

[8] The physician may not destroy medical records that relate to any civil, criminal, or administrative proceedings unless the physician knows the proceeding has been finally resolved. 22 Tex. Admin. Code § 165.1(b) (2008); Tex. Health & Safety Code Ann. § 241.103 (2007); 25 Tex. Admin. Code § 133.41(j)(8) (2008).

[9] Must maintain a record of a patient's health care information: for at least 1 year after receipt of authorization to disclose that health care information; and during the pendency of a request for examination, copying, correction, or amendment of that health care information. Wash. Rev. Code § 70.02.160 (2008); Wyo. Stat. Ann. § 35-2-615 (2008).

From HealthIT.gov: www.healthit.gov/sites/default/files/appa7-1.pdf

the state of New York will therefore have until the age of 21 to bring any legal action for injuries occurring during childhood.

Because individual states have different statutes of limitations for each type of legal action, the health services administrator will need to be concerned with the time periods of how long records need to be kept. Additionally, the health services administrator needs to continually monitor any changes to case law that may result in changes to the statutes.

OTHER TYPES OF DOCUMENTATION

Aside from the patient's medical record, a number of other types of documentation need to be maintained in a health care setting. These records include appointment schedules, maintenance records for the facility and any equipment owned or leased by the facility, financial records, and continuing medical education verification.

Additionally, an important database is the **master patient index**, which is a database containing a complete list of patients who have been treated at the health care organization. The master patient index is usually maintained electronically and encompasses all of the patients' current demographic information, including contact information. Routine audits of the master patient index should be done to eliminate patient duplicates, such as the same patients who have different names, different addresses, and even different Social Security numbers.

> **master patient index** a database containing a complete list of patients who have been treated at the health care organization.

LEARNING CHECKPOINT 5.1
The Medical Record

1. The patient's name is a type of:

   a. demographic data
   b. legal data
   c. financial data
   d. clinical data

2. The group number on the patient's insurance card is a type of:

   a. demographic data
   b. legal data
   c. financial data
   d. clinical data

3. The operative report is a type of:

   a. demographic data
   b. legal data
   c. financial data
   d. clinical data

4. A(n) _____ specifies who will make medical decisions for the patient and under what type of circumstances.

   a. master patient index
   b. advance beneficiary notice (ABN)
   c. advance directive
   d. medical proxy

▪ LEARNING CHECKPOINT 5.1—cont'd
▪ The Medical Record

5. A(n) _____ details the types and limits of care in the event that a patient is unable to communicate his or her wishes.

   a. advance beneficiary notice (ABN)

   b. advance directive

   c. discharge summary

   d. informed consent

▪ USES OF DOCUMENTATION

There are many reasons why documentation is necessary in a health care setting. Medical records serve primarily to monitor and track the patient's health and the received services. Additionally, medical records are used for billing, research, and legal purposes. This section discusses many of the key uses of the patient's health data collected by the health care organization.

Patient Care

One of the most important reasons for documentation is to facilitate the patient's **continuum of care**, or a system or process that supports the patient's health care over time. Being able to access the reasons for the patient's past medical visit, the medical history, laboratory and imaging procedures, and medications and treatment plan is critical in maintaining and continuing the patient's care.

   For example, a patient presents to the physician with dry, itchy skin. The patient thinks it may be because of the dryer air in the winter, but the lotions she has tried do not seem to be helping. The physician reviews the patient's medical record and notes that the patient has gained 20 pounds since she was at the clinic a year ago and that she has a family history of thyroid condition. Using this information in the patient's medical record, the physician suspects the patient's dry skin may be caused by hypothyroidism, or an underactive thyroid, which can be hereditary and would explain her weight gain and skin condition. The physician orders laboratory tests and discovers values that confirm the diagnosis of hypothyroidism. This diagnosis was made based on the physician being able to develop a clinical picture of the patient based on her presenting condition, laboratory test results, and the documentation of her past medical and family history.

Support of Litigation

There may be occasions when the patient's medical care can result in a legal matter. Patients who feel a provider's actions adversely affected their health may seek damages in a court of law. **Litigation** is the dispute of a matter in court. A patient's medical record is considered a legal document and may be used as evidence in court to either support the patient's case against the provider or help defend the provider's actions. Thus the health services administrator should ensure that every clinical staff member is trained in documenting in medical records and that the information is factually accurate and legible.

TAKE AWAY

Uses for medical documentation include patient care, support of litigation, reimbursement, administrative function, medical research, and more.

continuum of care the provision of care for a patient over a period of time.

litigation the dispute of a matter in court.

Reimbursement

Any services billed for payment must be supported by the patient's medical record. Medical billers and coders use the medical record to code the proper diagnoses and procedures, which are used to support the necessity of treatment on claim forms sent to health insurance payers. For example, if the patient is treated with antibiotics for strep throat, the diagnostic justification should include a patient history of a sore throat and a positive strep test. If not, the health insurance company may deny the claim and refuse to reimburse the health care organization for the services. Without proper documentation, no care is considered to have been performed and therefore will not be reimbursed.

Licensure, Accreditation, and Certification

As discussed in Chapter 1, adhering to standards set by professional organizations assures quality patient care. Documentation for credentialing and licensure is checked when employment application to the practice takes place and then throughout the health care professional's employment with the practice. Initially, the educational requirements need to be checked for validity to assure graduation or completion from a medical health care program and that the health care professional is in good standing. Licensure, board certification, and references need to be verified. For physicians, any gaps in medical practice need to be explained, and the disciplinary arm of the State Federation of Medical Boards needs to be checked for reports of malpractice or other disciplinary actions.

The health services administrator is often responsible for monitoring each health care professional's continuing education status and maintaining documentation. Failure to meet the continuing education requirements in the time allotted by the state medical board or licensing or credentialing body may result in suspension or denial of licensure renewal to practice.

Administrative Functions

As the health services administrator, you must evaluate the services in the health care organization to ensure efficiency and effective workflow. As discussed in Chapter 4, the evaluation of the organization's workflow and processes of documentation should routinely occur to adopt changes in regulations and laws, staffing, patient care, and equipment and technology.

Information from facility documentation is used to monitor how well the facility is functioning and to make decisions regarding services. For example, the health services administrator may perform an audit of denied claims and track them back to improper coding, which resulted in a loss of revenue for the clinic. The health services administrator may also use the data in medical records to track the number and types of patients seen in the clinic to help negotiate contracts with managed care companies and monitor the number of referrals to determine whether a particular in-house service is cost effective or not.

Research

○ **morbidity** disease.

○ **mortality** death.

Documentation is also important for research purposes, such as for monitoring **morbidity** (disease) and **mortality** (death) statistics. Once a patient's diagnosis is documented in the medical record, this information will be translated into a series of alphanumeric codes based on the International Classification of Diseases (ICD), which will be discussed in more detail in the next section. These ICD codes are used to report and monitor health data and are indicators of the overall health of a general population. Specifically, this coded information can be used in research to study disease patterns, manage health care, monitor outcomes, and allocate resources. For example, if data from the ICD codes show an increase in the **incidence** (new cases) of a sexually transmitted infection, such as syphilis, the state or county health department may increase funding to the health departments to hire more staff and provide free testing services to the community.

incidence the number of new cases of disease.

LEARNING CHECKPOINT 5.2
Uses of Documentation

1. The term _____ refers to a patient's medical care over time.

2. _____ is the dispute of a matter in a court of law.

3. The term _____ refers to the number of new cases of a disease.

TAKE AWAY

Information about patient care is collected by state and federal agencies to monitor public health and research treatments.

CODING

As briefly discussed earlier, coding refers to the translation of diagnoses and treatments into alphanumeric or numeric codes. These codes help to classify information into a distinct, specific, universal vocabulary to describe the patient's condition and the treatment and services the patient received. Additionally, as a result of the HIPAA mandate, these specific codes must be used to transmit information about patient diagnoses and treatments on health care claims to ensure accuracy and help standardize the reimbursement process. As we will see in the next section, the coding for diagnoses and procedures is contingent on accurate and factual documentation in the medical records.

International Classification of Disease, 10th Revision, Clinical Modification

In the health care setting, the patient's chief complaint and any diagnoses are coded with the **International Classification of Disease, 10th Revision, Clinical Modification (ICD-10-CM)**. It is an international coding system developed by the World Health Organization that has been modified by United States Department of Health and Human Services to accommodate national standards. The ICD coding system is used by health care providers, health organizations, researchers, health information managers, medical billers and coders, and policy makers in more than 117 countries and used to report and monitor health data.

The ICD has been revised and published in a series of editions to reflect changes in health care and medical services over time. The ICD is currently in its 10th revision, which increased the number of codes from 14,000 in its 9th edition (ICD-9) to more than 69,000 codes in ICD-10. This increase in codes helps health care providers better capture specificity and complexity of diseases when coding, which may support the provider's clinical decision making to a health insurer. The structure of ICD-10-CM is organized primarily by body system, and each code includes three to seven characters (Fig. 5.5).

International Classification of Disease, 10th Revision, Clinical Modification (ICD-10-CM) diagnosis coding system used on health care claims.

Healthcare Common Procedure Coding System (HCPCS)

Just as ICD is used for coding diseases and diagnoses, the Healthcare Common Procedure Coding System (HCPCS), often pronounced as "hic-picks," is used to code treatment, procedures, and other medical services. HCPCS was initially developed by the Centers for Medicare and Medicaid Services to process Medicare claims. However, HCPCS

Decimal placed after the first three characters

| X | X | X | . | X | X | X | X |

1st character ALPHA (A-Z)
2nd character NUMERIC
3rd through 7th characters ALPHA or NUMERIC

Figure 5.5 Construction of an ICD-10-CM code.

codes are now used to represent medical procedures and services to Medicare, Medicaid, and several other third-party payers. The HCPCS code set is divided into two levels:
- Level I: Current Procedural Terminology (CPT)
- Level II: codes not included in CPT, such as durable medical equipment (DME), medications, and supplies

The **Current Procedural Terminology (CPT)** coding system, or Level I of the HCPCS, is used to code and describe medical, surgical, radiology, laboratory, and anesthesiology services, tests, evaluations, and any other procedures performed by a health care provider on a patient. For example, the casting of a broken bone is a specific treatment that would be documented using a CPT code. The CPT code was developed in 1966 by the American Medical Association and is updated annually. There are approximately 7800 codes in the CPT coding system, and each code is a five-digit number ranging from 00100 through 99499.

Level II of the HCPCS is a coding system that is used primarily to identify products, supplies, and services not included in the CPT codes, such as ambulance services and durable medical equipment (DME), prosthetics, orthotics, and other supplies when used outside a physician's office.

CPT's Evaluation and Management Codes

In addition to codes that designate a specific procedure, CPT utilizes **evaluation and management (E/M) codes** to summarize the various levels of service provided. E/M codes are a method of representing the amount of time and skill needed to treat the patient at that particular visit. As might be expected, the higher the level of time and skill needed, the higher the reimbursement.

For example, CPT's E/M codes assign separate codes for new patients as opposed to established patients. New patients will require more time and documentation because the collection of demographic data, financial information, and medical history will be more extensive and time consuming. The CPT's E/M code includes the reimbursement formula to capture the additional work required for new patients as opposed to an established patient, who only needs to be queried for changes in any of the previous information, as well as the current reason for the visit. In general, established patients are defined as patients receiving medical services from the health care provider or another provider of the same specialty who belongs to the same group practice for the last 3 years.

When determining the level of service or the E/M code, seven components should be considered:
- History
- Examination
- Medical decision making
- Counseling
- Coordination of care
- Nature of presenting problem
- Time

The first three of these components—history, examination, and medical decision-making—are the key components in selecting the level of E/M services.

Current Procedural Terminology (CPT) a coding system that documents and reports medical, surgical, radiology, laboratory, anesthesiology, and evaluation and management (E/M) services.

evaluation and management (E/M) codes a subset of CPT coding that represents the amount of time and skill needed to treat the patient.

When documenting the patient's history, the E/M services are divided into four levels, from least to most amount of time expended: *problem focused, expanded problem focused, detailed,* and *comprehensive*. The documentation in the record must support the definition for the particular level. For example, a *problem-focused* history only documents the history of the patient's present illness. A *comprehensive* history needs to have documentation for an extensive history of the present illness along with a review of all body systems and complete family, social, and past medical histories. Regardless, each type of history should include a chief complaint (CC); history of present illness (HPI); an ROS; and past, family, and/or social history (PFSH).

For the examination, the levels of E/M services are based on four types of examinations:

- *Problem focused* – a limited examination of the affected body area or organ system
- *Expanded problem focused* – a limited examination of the affected body area or organ system and other symptomatic or related organ system(s)
- *Detailed* – an extended examination of the affected body area(s) and other symptomatic or related organ system(s)
- *Comprehensive* – a general multisystem examination or complete examination of a single organ system

The CPT's definition for a body area is the head, neck, chest, abdomen, genitalia, back, and extremities. Organ systems include the cardiovascular, musculoskeletal, and genitourinary systems. The extensiveness of the examination should be dependent on the presenting symptoms and the provider's clinical judgment. For example, if a patient presents with a suspected fracture of his arm, the examination is limited to one particular body area, and the extent of evaluation is *problem focused*. A *comprehensive* examination is generally a multisystem or complete examination that should include 8 of the 12 organ systems documented.

The third key factor to consider when determining E/M levels is the medical decision making required by the health care provider. The medical decision making reflects the complexity of making a diagnosis and developing a treatment plan for the patient. The levels of medical decision making are summarized as *straightforward, low complexity, moderate complexity,* and *high complexity*. In order for a visit to be classified as a particular type of medical decision-making, there must be sufficient documentation to support it, such as the number of potential diagnoses or treatment options, the amount and complexity of testing and results to be reviewed, and the risk of complications and comorbidities or mortality. The health services administrator should make it a routine practice to audit charts to assure that the documentation required is present for accurate billing.

CASE STUDY

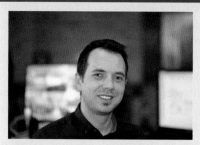

After reviewing a 10% sample of the patients from the previous week, Abel found two duplicates by running a list of birthdates and checking the other demographic information in the records. The office will work to combine these two records so that all of the patient's information is in one place, ensuring continuity of care and efficiency of administrative processes.

In addition, using a template of documentation requirements given to him by the clinic's health services administrator, Abel was able to report that in his sample he found one physician to have a large number of the highest E/M codes but with sparse documentation. Because documentation is required to support claims, inadequate records and documentation can result in denied claims and, ultimately, a loss in revenue. As a result, the health services administrator will request a meeting with this physician to discuss improving her documentation in patients' medical records. Abel was congratulated on a job well done!

REVIEW QUESTIONS

1. What are the four categories of information kept in medical documentation? What are examples of each type?

2. What is the statute of limitations for medical documentation in your state? Why do some states have different medical records retention requirements for minors as opposed to adults?

3. Besides medical records, what other types of documentation are kept by ambulatory facilities?

4. List three uses for medical documentation.

5. Why do health care professionals use codes to record information?

TECHNOLOGY

CHAPTER OUTLINE

INTRODUCTION
ELECTRONIC HEALTH RECORDS
    Benefits of EHR
      Technology

Health Information Exchanges
Challenges to Implementation
Incentives for Use

PRACTICE MANAGEMENT
    SOFTWARE
TELEHEALTH

VOCABULARY

algorithm
American Recovery and
    Reinvestment Act (ARRA)
audit trail
clinical decision support (CDS)
computer-assisted physician order
    entry (CPOE)
consumer-mediated exchange
contraindication
day sheet

directed exchange
electronic health record (EHR)
e-visit
health information exchange (HIE)
Health Information Technology for
    Economic and Clinical Health Act
    (HITECH)
interoperability
meaningful use
medical record

patient portal
practice management software
    (PMS)
protocol
query-based exchange
remote patient monitoring (RPM)
store-and-forward
superbill
telehealth

CHAPTER OBJECTIVES

After completing this chapter, the student should be able to do the following:

1. Define the electronic health record (EHR) and list its features.
2. Explain how EHR technology improves health care delivery.
3. Describe the function of health information exchanges (HIEs).
4. List the challenges and barriers to the implementation of EHRs.
5. Define the government's involvement in the promotion and oversight of EHR technology.
6. List the features of practice management software.
7. Define telemedicine and discuss examples of this technology used in health care.

INTRODUCTION

Innovative technologies have changed the way we live, learn, play, and work. This includes digital advances that allow us to locate, store, and receive information at the moment or in real time. Because health care is an industry that heavily relies on information delivered quickly, it should be no surprise that computers have become central to the work of the medical office and at other health care settings. This chapter examines the many ways computers and information technology aid health care professionals in both the clinical and administrative functions of the health care system.

ELECTRONIC HEALTH RECORDS

For most of modern medicine, medical offices and health care facilities have been maintaining medical information in paper files and charts (Fig. 6.1), and many providers still do. As computers and technology became more advanced and affordable, however, the health care industry has recognized the benefits of being able to record, store, and retrieve patient information electronically. As a result, more and more health care facilities are moving away from paper-based records to a digital or electronic format. This trend toward adopting electronic health records has been heavily boosted by incentives from federal and state governments.

An **electronic health record (EHR)** is a digital version of the patient's medical records and maintains demographic and clinical information about the patient that can be quickly retrieved and shared with multiple providers and staff. Oftentimes, the terms *electronic health records (EHRs)* and *electronic medical records (EMRs)* may be interchangeably used, although a distinction should be made. Similar to the EHR, the EMR contains the standard demographic and clinical data, but the information is gathered in one provider's office or during a specific encounter.

EHR technology is capable of much more than simply storing medical data. Current EHR systems are highly sophisticated and, for example, can send prescriptions directly to pharmacies, alert providers to potential drug allergies, order tests, and suggest treatment plans to providers. Box 6.1 lists the features of a fully functional EHR system.

electronic health record (EHR)
a system that maintains patient demographic and clinical information digitally and offers physician order entry, e-prescribing, and decision support.

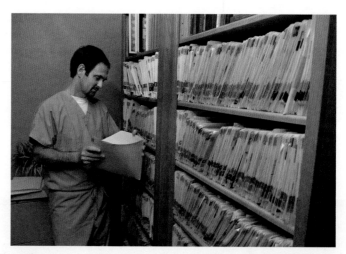

Figure 6.1 Paper files have been used for decades to store patient information, and it is still being used in many facilities.

○ CASE STUDY

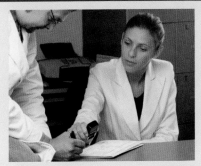

JoAnn is nearing her 1-year anniversary working at Dr. Roberts' walk-in clinic, providing administrative support at this privately owned, single-location enterprise. With clinic hours of 8 AM to 7 PM daily, Dr. Roberts is the primary provider, but he has a physician assistant to fill in part-time. The clinic has not transitioned to an EHR system and is still using paper medical charts. The clinic has used software to submit claims for Medicare and private insurance for decades, and laboratory tests are ordered using a webpage hosted by its laboratory services provider. Otherwise, Dr. Roberts has not seen the value in purchasing an expensive new EHR system and being trained on it. However, JoAnn recognizes that this technology can make the practice more efficient and effective. As you read this chapter, think about the benefits of EHR technology, even for a small organization like Dr. Roberts'. What benefits can JoAnn share with Dr. Roberts to convince him to adopt an EHR system?

BOX 6.1 FEATURES OF A FULLY FUNCTIONAL EHR SYSTEM

- Store, retrieve, transmit, and maintain patient records, including:
  - Demographic data (Fig. 6.2)
  - Financial information such as the patient's health insurer
  - Patient history, medication, allergy, and problem lists (Fig. 6.3)
  - Immunization records
  - Vitals signs (see Fig. 6.3)
  - Clinical documents and notes
- Order tests and medications (known as **computer-assisted physician order entry [CPOE]**) (Fig. 6.4)
- Suggest plans of care and treatment protocols to providers
- Print information for patients about specific diseases and treatments
- Generate care and discharge instructions specific for the patient
- Present results of laboratory and diagnostic testing (Fig. 6.5)
- Alert providers to drug allergies and interactions
- Prompt wellness screenings and other reminders for preventative medicine
- Assign and track tasks among various health care providers
- Facilitate messaging and communication between health care practitioners
- Generate correspondence to patients and their families
- Track authentication of the record and audit users who accessed the record
- Schedule patients
- Generate reports
- Support claims and reimbursement

○ **computer-assisted physician order entry (CPOE)** an electronic system in which a provider enters patient care orders to communicate to other members of the care team and which provides decision support and alerts.

Benefits of EHR Technology

There are multiple benefits and advantages to the EHR system for patients, the provider, and the health care facility. When patient data are stored digitally, health care professionals can view and update patient information in real time, from any computer with appropriate access to the facility's network. For instance, while the nurse is entering vital signs during intake, the physician can view the patient's previous diagnoses and treatments, and the medical biller can check the patient's account for any payment due. Because there is not a single paper medical chart in one physical location, multiple staff members

TAKE AWAY ○ · · · · · · · ·

Because the patient's health data are not kept in a physical paper file, the information can be used—and updated—from virtually anywhere, anytime.

Patient Demographics - Edit Patient   ✖

Fields in red need to be completed to save patient
Fields with * are required to complete the patient registration

| Patient | Guarantor | Insurance |

Last Name *:	Friedman	Address 1*:	837 W. 5th St.
First Name *:	Mitchell	Address 2:	
Middle Initial:	P	City *:	Hightown
Medical Record Number:	9663797	Country *:	United ▾ State/Province *: PA ▾
Date of Birth *:	03/26/1978 📅	ZIP/Postal Code *:	16870 -
Age:	38 Years 4 Months 22 Days	Email:	
Sex *:	⦿ Male ◯ Female	Home Phone *:	555 - 867 - 2368
SSN *:	221 - 16 - 8509	Driver's License:	
Emergency Contact Name *:	Leslie Friedman	Emergency Contact Phone *:	555 - 235 - 2357
Mother's Date of Birth:	📅	Father's Date of Birth:	📅
Mother's Work Phone:	- -	Father's Work Phone:	- -
Mother's SSN:	- -	Father's SSN:	- -
Patient Status:	☐ Single ☑ Married ☐ Other ☐ Employed ☐ Full-Time Student	Language:	
		Race:	

Fig. 6.2 Demographic data in an EHR system. (Courtesy of SimChart for the Medical Office, Elsevier, Inc, 2016.)

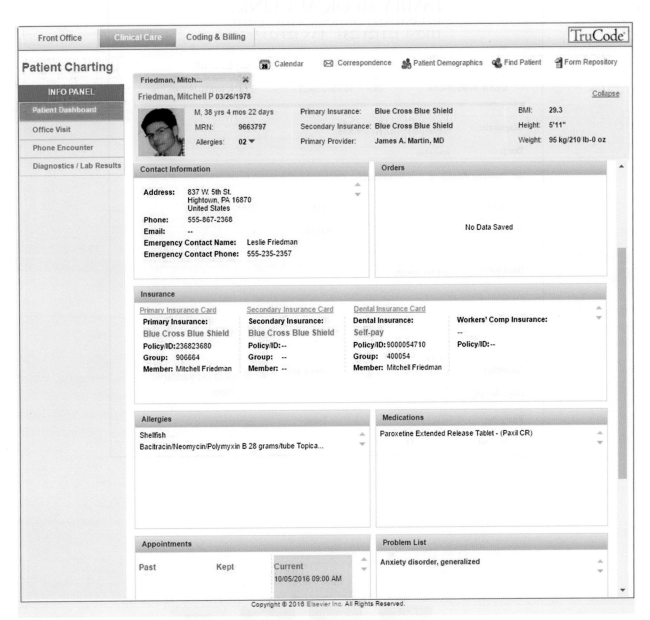

Fig. 6.3 Patient history, current medications, allergies, and vital signs in an EHR system. (Courtesy of SimChart for the Medical Office, Elsevier, Inc, 2016.)

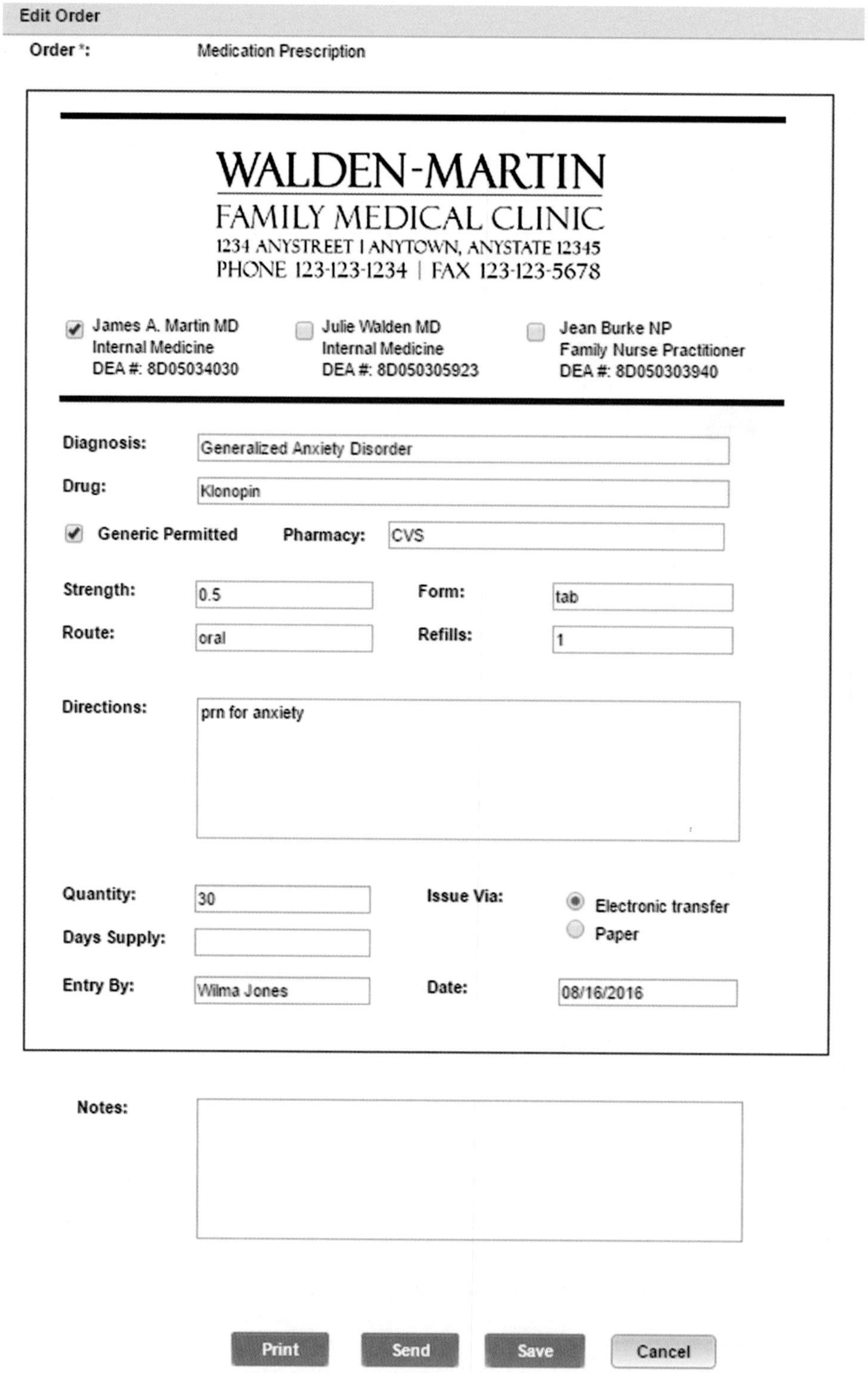

Edit Order

Order *:   Medication Prescription

WALDEN-MARTIN
FAMILY MEDICAL CLINIC
1234 ANYSTREET | ANYTOWN, ANYSTATE 12345
PHONE 123-123-1234 | FAX 123-123-5678

☑ James A. Martin MD   ☐ Julie Walden MD   ☐ Jean Burke NP
Internal Medicine   Internal Medicine   Family Nurse Practitioner
DEA #: 8D05034030   DEA #: 8D050305923   DEA #: 8D050303940

Diagnosis: Generalized Anxiety Disorder

Drug: Klonopin

☑ Generic Permitted   Pharmacy: CVS

Strength: 0.5   Form: tab

Route: oral   Refills: 1

Directions: prn for anxiety

Quantity: 30   Issue Via: ⦿ Electronic transfer
                                                   ○ Paper
Days Supply:

Entry By: Wilma Jones   Date: 08/16/2016

Notes:

[Print]   [Send]   [Save]   [Cancel]

Fig. 6.4 A medication order being input into an EHR system. (Courtesy of SimChart for the Medical Office, Elsevier, Inc, 2016.)

can access the patient's record at the same time, improving coordination of care. Patient information can also be updated and accessed almost instantly, which helps with efficiency and productivity of the provider and health care facility.

Additionally, accuracy can literally be a matter of life and death in health care. Mistaken or misread dosages, times, and other critical information can result in fatal errors. Using

Front Office	Clinical Care	Coding & Billing		TruCode

Correspondence   📅 Calendar   ✉ Correspondence   👥 Patient Demographics   🔍 Find Patient   📋 Form Repository

INFO PANEL
Emails
 Appointment Reminder
 Blank Email
 Memorandum
 Missed Appointment
 New Patient Welcome
 Normal Test Results
 Patient Termination
Letters
Phone Messages

Normal Test Results
Please perform a patient search to find a specific patient.

To: n.rodriguez@anytown.mail
Cc:
Subject: Lab results

[Attach File]

WALDEN-MARTIN
FAMILY MEDICAL CLINIC
1234 ANYSTREET | ANYTOWN, ANYSTATE 12345
PHONE 123-123-1234 | FAX 123-123-5678

08/22/2016

Rodriguez, Noemi N

441 Hyacinth Way
Anytown, AL 12345-1234
United States

Dear Noemi Rodriguez ,

This letter is to inform you of recent test results. Your procedure Urinalysis performed on, October 31, 2016 was within normal limits.

If you have any additional questions or are still experiencing problems related to this test, please call our office at 123-123-1234 as soon as possible to speak with the Medical Assistant.

Thank you for choosing Walden-Martin Family Medical Clinic for your healthcare needs. Our office is open Monday-Friday 8-6pm.

Sincerely,

Walden-Martin Family Medical Clinic

Nicole Ronson

[Patient Search] [Print] [Send] [Cancel]

Fig. 6.5 The EHR system can send the results of tests to patients electronically. (Courtesy of SimChart for the Medical Office, Elsevier, Inc, 2016.)

an EHR system, certain safeguards ensure the data entered into the medical record are accurate and standardized. Administrative and clinical staff do not freely type into the computer system, but rather select entries through the use of dropdown menus and buttons, greatly reducing errors caused by illegible handwriting or incorrectly inputted information. Most EHR systems set a range of valid values for text entry fields to prevent staff from entering erroneous information into a patient's record. For example, the system may not allow a patient's body temperature to be entered as 201°F when it is actually 102°F.

Software for EHR systems also aids providers through prompts and alerts. For instance, when entering prescriptions, the EHR can alert the provider of any **contraindications**, such as drug allergies or drugs that cannot be taken because of a current treatment regimen. It can flag other inappropriate orders, such as if a male patient is scheduled for a Pap smear. EHR software also helps make sure the medical record is complete through automated reminders and prompts to fill in missing information.

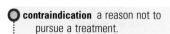
contraindication a reason not to pursue a treatment.

protocol a guideline for the treatment of a disease or disorder.

algorithm a structured path of decision making.

clinical decision support (CDS) a function of the EHR that recommends approaches for diagnoses of specific diseases, guides selection of the correct diagnostic tests, and assists in the treatment and monitoring of patients.

More comprehensive EHR systems will include tools and applications that can help reduce potential errors and standardize delivery of health care. Using scientific evidence, patient data, and standards of care, the medical field has developed specific guidelines to follow for a given disease or disorder, called clinical **protocols**. These protocols aim to standardize the plan of care for patients using a structured path of decision making called a medical **algorithm** (Fig. 6.6), which can reduce unnecessary testing and accelerate the diagnostic process. These medical algorithms are included in the EHR's **clinical decision support (CDS)** system and can recommend approaches for diagnoses of specific diseases, guide selection of the correct diagnostic tests, and assist in the treatment and monitoring of patient care.

For example, a patient presents with indigestion—a thorough patient history is taken and a physical examination performed. The patient's information is entered into the EHR system, which will then determine the next steps in the diagnostic process. If the patient has other signs or symptoms, such as vomiting, bleeding, unintentional weight loss, and family history of esophageal or gastrointestinal cancer, the EHR's CDS system will recommend an endoscopy with biopsy to detect the presence of the bacteria *Helicobacter pylori*. If the patient has no other symptoms besides indigestion, the EHR's CDS system will determine the next step in evaluation based on the patient's age. For a patient 54 years old and younger, a urea breath test or a stool antigen test for *H. pylori* will be recommended. For a patient older than 55 years, an endoscopy with biopsy will be recommended.

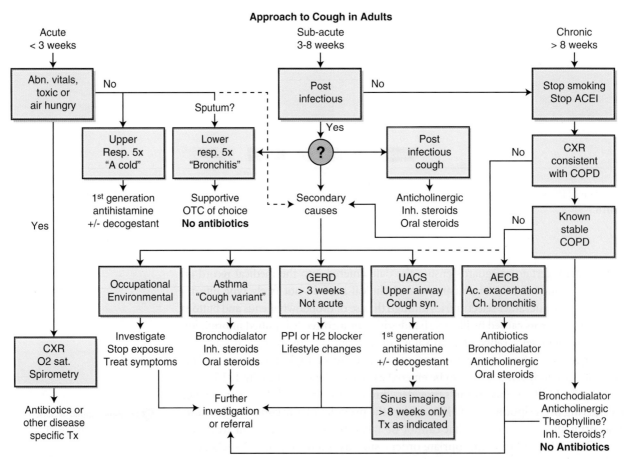

Figure 6.6 An illustration of a medical algorithm to advise on the treatment of a patient who presented with a cough. (Courtesy of Dr. Richard Rathe, Gainesville, FL.)

Another advantage of an EHR system is that it is more secure than a paper medical record. Because the content is digital, it eliminates the space needed for paper files and the security concerns that go along with having so much sensitive information in one filing room. Many facilities utilize special monitors that can only be viewed by a person facing it directly, preventing others from being able to see the information on the screen. Of course, each workstation in the medical office requires a login and password to access the EHR system. These user names and passwords are unique to every employee in the facility, and passwords are usually changed frequently. Office policy will also require staffers to log out of the system immediately, or the terminals should log the user out automatically after a period of inactivity. Furthermore, the EHR system tracks the identity and time each user viewed the medical record, called an **audit trail**. This traces the individuals who accessed a medical record to ensure its contents are only viewed and updated by authorized persons (Fig. 6.7).

audit trail a feature of the EHR system that tracks users who accessed a patient record and when they did so.

Health Information Exchanges

To ensure the most efficient and effective patient care and continuity of care, health care professionals need access to the patient's medical history, as well as the ability to share patient information with other health care providers. This includes information sharing not only among the clinicians and administrative professionals in the same medical office or practice, but also providers from different organizations. However, sharing patient data between different providers is not the simple and straightforward process it could be because different health care organizations may use different software that may not always be compatible. Accessing and sharing data are not possible unless these different software systems are **interoperable**, or have the ability to communicate, exchange data, and use the information that has been exchanged across health care providers, laboratories, hospitals, pharmacies, and patients, regardless of the EHR system.

interoperability the capacity for different computer systems to communicate, exchange data, and use the information that has been exchanged.

CURRENT TRENDS IN HEALTHCARE

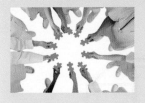

A 2014 survey by the health data warehousing firm Premier, Inc., found that of the 62 accountable care organizations they asked, 100% said accessing data from external sources was challenging.

https://www.premierinc.com/aco-interoperability-survey-9-24-14/

	A	B	C	D	E	F
1	**Username**	**Last**	**First**	**Date/Time**	**MRN**	**Action**
2	TFINN	Finn	Timothy	04/24/2018 12:10	12485635401	Submitted dictation file
3	TFINN	Finn	Timothy	04/24/2018 12:12	12485635401	Played dictation file
4	PSTENNET	Stennet	Phillip	04/24/2018 14:25	12485635401	Played dictation file
5	PSTENNET	Stennet	Phillip	04/24/2018 14:28	12485635401	Countersigned dictation
6	SCODY	Cody	Scott	04/27/2018 14:03	12485635401	Edited patient demographics information
7	TFINN	Finn	Timothy	04/28/2018 7:10	12485635401	Submitted transcription file
8	SCODY	Cody	Scott	04/28/2018 11:11	12485635401	Viewed record
9	SCODY	Cody	Scott	04/28/2018 18:50	12485635401	Edited patient financial information

Figure 6.7 The audit trail shows who accessed the medical record and when.

Both private and governmental agencies have recognized the benefits of widespread interoperable EHR systems. Such a network would save money spent on printing, scanning, and faxing; it would save the time it takes to mail documents; and it would reduce inefficiencies like duplicate tests and imaging. To work toward interoperability, many organizations have advocated for **health information exchanges (HIEs)**, which are groups of providers whose computer systems are networked to form a secure, accessible database of patient records (Fig. 6.8). By joining an HIE, health care organizations, such as laboratories, pharmacies, clinics, hospitals, and other facilities, are able to access and add information about a patient when needed.

There are three different forms of HIEs: directed exchange, query-based exchange, and consumer-mediated exchange. **Directed exchange** is simply the ability for one provider to send information to another in a secure fashion. For example, when referring a patient to a specialist, a PCP can send the patient's laboratory test results and other data to the specialist's office. Most health care providers who have a business relationship with other providers or health care facilities are using this type of exchange. In a **query-based exchange**, a provider can search the database of another provider to bring up a patient's record. Usually, this type of exchange is used for unexpected situations, such as an emergency department (ED) visit. If a patient arrives at the ED with dyspnea (difficulty breathing), physicians can search the database of the patient's primary care provider to view a recent chest x-ray. Lastly, a **consumer-mediated exchange** lets patients send information to other providers. Patients can log onto a website, often referred to as a **patient portal,** to request their information be sent to a specific provider, edit demographic and billing information, view laboratory test results, and track and monitor information regarding their personal health.

Challenges to Implementation

There are several challenges to implementing an EHR system within a health care organization, including having the time, resources, and cooperation from the entire medical staff. The medical staff must be trained to use the EHR system, and this can be a frustrating experience. Some may feel that entering data into an EHR is

health information exchange (HIE) groups of providers whose computer systems are networked to form a secure, accessible database of patient records.

directed exchange a type of HIE with the ability for one provider to send information to another securely.

query-based exchange a type of HIE in which one provider can search the database of another.

consumer-mediated exchange a type of HIE in which patients can request their information be sent to another provider.

patient portal a website on which a patient can interact and communicate with their provider; view laboratory test results; and track, monitor, and send information regarding their personal health.

TAKE AWAY

Interoperability among different users of a patient's medical record is the key to unlocking the potential of the EHR.

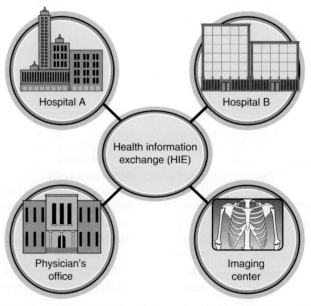

Figure 6.8 Different providers share patient information in an HIE.

BOX 6.2	COMMON CHALLENGES TO USING EHR TECHNOLOGY

- Expensive
- Requires training
- Concern for data security and privacy
- Poor design interface
- Not enough staff empowerment

- Needs more flexible data input
- Data inaccessible to other systems
- Lack of EHR/patient support
- Lack of user input in the system design

cumbersome and time consuming and may be reluctant to change and learn a new system. Privacy and ensuring confidentiality may be a concern for some health care providers and patients when using EHRs. Implementing an EHR system is also quite costly. Small and solo practices may not be able to invest in the technology, especially because the return on investment is uncertain and may take years to see. Box 6.2 lists some common challenges and concerns expressed by health care organizations with regard to using EHRs.

TAKE AWAY

Cost is the biggest barrier to using new health information technology.

LEARNING CHECKPOINT 6.1
Electronic Health Records

1. Which function of the EHR allows a provider to order an x-ray?

    a. the patient portal
    b. health information exchange (HIE)
    c. computerized physician order entry (CPOE)
    d. clinical decision support (CDS)

2. A structured path of decision making is called a(n) _____.

    a. algorithm
    b. contraindication
    c. audit trail
    d. patient portal

3. The directed exchange and the consumer-mediated exchange are each types of _____.

    a. EHRs
    b. medical records
    c. HIEs
    d. patient portals

4. Which is a function of the patient portal?

    a. e-prescribing
    b. ordering labs
    c. viewing the audit trail
    d. viewing lab results

5. A _____ exchange allows one provider to search the patient database of another.

Incentives for Use

The benefits of a fully functional, secure, and interoperable EHR system has the potential to improve safety, quality, efficiency, and costs in the delivery of health care. One of the biggest challenges to implementing an EHR system is the cost. The expense to abandon paper recordkeeping and use this new technology has been prohibitive for many health care organizations, especially small medical practices. Recognizing the prohibitive costs, as well as other barriers to adoption, the federal government has established legislation to support the adoption of an EHR system for the nation's health care system.

As early as 2004, the Bush administration created the Office of the National Coordinator for Health Information Technology (ONC) and allocated $100 million to develop information exchange standards and certifications and to improve security. In 2009, the United States Congress passed the **American Recovery and Reinvestment Act (ARRA)**, commonly known as the *Recovery Act*. A portion of ARRA included a stimulus bill called the **Health Information Technology for Economic and Clinical Health Act (HITECH)**, which approved nearly $30 billion in spending to promote health information technology.

Both federal and state governments created several incentive programs to encourage health care providers to purchase and utilize this new computerized technology, including the development of EHRs and HIEs. To benefit from these incentive programs, health care providers had to adopt technology with certain functions that would enhance the overall quality of care to patients. Specifically, the government did not want to merely incentivize the computerization of health records, but rather encourage the *meaningful use* of EHR systems. **Meaningful use** refers to the set of benchmarks created under the HITECH Act to measure the capabilities of EHR technology in use by health care providers and therefore qualify them for the financial incentives of the program. At the minimum, this means that the health care provider must purchase an EHR system with the capabilities to e-prescribe, report quality data, and exchange data with other health care providers.

Another incentive program, the Medicare and Medicaid EHR Incentive Program, allowed health care providers to receive increased reimbursements from services to Medicare and Medicaid patients from 2011 to 2015 if they implemented this technology with specific capabilities. Health care providers who did not adopt this technology, however, would be penalized with reduced payments for their Medicare and Medicaid patients. Additionally, health care organizations that adopted and began using EHRs earlier received higher financial incentives than those that waited. Eligibility for the program was based on completion of three stages, each taking at least 2 years and having documented proof of completion. Upon completion of the program, health care providers with at least 30% of Medicare patients and Medicaid patients could receive up to $44,000 and $63,750 in total incentives, respectively. Currently, more than 479,000 health care providers participate in the Medicare and Medicaid EHR Incentive Program.[1]

By encouraging the adoption of EHRs, the Centers for Medicare and Medicaid Services (CMS) aimed to create a computerized infrastructure that would modernize the system of communication among health care entities across the nation. This interoperability was designated as a critical health care goal, with the EHR technology having the following functionalities:

- Protect patient health information with risk management processes and through technical and physical safeguards

American Recovery and Reinvestment Act (ARRA) the 2009 legislation providing federal funding in science, research, and infrastructure, including a portion called HITECH to promote health information technology.

Health Information Technology for Economic and Clinical Health Act (HITECH) the portion of the 2009 ARRA that funded and mandated health information technology initiatives.

TAKE AWAY

Government incentives seek to offset the high cost of EHR implementation.

meaningful use the set of benchmarks created under the HITECH Act to measure the capabilities of EHR technology and provide financial incentives to health care providers.

[1]https://www.cms.gov/regulations-and-guidance/legislation/ehrincentiveprograms/basics.html

- Electronic prescribing
- CDS to guide providers in the care and treatment of patients
- CPOE allowing practitioners to order laboratory analysis, diagnostic imaging, and medications electronically
- Provide patients with electronic access to health information
- Coordinate care by offering patients educational materials
- Create a summary of care for patients and make it available through an HIE
- Report immunization data and syndromic surveillance data to public health and clinical data registries

In 2016, CMS announced it would end the "meaningful use" EHR Incentive Program and would propose a series of changes to the last stage of the program. At the time of publication, its successor program has not yet been announced, but it is expected to adapt the tenets of meaningful use to a value-based model of health care, include payment adjustments, and have hardship exemptions.

LEARNING CHECKPOINT 6.2
Challenges and Incentives

1. Which program provided financial incentives for providers who use health information technologies?

   a. meaningful use
   b. HITECH
   c. ARRA
   d. Medicaid

2. The Office of the National Coordinator for Health Information Technology (ONC) was created under which president?

   a. Ronald Reagan
   b. William Jefferson Clinton
   c. George W. Bush
   d. Barack Obama

3. Which legislation was commonly known as the Recovery Act?

   a. ARRA
   b. HITECH
   c. HIPAA
   d. none of these

PRACTICE MANAGEMENT SOFTWARE

Computer software is instrumental to efficient workflow on the administrative side of the medical office. In fact, most of the tasks performed by front-office personnel are aided by **practice management software (PMS)**, used to facilitate the day-to-day operations of the medical office. When selecting a PMS for the medical office, it is important that it is compatible with the EHR system. Some PMSs operate on a completely separate software suite, which may or not be able to *interface,* or share data, with the facility's EHR system. However, other PMSs are *integrated* with the EHR system,

○ **practice management software (PMS)** software used to facilitate the day-to-day operations of the medical office.

meaning that they are different applications of the same piece of software and are constructed to share data with each other. Integrated or interfaced systems are ideal in that they reduce the work of entering patient and provider data into two separate software systems.

Among the functions of the PMS, the most important is the tracking and storing of the demographic and financial information of each patient treated by the office. Collected during the patient registration, this includes the individual's contact information, date of birth, gender, race and ethnicity, Social Security number, and employer and insurance information. Many systems also store an image of the patient and his or her insurance card.

This information is crucial for billing the patient and to identify the patient for appointments and scheduling. PMS systems use a calendar interface to help front-office staff schedule patients (Fig. 6.9), which shows daily, weekly, or monthly views. The graphical interface can manage the different types of scheduling functions discussed in Chapter 4. It can schedule appointments with every provider in the office, avoid double-booking patients, and block off times for walk-in appointments or times

TAKE AWAY

The PMS maintains patient demographic information for scheduling and billing purposes.

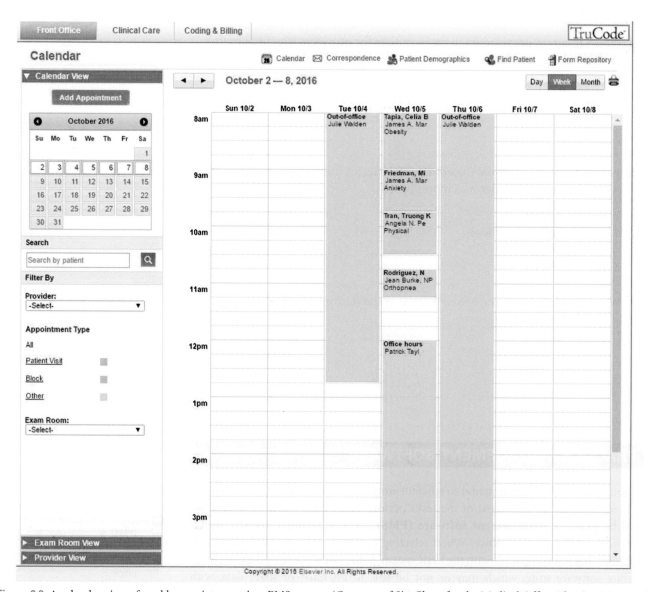

Figure 6.9 A calendar view of weekly appointments in a PMS system. (Courtesy of SimChart for the Medical Office, Elsevier, Inc, 2016.)

a provider is out of the office. Usually the appointment itself is categorized into one of several broader reasons for the visit, such as whether this is a new patient visit, follow-up for a previous concern, an annual physical, or an urgent visit. In the scheduling matrix, the PMS lists the patient's name, chief complaint, and the provider the patient will see. Patient registration staff can also specify which exam room will be used.

Once an appointment is set, the PMS can automatically generate reminders for the patient as the time of the appointment and date approach. The PMS can print these reminders on paper or postcards to be sent in the mail, sent as an email or text message to the patient, or it can place an automated phone call.

The PMS system makes it easy to generate the forms commonly used in the medical office, discussed in Chapter 5. Forms can be personalized, printed, and signed by the patient, such as an advance directive form shown in Fig. 6.10. After it is signed, the form can be scanned so that the image is saved with the patient's record. Other types

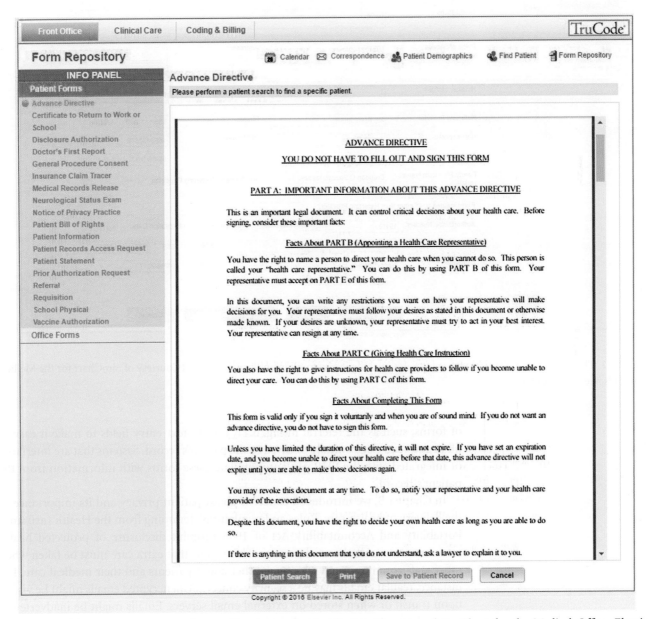

Figure 6.10 The PMS can generate advance directives and other forms. (Courtesy of SimChart for the Medical Office, Elsevier, Inc, 2016.)

| Front Office | Clinical Care | Coding & Billing | | | | | | TruCode |

Form Repository

Calendar   Correspondence   Patient Demographics   Find Patient   Form Repository

INFO PANEL

Patient Forms

Referral

Please perform a patient search to find a specific patient.

Advance Directive
Certificate to Return to Work or School
Disclosure Authorization
Doctor's First Report
General Procedure Consent
Insurance Claim Tracer
Medical Records Release
Neurological Status Exam
Notice of Privacy Practice
Patient Bill of Rights
Patient Information
Patient Records Access Request
Patient Statement
Prior Authorization Request
Referral
Requisition
School Physical
Vaccine Authorization

Office Forms

Diagnosis/Code: S62.605A

Surgical Procedure/ Date: 2W0FX1Z

Significant Clinical Information/Symptoms: Injury to left hand 4th digit

Previous Clinical Treatments: N/A

Allergies: None

Medications: None

Place of Service: ME Frenchtown

Number of Visits: 1

Referring Provider: ME Frenchtown

Name (print): Josiah Daulis

Signature: Josiah Dailis

Family Physician Name (print): Brendan O'Shaughnassey

Patient Name: Willis, Erma I

Address: 33 Pacific Avenue Anytown, AL 12345-1234 United States

Patient Phone: 123 - 567 - 2689

Alternate Contact:

Date of Birth: 12/09/1947   Health ID: 168410

Diabetic: ○ Yes ● No

Address:

Length of Stay:

Phone: 555 - 123 - 1231

NPI Number: 1852432578

Date: 08/06/2017

☐ Same as Referring Physician

Form initiated by (if other than Referring Provider):

Authorization Number: 15110   Effective Date: 08/06/2017   Expiration Date: 08/13/2017

Name (print), Position: Nancy Slacks, Medical Assistant   Phone: 555 - 123 - 1231

Signature: Nancy Slacks   Date: 08/06/2017

| Patient Search | Print | Save to Patient Record | Cancel |

Figure 6.11 The referral form features text-entry fields, making it easy to fill in and print or send. (Courtesy of SimChart for the Medical Office, Elsevier, Inc, 2016.)

of forms, such as the referral in Fig. 6.11, feature text-entry fields to make it easy to fill in and send electronically or saved to the patient's record. Systems that are interfaced or integrated with the EHR can autopopulate these forms with information from the patient's record.

In Chapter 3, we introduced concerns about patient privacy and its importance in the delivery of health care. Rules and regulations stemming from the Health Insurance Portability and Accountability Act of 1996 prohibit disclosure of protected health information to unauthorized persons. This means that extra care must be taken when office staff communicate with one another about patients and their medical care. For instance, regular emails may be a security concern. Unencrypted emails might be visible upon transit or when stored on external email servers. Emails might be inadvertently sent to the wrong patient as well. PMS systems provide the tools for health care professionals to send secure messages to patients and communicate about specific patients to other health care providers. They can also generate interoffice memos and convey phone messages from patients to providers (Fig. 6.12).

The PMS system can also facilitate the billing tasks needed to complete the patient encounter, as well as the following:

- Create entries in financial ledgers to track moneys owed to the practice
- Look up diagnosis and procedure codes (Fig. 6.13) to prepare the **superbill**, a summary of the patient's visit and charges incurred (Fig. 6.14)
- Submit claims for reimbursement to third-party payers (Fig. 6.15)

> **superbill** a summary of the patient's visit and charges incurred.

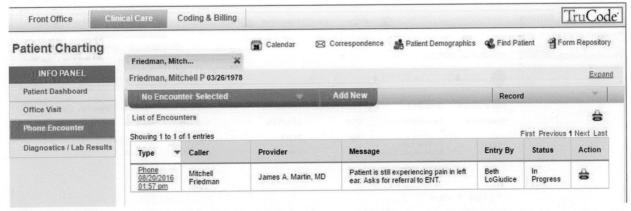

Figure 6.12 The PMS system logs and delivers phone messages for the provider. (Courtesy of SimChart for the Medical Office, Elsevier, Inc, 2016.)

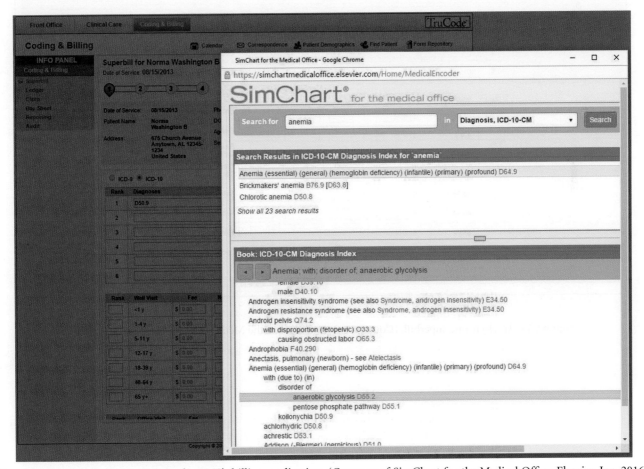

Figure 6.13 A code lookup screen in the PMS's billing application. (Courtesy of SimChart for the Medical Office, Elsevier, Inc, 2016.)

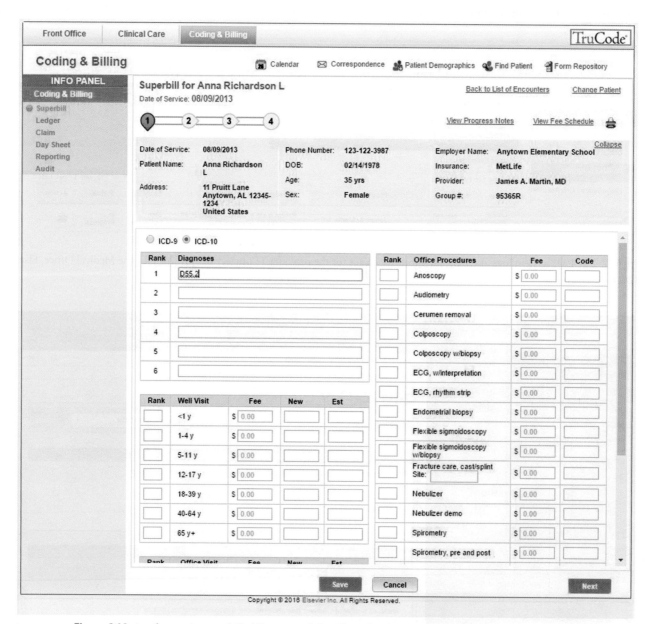

Figure 6.14 An electronic superbill. (Courtesy of SimChart for the Medical Office, Elsevier, Inc, 2016.)

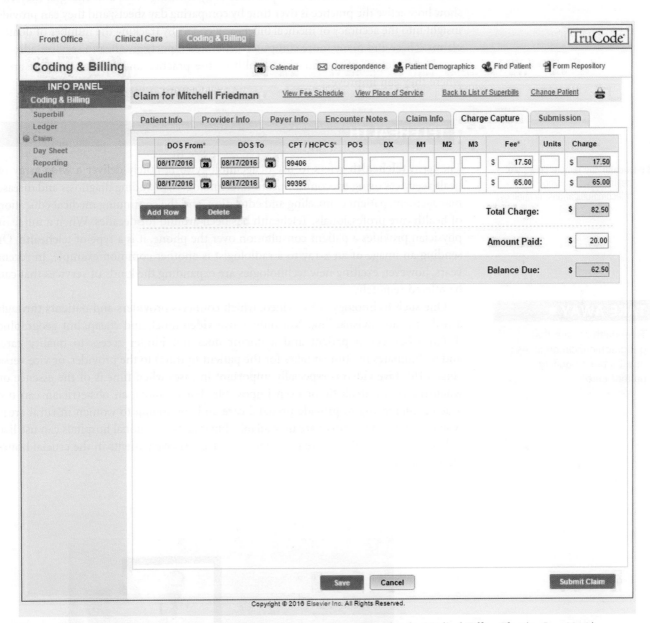

Figure 6.15 Submitting a claim to a payer. (Courtesy of SimChart for the Medical Office, Elsevier, Inc, 2016.)

day sheet a summary of the provider's charges and payments received in a single day.

- Prepare patient statements to bill patients
- Document activity in a **day sheet**, which summarizes charges and payments in a single day

Lastly, PMS systems usually offer several reporting tools to help make decisions in regard to the business aspect of the medical office. For instance, they can generate reports about the types of services the office is providing by indexing procedure codes; they can show how efficient each provider is by tracking visits and charges; they can show how active the practice is over time by comparing day sheets; and they can provide insight into the accuracy of medical billers and coders by tracking the number of denied claims. These and many more computer-generated reports give health services administrators a picture of the financial health of the practice and inform them of areas where they can improve.

TELEHEALTH

telehealth the remote delivery of health services using telecommunications technology.

The term **telehealth** refers to use of technology to remotely deliver a wide array of health services using telecommunication technologies, including diagnosis and disease management, patient counseling and education, and the continuing medical education of health care professionals. Telehealth has been around for decades. When a nurse or physician provides a patient consultation over the phone, it is a type of telehealth. Or sending an image of an x-ray to a radiologist is another common example. In recent years, however, exciting new technologies are expanding the kinds of services that can be offered remotely.

One such technology is live video, which connects providers and patients through a real-time audiovisual link. Not only is live video quick and cheap, but geographic distance between a patient and a doctor does not hinder access to quality care, and it eliminates the time it takes for the patient to travel to the provider, or vice versa (Fig. 6.16). Live video is especially important in cases when time is of the essence or when travel is unrealistic or even impossible. For example, an obstetrician can use video conferencing to provide prenatal care and counseling to women in rural areas where obstetrical resources are unavailable. Physicians at regional hospitals can use live video to consult with remote neurologists to treat stroke patients in the crucial hours after a stroke.

TAKE AWAY

Telehealth means that geographic location is less of a barrier to quality patient care.

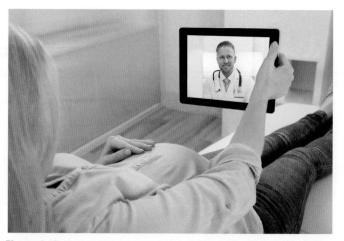

Figure 6.16 A patient communicates with a provider via live video.

The use of live video is not limited to matters of life and death, of course. Today, nearly every smartphone, laptop, and tablet sold is equipped with a video camera and a microphone capable of connecting a patient to a health care provider. This makes it possible for providers in primary and urgent care to offer **e-visits** for acute, nonemergency situations. Providers can use e-visits to diagnose the most common ailments seen in medical office, such as conjunctivitis (pinkeye), sinusitis, upper respiratory infections, and urinary tract infections. This functionality makes the delivery of health care available nights and days, weekends, and holidays.

Other types of services may utilize **store-and-forward** technology, where images or video of a patient is recorded to be viewed by a specialist later. This type of technology is useful in less time-sensitive instances and when the physician does not necessarily need to communicate with the patient. For example, a primary care provider can take a photograph of a rash or other skin condition and send it to a dermatologist via telehealth technology, who can then diagnose the condition remotely.

e-visit a patient interaction with a provider using telecommunications technology.

store-and-forward a type of telemedicine in which images or video of a patient is recorded to be viewed by a specialist at a later time.

CURRENT TRENDS IN HEALTH CARE

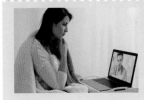

Although the technology to deliver telehealth has been available for quite some time, its implementation has suffered in large part because of reimbursement issues. Except for store-and-forward services, Medicare will not cover telehealth expenses unless the patient is in a rural area or an area with a shortage of health care professionals. Coverage of telehealth under private plans varies greatly.

Remote patient monitoring (RPM) is another important telehealth technology that transmits physiologic health data from a patient outside of a health care setting (such as at home) to a provider. By tracking blood pressure, oxygen saturation, and blood glucose levels, RPM allows patients with chronic diseases like diabetes or heart disease to manage their illnesses outside of the hospital setting. At the same time, their biometric data are carefully monitored for signs of any impending problem. Some systems even run the data through a CDS algorithm to alert health care professionals of a change in status or standard of care. RPM technology lowers costs and increases quality by keeping patients out of the hospital, reducing readmission rates, and reducing the number of office visits.

remote patient monitoring (RPM) a type of telemedicine in which the patient transmits physiologic health data outside of a health care setting (such as at home) to a provider.

● CASE STUDY

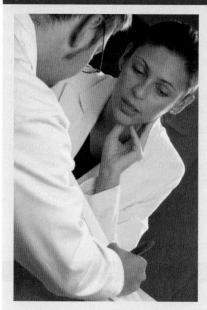

JoAnn makes the case to Dr. Roberts that with an EHR system, medical records can be kept digitally, with information viewed and updated in real time for multiple locations. In addition, the data are of a higher quality because they are standardized, greatly reducing errors caused by illegible handwriting or incorrectly inputted information. The software can also help provide CDS and alerts the physician of any contraindications. Furthermore, because the records are digital, the process of referring patients (and sending their records) to other providers is streamlined.

REVIEW QUESTIONS

1. What are three features of an electronic health record (EHR)?

2. List three ways EHR technology improves the delivery of health care.

3. What is a health information exchange (HIE)?

4. What are the challenges and barriers to the implementation of EHRs?

5. Why did the federal government develop programs to hasten the implementation of EHRs?

6. How is practice management software (PMS) different from the EHR?

MANAGING SUPPLIES AND INVENTORY

Pat DeVoy and Carol Colvin

CHAPTER OUTLINE

INTRODUCTION
MANAGING INVENTORY
   Duties and
      Responsibilities

Inventory Loss
   Employee Theft
ORDERING
   Preparing a Purchase Order

RECEIVING
BEST PRACTICES

VOCABULARY

lead time
par level
purchase order (PO)

real cost
shelf life
shrinkage

stock-out
vendor

CHAPTER OBJECTIVES

After completing this chapter, the student should be able to do the following:

1. Explain how a budget for supplies and services is determined.
2. Explain how office staff manage inventory.
3. Define shrinkage and list the ways it can be reduced in the medical office.
4. Describe the evaluation of vendors.
5. Explain how to prepare a purchase order.
6. Discuss the receipt of new shipments.
7. List best practices for inventory management.

INTRODUCTION

Similar to any business, the medical office needs a wide range of supplies and equipment to operate and provide its services. Imagine the supplies used at your last visit to a medical office. For example, the medical office needs pens and paper, toner for the copy machines and printers, paper cups for the water cooler, and magazines in the reception area. Each examination room will have bandages and tongue depressors, cotton swabs and alcohol swabs, syringes, and gloves (Fig. 7.1). Some medical offices might need a laundry service for patient gowns and scrubs or a software vendor who provides and maintains the software for billing, coding, and electronic health records (EHR). Additionally, health care providers need a consistent supply of syringes and medication, which needs to be ordered, received, inventoried, and reordered.

In this chapter, we will look at how successful medical offices obtain and monitor the inventory on hand to make sure they have the right supplies, at the right time, in the right quantity, and at the right cost.

CASE STUDY

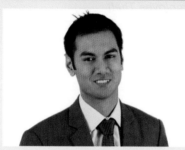

Han is the health services administrator at Med+Care, a local retail health care clinic. He has been tasked with selecting a new vendor for medical supplies. This includes items such as automatic blood pressure cuffs, thermometers with disposable ends, saline solution, hand sanitizer, disinfectant wipes, sterile gauze sponges, bloodwork trays, tech trays, non-latex gloves, and various other consumable products. In the past, supplies were purchased from various vendors. But Han is hoping that he can streamline the purchasing process by ordering from one major vendor who can offer these items at a reduced cost. This will help him standardize and simplify the ordering process, as well as the management of inventory needed for the daily operation of his facility. As you move through the chapter, take note of some things Han should consider when searching for a new vendor.

MANAGING INVENTORY

stock-out the state of being out of an item.

The practice of managing inventory is a critical part of operating a successful business and being able to provide quality care to patients. The key to managing inventory is being able to balance having a sufficient supply while avoiding an oversurplus. Being out of an item, called a **stock-out**, is frustrating to both patients and providers, especially

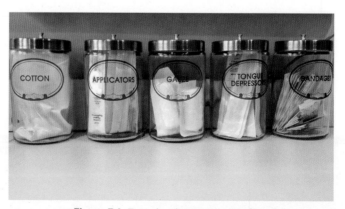

Figure 7.1 Examination room supplies.

if the item is needed for patient care. Without the supply or equipment on hand, the provider may not be able to perform a procedure, resulting in a loss of revenue and potentially the patient. On the other hand, keeping too much of an item in inventory is problematic because it may tie up needed funds and result in inventory waste. Therefore the process of inventory management has an effect not only on patient care, but also on the financial flow of the business.

How does the medical office know how much money to spend and how much of any particular item to order? One of the first things the medical office must decide is its buying cycle for each item. How often will the item need to be ordered—weekly, monthly, quarterly, etc.? Although this depends on utilization and storage space, most offices should order supplies weekly or monthly.

Next, the amount of each item typically used during each buying cycle needs to be determined. When ordering, quantities and monies budgeted are usually determined by the amount that was ordered in the past. The amount of supplies used daily, such as soap, paper towels, toilet paper, and table paper, will generally stay the same month to month. For example, if the medical office spent $100 each month for the past year on examination gloves, the medical office could reasonably budget that same $100 for gloves in future months. Supply budgets may slightly alter, sometimes as a result of an increase in the price of supplies or services and/or a growth in the number of patients. The staff member who is responsible for the ordering should be aware of any price changes in supplies and budget accordingly. If the medical office begins to offer any new services, this may mean an increase in the supplies and budget needed. In general, enough of each item should be purchased for at least two buying cycles, except for items with expiration dates or seasonal items such as flu vaccine.

Duties and Responsibilities

In any medical office, the process of identifying what supplies need to be ordered, how these supplies should be ordered, and who is responsible for ordering is found in the office policy and procedures manual. Usually, it is best to have one staff member in charge of managing the inventory to streamline and organize the process. If the medical practice is larger, two or more staff members may be needed, with one responsible for administrative supplies and the other clinical supplies. The overall management of inventory is often the function of the medical office manager, the health services administrator, a medical assistant, or whichever staff member is directly responsible for the health care facility's budget. We will refer to the staff member in charge of inventory management as the health services administrator for the remainder of the chapter.

In addition to the ordering, the health services administrator may be responsible for receiving and maintaining inventory; if not, he or she must appoint another staff member to perform this function. For example, the health services administrator places an order for paper patient gowns. Two days later, the boxes of patient gowns are delivered to the medical office. How does the health services administrator know that the shipment has arrived? Who checks to make sure the correct gowns were received? How do the gowns get to the storage area and placed in the exam rooms where they are needed? The health services administrator or whoever is in charge of receiving supply orders needs a system to record the new supplies and make sure they are available for use (Fig. 7.2). The medical office should have a method in place to track what new supplies have arrived and update the current counts of how much of any item are "on hand."

The health services administrator must be on alert for any extreme variations in the usage of supplies. In general, the medical office should not suddenly use twice as many pregnancy tests as it did in the previous months. Monitoring for situations like this

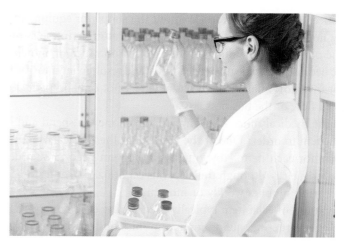

Figure 7.2 A laboratory assistant stocks glassware in the lab.

can alert the health services administrator to changes in the patient population and the services being offered, or the possibility of theft.

There are many types of inventory systems, but the most common approach is to use an inventory spreadsheet that lists all of the supplies needed in the medical office. The spreadsheet lists the **par level**, or reorder point, which is the quantity of an item that must be kept on the premises before a new order needs to be placed. This spreadsheet should also be used to determine the periodic ordering of supplies. An example of such a spreadsheet is shown in Fig. 7.3. Larger health care facilities may use automated software to keep track of supplies.

par level the quantity at which supplies are reordered.

Inventory Loss

One might wonder why the medical office just does not order more supplies at one time. Would it not be better to order large quantities of every item than risk running out? There are many reasons why this is not a good business practice. First, ordering large quantities of supplies affects the supply budget and the cash flow of the medical office. Medical offices maintain their financial health by balancing the amount of money taken in and paid out each month. The medical office must earn enough each month to meet all of its financial obligations, including payroll, rent, and, of course, the purchase of supplies. If too much cash is used to purchase unneeded supplies or supplies that will not be used for several months, it will reduce the flow of cash for that month and ultimately compromise other financial obligations of the medical office.

TAKE AWAY •·········

Ordering too much inventory wastes money and space.

Second, by ordering large quantities of supplies, more space is needed for storage. Most medical offices are limited in the amount of space they have available for storage. This is especially true of inventory that must be kept in locked cabinets or refrigerated, such as culture media, vaccines, antibiotics, and other medications.

Lastly, many products used in a medical office have an expiration date, particularly items used for patient treatments or procedures, such as medications, and items that need to maintain sterility, such as sterile gauze. An expiration date for an item is determined by the manufacturer, and it guarantees the product is safe and effective for use until that date has expired. The amount of time an item may be stored before use is called its **shelf life**. Supplies should never be used past its shelf life because it puts both the medical office staff and the patient in jeopardy because the supply is no longer considered safe to use and/or is no longer effective. Because of this, any supplies in the office that are beyond the expiration date must be thrown out or destroyed.

shelf life the amount of time an item may be stored before use.

	A	B	C	D	E
1	Item	Units	Par level	On hand	Qty to order
2	Disposable gowns	50/CS	2 CS	2 CS	3 CS
3	Disposable drapes	100/CS	3 CS	3 CS	4 CS
4	Gloves, latex-free, vinyl, small	1000/CS	1 CS	2 CS	1 CS
5	Gloves, latex-free, vinyl, medium	1000/CS	1 CS	3 CS	0
6	Gloves, latex-free, vinyl, large	1000/CS	1 CS	3 CS	0
7	Urine collection cups	200/CS	1 CS	1 CS	3 CS
8	Urine test strips	600/CS	2 CS	2 CS	1 CS
9	Lancets	2000/CS	1 CS	1 CS	1 CS
10	Glucose test strips	1800/CS	1 CS	1 CS	1 CS
11	Alcohol prep pads	1000/CS	1 CS	1 CS	2 CS
12	Iodine swab sticks	50/CS	1 CS	1 CS	2 CS
13	Triple antibiotic ointment	1728/CS	1 CS	1 CS	1 CS
14	Tongue depressors	1000/CS	1 CS	1 CS	1 CS
15	Hand sanitizer, 1000 ml	8/CS	3 cases	1 cases	2 cases
16	Exam table paper	12/CS	6 cases	2 cases	4 cases
17	Paper towels	24/CS	2 CS	1 CS	1 CS
18	Biohazard waste bags	100/CS	1 CS	2 CS	0
19	Sharps container	32/CS	1 CS	1 CS	1 CS

Figure 7.3 Inventory tracking spreadsheet.

Any time a piece of inventory must be thrown away or destroyed or goes missing, it is considered loss. The loss of inventory is called **shrinkage**. Sometimes, shrinkage is unavoidable in the medical practice. For example, a retail clinic may want to keep a supply of insulin in stock because this is a common medication to manage patients with diabetes. The clinic orders only 10 vials of insulin each month. Standard guidelines recommend that a vial of insulin should not be used past 28 days, and it needs to be discarded and reordered each month. If the clinic only administers eight vials of insulin in a particular month, the remaining two vials will expire and must be discarded as shrinkage. However, despite this inventory waste, given the revenue earned from administering the insulin, it makes financial sense to order more than needed, even if some of the insulin is lost as shrinkage.

Let us assign some prices and costs to this scenario as an example. The clinic orders 10 vials of insulin, and each vial costs $300 for a total of $3000. Because two vials are discarded, what is the *real cost* per unit? Even though only eight vials were used, the

● **shrinkage** the loss of inventory.

clinic paid a total of $3000, which gives the real cost to the clinic as $375 per vial ($3000 ÷ 8 vials), not $300. Accounting for loss is part of the total cost of any particular item or service, or its **real cost**: the cost of an item including the cost of all resources used to offer the good or service. The clinic missed $600 of potential revenue due to the loss of two vials of insulin.

A manual inventory of supplies performed on a regular basis is the best defense against loss. This will establish the current and accurate count of supplies on the premises and help determine if supplies are being used efficiently or if waste or theft has occurred. The manual inventory is a physical hand count of all supplies, which is recorded on a spreadsheet or computer software system. This physical count is then checked against the quantities on the spreadsheet, and any discrepancies are noted. Hopefully, as the inventory is performed, the numbers are either exact or very similar. If an inventory is conducted and unusual amounts of supplies are missing, the health services administrator must conduct an investigation to determine the reason for the missing supplies.

Supplies should be replenished in the administrative areas and patient exam rooms daily. This is to not only provide quality patient care, but also to ensure that inventory counts are accurate. This task should be designated to one staff member to ensure that the needed supplies are readily available at all times.

Employee Theft

One of the most common causes of shrinkage is employee theft. Unfortunately, employee theft occurs in every type of business (Fig. 7.4). Having too much inventory on hand may provide a perceived opportunity for employee theft. Employees may steal because they have personal financial pressures or because they feel like they are treated unfairly. It is the health services administrator's responsibility to be aware of any of these situations and intervene when possible.

Managers can take a number of steps to deter employee theft. First, the office should keep a current and accurate inventory spreadsheet in place. Do not over-order supplies, particularly high-priced items. All deliveries should be inventoried and stocked as soon as possible, and all supplies should be accounted for.

Second, work to maintain a positive environment in the medical office. Poor morale toward the organization or its management can make theft more likely. If the health services administrator becomes aware of an employee's gambling, alcohol, or drug problem, it is in the best interest of both the employee and the medical office to refer the employee for personal counseling.

real cost the cost of an item, including the cost of all resources used to offer the good or service.

TAKE AWAY ●··········

One of the most common causes of shrinkage is employee theft.

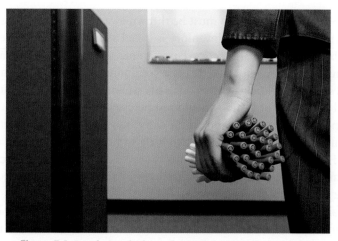

Figure 7.4 Employee theft can happen in any place of work.

When an employee is stealing supplies for his or her own personal use, the health services administrator must immediately address this situation. The first step is to conduct a staff meeting to make employees aware that supplies from the medical office are being removed from the premises illegally and that this will not be tolerated. Then, the health services administrator may want to speak with the employee directly. In some organizations, an employee may continue working after correction and some disciplinary action. In other organizations, policies may dictate a release from employment or the employee being criminally prosecuted.

LEARNING CHECKPOINT 7.1
Managing Inventory

1. The medical office runs out of diabetic test strips. This is called a(n) _____.

2. The clinic never wants to run out of hydrogen peroxide, so it sets a(n) _____ of twelve 1-liter bottles.

3. True or False. Sterile gauze has an expiration date.

4. True or False. The amount of time an item may be stored before use is called shrinkage.

ORDERING

The medical office relies on business relationships with other entities to provide the materials, equipment, and outsourced services that make it possible to conduct business and provide patient care. The products and services provided by these outside organizations, or **vendors**, are essential to the success of the health care facility.

It is important for the health services administrator to make the medical office's supply budget go as far as possible. Just as you would try to find the best prices when you buy things for yourself, the same is true in the medical office. The health services administrator should routinely compare prices of medical supplies and services and let the vendors know that their prices are being compared. If a better price is found for a product, the health services administrator may want to switch vendors or notify the current vendor that a better price is available. Oftentimes, vendors will match a competitor's prices.

Fortunately, due to technology, even the smallest medical practices have more options for supply and services than ever before. Medical offices are able to research and compare prices and can select vendors that provide the best-quality products at the lowest cost. As a result, this has increased the level of competition among the different medical vendors, giving buyers more power, options, and flexibility.

Directly working with vendors can help not only with basic prices but also the services the vendor will provide. For example, the vendor may offer a faster **lead time**, or the amount of time it takes to receive an order once placed, or offer a more flexible return policy. The Internet also provides for better tracking of the placed order and shipment of supplies. In general, the use of technology in the medical office has had a positive impact on the organization's bottom line. Box 7.1 offers considerations for the health services administrator when selecting a vendor.

vendor an outside organization that provides products or services to the medical office.

lead time the amount of time it takes to receive an order once placed.

CURRENT TRENDS IN HEALTH CARE

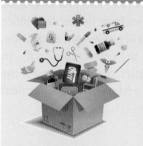

To meet the demand for efficiency and cost saving for medical practices, more medical supply vendors are moving to a new trend called *convergence*. Medical supply vendors used to be specific in the supplies they offered. For example, pharmaceutical companies supplied medications, and office supply companies supplied paper, pens, and paperclips. Now, the lines are becoming blurred between specialized medical supply companies and the new "department store" supply vendors. These "department store" supply vendors are companies providing a wide array of supplies, equipment, and even services. This is a great benefit to the health services administrator because it provides the opportunity to easily compare prices between generic and name-brand items and allows for the ordering of all or most supplies from one vendor versus multiple vendors.

BOX 7.1   SEVEN C'S FOR SELECTING A VENDOR

Conducting a comparative analysis of various vendors that offer the same services or supplies allows the health services administrator to choose the best fit. The following are the Seven C's to look for when selecting a vendor:

1. Competency – Determine the vendor's competency level. Health services administrators should conduct a thorough assessment of each potential vendor's capabilities and compare those abilities to the needs of the organization. Health services administrators should also consider the level of customer satisfaction of the vendor's previous and/or current clients. The Internet has made it easy to access information on how local health care organizations rate the vendor. If there is no public information available regarding the satisfaction of other customers, the health services administrator can always ask for references from current and past customers.

2. Consistency – While collecting customer feedback, ask about the consistency of the vendor. The vendor's approach to the creation and development of goods and services can provide insight about the vendor as an organization. If a vendor is focused on low cost, with no mention of quality assurance or control, consistency in the supply of goods or services may not be provided.

3. Commitment – Determine the level of commitment to providing a high-quality product. When organizations are at the top of the market, they typically do not hesitate to advertise it. Letting the world know that they produce high-quality goods provides a marketing edge and creates brand or company recognition. Health services administrators must make a determination about how committed the vendor will be to providing consistent quality products or services over the life of the relationship.

4. Control – Does the vendor control all aspects of the manufacturing of the supplies? Do they ensure their own vendors are responsible? Do they comply with industry regulations? Understanding how much control a vendor has over their own supply chain can help paint a picture about the full process and risks involved should resources become scarce.

5. Cost – Determine if the cost is comparable to other vendors. Although cost is not the only factor when seeking a vendor, health services administrators want to ensure that they are getting a fair price. When quality is comparable between vendors, it is important to then seek the best price available.

6. Capacity – Determine if the vendor will be able to handle the medical office's requirements. Does the vendor have the resources such as personnel, materials, equipment, delivery capabilities, and storage to provide the supplies needed?

7. Communication – Determine how the vendor plans on communicating with the health care organization. Communication is the key to a successful relationship between any organization and its vendors. Health services administrators should find out how the vendor plans on keeping them abreast of situations that can affect the organization and have a point of contact. A written plan of communication should be established for changes that occur in price, production schedule, delivery, or changes in product specifications. Health services administrators should specify in the contract with a vendor that any disruption in the delivery of a good or service be brought to their attention within a specified time frame once the delay becomes evident.

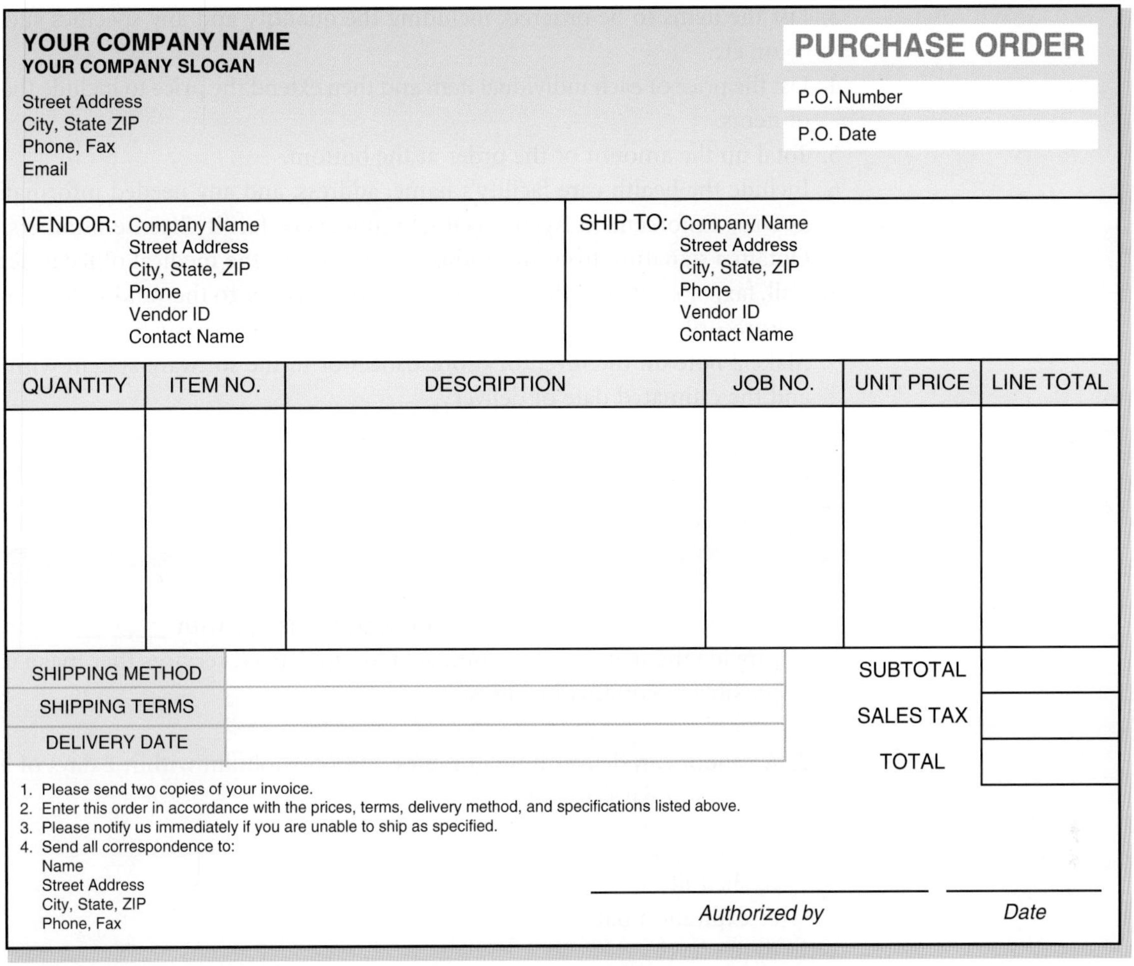

YOUR COMPANY NAME
YOUR COMPANY SLOGAN
Street Address
City, State ZIP
Phone, Fax
Email

PURCHASE ORDER
P.O. Number
P.O. Date

VENDOR: Company Name
Street Address
City, State, ZIP
Phone
Vendor ID
Contact Name

SHIP TO: Company Name
Street Address
City, State, ZIP
Phone
Vendor ID
Contact Name

QUANTITY	ITEM NO.	DESCRIPTION	JOB NO.	UNIT PRICE	LINE TOTAL

SHIPPING METHOD		SUBTOTAL	
SHIPPING TERMS		SALES TAX	
DELIVERY DATE		TOTAL	

1. Please send two copies of your invoice.
2. Enter this order in accordance with the prices, terms, delivery method, and specifications listed above.
3. Please notify us immediately if you are unable to ship as specified.
4. Send all correspondence to:
   Name
   Street Address
   City, State, ZIP
   Phone, Fax

Authorized by   Date

Figure 7.5 Example of a purchase order.

Preparing a Purchase Order

A purchase order is often needed when supplies are ordered from a vendor. A **purchase order (PO)** is a form listing the items, quantities, and agreed prices for products or services needed from a specific vendor. It lists the name and contact information of the vendor and the medical office, and each PO is assigned a unique number (Fig. 7.5). Usually, a PO contains a signature line for the individual who authorizes the order. The completed PO offers both the medical office and the vendor a legally binding document of the supplies being requested, the amounts and the price, the delivery date, and the terms of the payment.

purchase order (PO) a form listing the items, quantities, and agreed prices for products or services needed from a specific vendor.

When ordering, be aware that items come in quantities of all types and sizes. Some supplies may be ordered individually, whereas others may come in counts of two, five, ten, by the dozen, and much more. Items may be shipped by the box, by the carton, or by the case. It is important to know how many individual items are in each unit ordered. If a case contains more items than needed, especially if the items have an expiration date and not all of the items will be used before then, contact the vendor to see if the item can be purchased in smaller amounts. If that is not possible, contact another vendor.

The procedure for preparing a PO includes the following:

1. Review the inventory of the medical office and determine the items needed.
2. Fill out the date of the order.

3. List the items to be ordered, including the quantity and any specifics such as size, color, etc.
4. List the price of each individual item and then extend the price to include the number of items.
5. Total up the amount of the order at the bottom.
6. Include the health care facility's name, address, and any needed information such as Drug Enforcement Agency (DEA) numbers or facility/license numbers.
7. Obtain a signature from the authorized person in the medical office if needed.
8. Call, fax, or electronically submit the purchase order to the vendor. Keep a copy for your records and any verification provided by the vendor, such as an order number.
9. Make a note on the inventory spreadsheet or in the software system with the PO# and the estimated date of delivery.

LEARNING CHECKPOINT 7.2
Ordering

1. The medical office relies on business relationships with _____ to provide the materials, equipment, and outsourced services that make it possible to conduct business.

2. A vendor can deliver human rabies immunoglobulin within 2 days of an order. Two days refers to:

   a. lead time
   b. shelf life
   c. expiration date
   d. par level

3. True or False. A purchase order lists the prices of the items ordered.

RECEIVING

TAKE AWAY ●·········

When receiving inventory, each item should be identified and compared with the packing slip to verify that the correct item and quantity were shipped.

When an order arrives, the health services administrator or designated staff member needs to know that new inventory has arrived. Each package should have a packing slip, which is a list of items ordered and included in the shipment. The packing slip is either affixed to the outside of the box or inside with the items. Each item should be identified and compared with the packing slip to verify that the correct item and quantity were shipped. The packing slip should also be checked for any additional information, such as an item being backordered or shipped separately. The packing slip should also be compared with the order form to verify that the items shipped match the items ordered and that the prices are correct. If there are any discrepancies, the vendor must be contacted immediately. If the shipment is correct, the receiving staff member will usually initialize, date, and file the packing slip.

Electronic inventory management systems often use bar codes for tracking inventory. As supplies are delivered, the staff member is able to scan the items with a bar code reader, which inputs the updated quantity into the system (Fig. 7.6). This allows the staff member to know exactly how much of the item the facility has on hand. Electronic systems can also provide automatic notifications when supplies need to be ordered.

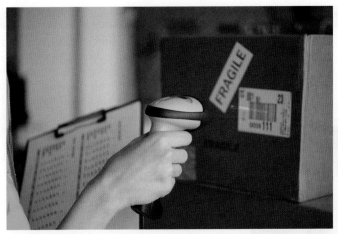

Figure 7.6 A staff member scans new inventory into stock.

After the shipment has been checked in, it must be properly stocked. Inventory should always be rotated so that any old items are used before newer supplies. This usually means stocking the new items behind the old items on shelves and in cabinets.

BEST PRACTICES

There are a number of goals for effective inventory management. Table 7.1 lists specific goals and how they affect business.

TABLE 7.1	
PRIMARY AND SECONDARY GOALS OF SUPPLY MANAGEMENT	
Goal	**Explanation**
Reduced investment in inventory	Keep costs low. Identify and determine exactly what supplies need to be purchased. Plan quantity needed and timeline to have the supplies available for use. If deeper discounts are available when ordering supplies in greater quantities, a manager must weigh the costs and benefits of ordering a higher quantity at a time. Some factors to be considered in this situation include the shelf life or expiration of the supplies, continuity of demand, cost of storage, and the risks of shrinkage.
Relationships with vendors	Vendors prefer to maintain existing relationships that have consistently produced income than to have to secure new business. In addition, if supplies are needed on short notice, an existing relationship with a vendor may expedite the delivery of an order. Having a good relationship with a reliable and consistent vendor could be the difference between staying in business and going out of business.
Continuity of supply	Track inventory. Whether due to regular business usage or fluctuations in patient care, which are causing changes in demand, running out of an item is unacceptable to providers and their patients.
Reduction in real cost	Reducing real costs increases the bottom line, which may lead to lower costs to customers. Put into place systems to prevent loss, theft, or misuse of supplies.

⬤ CASE STUDY

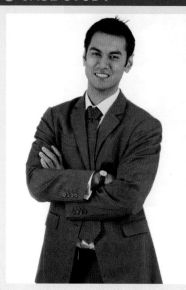

After doing some comparison shopping, Han was able to find a vendor that offered lower prices on most of the consumable items the office needs. Using the vendor's website, Han is able to track his order history, so he is able to quickly see what the office has ordered in the past. In addition, this new vendor supplies many of the things he needs for the front office, such as memo pads, paperclips, and copy paper. Han plans to talk with the sales representative from the vendor that currently supplies the front office about getting better prices.

REVIEW QUESTIONS

1. What are some ways the medical office manager knows how much of an item to order?

2. How is inventory tracked in a medical office?

3. List some reasons employees may steal from the organization.

4. List three qualities to look for when selecting a vendor.

5. Why do medical offices use purchase order forms when ordering supplies?

6. How does a bar code reader streamline inventory management?

7. What are three goals when managing inventory?

BASIC FINANCE AND HEALTH CARE ACCOUNTING

Carol Colvin

CHAPTER OUTLINE

INTRODUCTION
FINANCIAL STATEMENTS
    Balance Sheets
        Current Assets
        Fixed Assets

Liabilities
Net Worth
Income Statements

BUDGETING
    Capital Budget
    Operational Budget
        Variance

VOCABULARY

accounts payable (AP)
accounts receivable (AR)
accrual basis accounting
asset
balance sheet
capital expenditure
cash basis accounting

depreciation
fiscal year
fixed costs
gross income
income statement
liability
net income

net worth
operational budget
payback period
revenue stream
variable costs
variance

CHAPTER OBJECTIVES

After completing this chapter, the student should be able to do the following:

1. Understand the parts and functions of balance sheets for a health care business.
2. Recognize the key parts of an income statement, identifying revenue streams and choosing an accounting method (cash or accrual).
3. Compare the operational budget with the capital budget, describing the use of each in the organization.

INTRODUCTION

As discussed in the previous chapter, managing a health care facility requires an understanding of the business side of medicine. The health services administrator should have a solid foundation in all functional areas critical to the operation of the health care facility, including financial management. This chapter examines basic accounting and financial management and their importance in the operations of a successful medical practice.

● CASE STUDY

Evergreen Health is weighing the pros and cons of purchasing new equipment to offer additional services to its patients. Dr. Lane founded the practice and has been a primary care physician in the community for more than 25 years. Ten years ago, he expanded his office to include three other primary care physicians due to the demand for primary care providers in the area. Dr. Lane has also been partnering with other medical facilities that provide ancillary services, such as echocardiograms. Echocardiograms could be ordered the same day, with results returned within 48 hours.

However, during the past year, Dr. Lane has noticed that his nearest provider of echocardiogram services takes as long as 3 weeks to schedule a test. Not only is this frustrating to patients, but it delays diagnosing patients, scheduling interventional surgeries, and prescribing or monitoring medication and treatment. Dr. Lane has also heard his patients complaining about the long wait times when they arrive at the facility and about having to drive more than 15 miles to this facility.

Last week, Dr. Lane called a meeting with his staff to discuss these problems. He

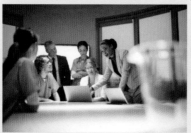

asked that the other physicians in the practice attend, along with Brittney, the heath care administrator, and Kyleigh, the patient registration representative. Brittney made the following notes from the meeting:

- All three physicians expressed the same frustration—having to wait days and sometimes weeks to schedule an echocardiogram for their patients.
- Kyleigh reported that appointments for patients referred out for this service were rescheduled more than 50% of the time due to results not being received in the expected time frame. Multiple requests had to be submitted before receiving the results.
- Brittney provided data showing that over the past 6 months, an average of 8 to 10 patients per week were scheduled for echocardiograms at the referral facility. Patients referred for an echocardiogram generally had return appointments to discuss results 23 days after the test was ordered.
- All meeting attendees agreed that there was a need for action. One of the fellow physicians stated that, in his previous office, echocardiograms were provided in-house for both the convenience of the patient and because the provider could obtain test results almost immediately.
- Dr. Lane tasked Brittney with gathering the following data:
  - What will performing echocardiograms in-house cost, taking into account the purchase of the equipment and paying a technician to perform the test?
  - Will it be more cost effective to purchase or lease the equipment?
  - What is the annual cost to maintain the echocardiogram equipment, and how often will the equipment need to be updated?
  - Will the addition of the equipment lead to additional staffing needs, or can current staff be trained? Also, if current staff can be trained, do they have the time?
- Dr. Lane asked the group to reconvene in 1 week to discuss the results of Brittney's research.

FINANCIAL STATEMENTS

To successfully manage any health care facility, the health services administrator must be able to make decisions based on having an accurate picture of the financial position and performance of the health care facility. This information can be found in the financial statements, or financial reports, which provide a record of the financial activities of a business. Financial statements are the primary documents needed for financial analysis and to determine the overall financial health of the facility. The most common types of financial statements prepared are *balance sheets* and *income statements*.

Balance Sheets

The **balance sheet** shows how much an organization is worth. It includes the *assets* of a company, the *liabilities* associated with those assets and the general business operation, and the company's *net worth*. **Assets** are resources that are owned by a company, such as the equipment, cash, and cash receivables or income of the company. Assets create value in the company and benefit the overall business operation. For instance, an x-ray machine would be a necessary asset in order for a medical office to generate income for billing from x-ray services. **Liabilities** are the debts or other financial obligations that are incurred during the operation of the business. Examples of liabilities are employee salaries and wages and money owed (accounts payable) to the supplier of the paper products for the office.

A balance sheet has two sides (Fig. 8.1). On one side (the left), you have assets; on other the other side (the right), you have liabilities and net worth. The two sides must be equal to each other; this is where the form gets the name *balance sheet.* It must balance in order to calculate a business's net worth. The equation to calculate net worth is:

$$\text{Assets} = \text{Liabilities} + \text{Net Worth}$$

A balance sheet is usually updated at the end of each year for accounting purposes and to help in planning and budgeting for the upcoming year. Some health care facilities will choose to maintain a more current balance sheet, such as monthly, whereas others choose to update annually.

balance sheet a financial statement listing an organization's assets, liabilities, and net worth.

asset resources owned by an organization.

liability a debt or other financial obligation incurred during the operation of the business.

Assets = Liabilities + Net Worth

Smalltown Health Balance Sheets for FYs ending Dec 31

ASSETS	2018	2017	LIABILITIES	2018	2017
Cash	$ 20,478.00	$ 18,795.00	Accounts payable	$ 1,115.00	$ 2,154.00
Accounts receivable	$ 61,245.00	$ 75,212.00	Current portion of long-term debt	$ 14,400.00	$ 16,000.00
Inventories	$ 3,562.00	$ 3,782.00	Taxes payable	$ 12,452.00	$ 12,452.00
Prepaid expenses	$ 2,000.00	$ 2,000.00	Total current (short term) liabilities	$ 27,967.00	$ 30,606.00
Total current assets	$ 87,285.00	$ 99,789.00	Mortgage (minus current portion)	$ 100,000.00	$ 110,000.00
Building	$ 201,000.00	$ 199,000.00	Equipment loans	$ 27,967.00	$ 20,606.00
Equipment	$ 75,000.00	$ 62,000.00	Total long-term liabilities	$ 127,967.00	$ 130,606.00
Depreciation	$ (16,000.00)	$ (14,000.00)	Total liabilities	$ 155,934.00	$ 161,212.00
Net property and equipment (fixed assets)	$ 260,000.00	$ 247,000.00	Net worth	$ 191,351.00	$ 185,577.00
Total assets	$ 347,285.00	$ 346,789.00	Total liabilities and equity	$ 347,285.00	$ 346,789.00

Figure 8.1 Balance sheet.

Assets are broken down into two categories: current and noncurrent (fixed) assets. *Current assets* are those that will be used up within 1 year. In a medical office, current assets usually include cash, accounts receivable, and inventory. *Noncurrent,* or *fixed, assets* are assets that are expected to offer value to the company for more than a year. This would include the building or the facilities, equipment, furniture, and other items in a medical office that are considered fixtures.

Current Assets

What does it mean to be a current asset and to be used within 1 year? This definition may be a little tricky at first, but keep in mind that just because an asset can be used up within 1 year does not necessarily mean that it will be. Many times students get confused looking at a cash balance on a balance sheet and question how quickly it will be used. Even though some cash may be retained from year to year—for instance, an investment account where excess cash is held, such as a certificate of deposit or savings account—it is available for use should the company need it.

Consider current assets from a more personal view. Imagine that you have a savings account with a balance of $500. During the year, you manage to control your spending and only use the cash that you make from working to finance your needs. At the end of the year, you still have the $500 in savings and now have the interest that was accrued on it throughout the year. However, you know that should you have needed it for an unexpected expense, it was available to be used at any point in time during the year.

Current assets also include receivables, inventories, and prepaid expenses. **Accounts receivable (AR)** are accounts where money is owed to the company. In a health care facility, most accounts receivable are made up of customer accounts where services have been performed but not yet paid for. Because most patients pay for their health care with third-party payers, such as health insurance, Medicare, or Medicaid, most patients will have an account with the health care facility. It is expected that payment for the service will be submitted to the office within an acceptable amount of time (usually within 30 days of billing) but will vary from office to office based on billing procedures, payment collection processes, and the mix of third-party payers.

Inventories are items kept on hand for use in the practice that are expected to revolve and need to be replenished in the normal operation of the business. As discussed in Chapter 7, a few examples of some inventory items in a medical office are alcohol swabs, disposable thermometer shields, paper towels, and pens. *Prepaid expenses* are expenses that will be incurred within a year but have already been paid for. Prepaid expenses may include insurance, which is usually paid for in 6-month increments, filtered water delivery, or prepaid utility bills.

Fixed Assets

Fixed assets are items owned by a company that are used to generate income in the general operation of the business and are not expected to be used up or consumed within a 1-year time frame. Fixed assets are items that are not for resale. They include real estate (the office building), furniture, and fixtures (lobby chairs and tables, desks, exam room tables, medical technology equipment, office machines, computers). As fixed assets age, their value decreases over time, called **depreciation**. To account for this, the balance sheets show the accumulated depreciation, which is calculated over the lifespan of the fixed-asset item. For example, if a medical exam table is expected to be in use for 5 years and costs $5000 at the time it was purchased, the depreciation would be calculated evenly over the 5-year period ($5000/5 years= $1000 per year

accounts receivable (AR) monies owed to an organization.

depreciation the cost of an asset over time.

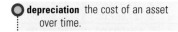
TAKE AWAY

Current assets are expected to be used within 1 year, whereas fixed assets are consumed over a longer time period.

depreciation). This is figured as a negative number on the balance sheet and reduces the value of the asset. It would appear on the balance sheet as seen here:

Exam table	$5000
Depreciation on exam table	($3000)
Net value of exam table	$2000

Liabilities

Liabilities are found on the other side of the balance sheet, opposite to assets. They include loans, mortgages, accrued expenses, and **accounts payable (AP),** or money owed to vendors and other businesses.

accounts payable (AP) money owed to vendors and other businesses.

Liabilities are divided into two categories: *short-term* and *long-term liabilities.* Short-term liabilities are current and consist of debts that are due within 1 year. This amount also includes any portion of long-term debt that is due within the coming year. For example, if a medical office has a mortgage totaling $1.5 million, consisting of monthly payments of $5000, the short-term liability amount on the balance sheet would be $60,000, or the amount of 12 monthly payments on the mortgage. Long-term liabilities are fixed and are the debt obligations that are due more than 1 year in the future, such as a bank loan.

Net Worth

Net worth is the amount by which assets exceed liabilities, as indicated in the following equation: assets = liabilities + net worth. The net worth is the balance difference between assets and liabilities. This means that to calculate net worth, the equation could also be written as:

net worth the amount by which assets exceed liabilities.

$$\text{Net Worth} = \text{Assets} - \text{Liabilities}$$

For example, if the total assets is $250,000 and the total debt (liability) of the company is $75,000, the net worth of the company is $175,000 ($250,000 − $75,000).

Income Statements

An **income statement** shows a company's financial performance over a specific period of time. This is calculated by showing the revenue coming into a company and the expenses that are incurred in the normal operation of business and any other expense incurred during the given time period. Income statements are often referred to as *profit and loss* statements because they show the profit made during the year compared with the losses accounted for during that same time frame. An example income statement is shown in Fig. 8.2.

income statement a financial statement showing an organization's revenue and expenses over a time period.

An income statement includes all revenue streams in the company. A **revenue stream** is a source of income for a company that is usually produced by a product or service offered. In a medical office, the majority of all income will come from the billing of patient care services. However, many medical offices and providers choose to add revenue streams, such as having an onsite pharmacy or selling products (t-shirts, vitamins, and nutritional kits). Regardless of the source, all income will be accounted for on the income statement.

revenue stream a source of income for a company.

Income statements are important in the financial management of a health care facility. The income statement gives a quick overview of income vs. outflow. It shows the profitability of the medical office, and, depending on the amount of detail shown on the statement, it can help isolate unprofitable revenue streams, or cash flow drains. Typically, medical offices use one of two methods for tracking income

Evergreen Health Income Statement For the year ended December 31, 2015	
Total revenue	
Total sales	$1,672,000
COGS	$0
Gross profit	$1,672,000
Operating expenses	
Salaries	$293,000
Current portion debt	$60,000
Depreciation	$30,000
Office supplies	$75,000
Utilities and maintenance	$125,000
Advertising	$10,000
Insurance	$80,000
Doctors' salaries	$526,000
Other operating expenses	$38,000
Total operating expenses	$1,237,000
Net operating profit	$435,000
Income tax expense	$157,000
Net profit	$278,000

Figure 8.2 Income statement.

and reporting on an income statement: *cash basis accounting* and *accrual basis accounting*.

- **Cash basis accounting** reports income as it comes in. For instance, when a patient comes in to see the provider or to have a test completed, the income from that patient visit is not reported until the insurance company pays. Expenses are reported as they are paid. Inventory costs are expensed when the payment for the inventory is made.
- **Accrual basis accounting** reports income as the services are rendered and expenses when they occur. In a medical office, income would be reported when the patient comes in and expenses are incurred during that visit.

The income statement reports total income. When the basic operating expenses associated with the medical operation are expensed off the income statement, the equation is:

$$\text{Total Income} - \text{Cost of Goods Sold} = \text{Gross Income}$$

Gross income is the total income of the company minus the costs of the goods sold (COGS). Because most medical facilities do not sell inventory items, there is usually no COGS. From the gross income, operating expenses are taken out and produce the *net operating income (NOI)*. The NOI shows the total profit of the company before taxes and before any loan payments or capital expenditures, which are discussed later in this chapter. In a medical office, physicians will often split the NOI, or a percentage of it, after taxes and other expenses are paid. Some physicians may have a partnership agreement where they keep a portion of the NOI in the medical office and do not take it as personal income.

Net income is the total income for the company after subtracting COGS, operating expenses, taxes, shareholder distributions, and other expenses.

cash basis accounting a method of tracking finances in which transactions are recorded at the time when cash is exchanged.

accrual basis accounting a method of tracking finances in which transactions are recorded when goods or services are exchanged, rather than when cash is exchanged.

gross income the total income of the organization minus the costs of the goods sold.

net income the total income for the company after subtracting costs of goods sold, operating expenses, taxes, shareholder distributions, and other expenses.

CURRENT TRENDS IN HEALTH CARE

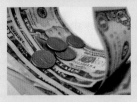

According to *Health Care News,* most medical offices use the cash method of accounting, or cash accounting, versus the accrual method. The cash method records income or revenue only when cash is received and expenses only when they are paid in cash. The advantages to the cash method are:

- Income taxes are only paid as the income is collected. In the accrual method, income tax is paid as income is earned, whether or not the service is ever paid for.
- It allows for expenses to be recorded as they are paid for.

http://healthcarenews.com/is-your-practice-properly-accounting-for-inventory-and-prepaid-supplies/

In managing a medical office, it is important to be able to read the income statement and to know how certain business decisions will affect the income statement. It is also beneficial to be able to see trends occurring in the income statement or items that are not in line with previous years. For example, at a medical office, employee salaries usually account for 27% of total revenue each year. But in the current year, it now accounts for 51% of total revenue. This increase might be a cause for concern and require further investigation by the health services administrator. In addition, a medical office that shows a trend of decreasing net income over the last several years would be a concern, and the health services administrator should research, analyze, and plan for action.

Take Learning to the Next Level

Assets = Liabilities + Net Worth

It seems simple enough, but sometimes financial statements can be overwhelming. For a better understanding of the balance sheet and its various parts, go to the video links from Investopedia listed here, which provide a detailed explanation and examples of the different parts of a balance sheet:

Fixed Assets
http://www.investopedia.com/terms/f/fixedasset.asp
Depreciation
http://www.investopedia.com/terms/d/depreciation.asp
Balance Sheets
http://www.investopedia.com/terms/b/balancesheet.asp
Liabilities
http://www.investopedia.com/terms/l/liability.asp
Net Worth
http://www.investopedia.com/terms/n/networth.asp
Income Statement
http://www.investopedia.com/terms/i/incomestatement.asp

LEARNING CHECKPOINT 8.1
Financial Statements

1. A resource owned by a company is a(n) _____.

2. The decrease in value of a fixed asset over time is called _____.

3. What balance sheet item reflects money owed to the company? _____

4. _____ income is the income for the company after subtracting costs of goods sold, operating expenses, taxes, shareholder distributions, and other expenses.

BUDGETING

When budgeting for a household, families must make sure the money they earn covers their monthly bills and expenses. Additionally, a family might set aside extra money if it hopes to buy a new television or car. In proper financial planning, the medical office or any business must monitor its funds in much the same way. It budgets for fixed monthly expenses and must set aside funds for additional expensive purchases or expenditures, such as new equipment or a remodeled waiting area. To help the organization maintain healthy finances, the health services administrator will prepare two kinds of budgets: the *capital budget* and the *operational budget*.

Capital Budget

capital expenditure money set aside for large purchases over a certain dollar amount whose use will span multiple fiscal years.

Capital expenditures ("capex") are large, one-time purchases, such as new computers or an x-ray machine. The dollar value or amount considered as a capital expenditure varies from organization to organization. For example, one medical office may consider anything over $1000 as a capital expenditure, whereas another medical office may decide that a capital expenditure is a purchase more than $5000.

To ensure money is being spent wisely, capital expenditures are often planned years in advance and are subject to a process of proposal and approval. Often the process begins with the submission of a capital expenditure request (CER) form (Fig. 8.3).

Note that the CER form asks specifically for the requester to justify the purchase. The form should explain the reasons why monies should be expended and the benefit the purchase will have on the operation of the facility. Some capital expenditure purchases will add to the facility's aesthetic or improve the quality of the patient's experience, such as repainting the building or buying a new television for the waiting room. In other instances, the capital expenditure will add to the office's revenue stream by either bringing in new patients or reducing the amount of staff time spent on a task. For example, imagine a clinic usually refers patients to a podiatrist to treat onychomycosis (toenail fungus) and verrucae (warts). This clinic might consider the purchase of a compact laser that will allow it to perform onsite treatment. This means a financial justification can be made in the form of a **payback period**, or the length of time it will take to recover the expense of the equipment. The formula for the payback period is:

payback period the length of time for the savings or revenues generated by a purchase to pay for the purchase itself.

$$\text{Payback period} = \frac{\text{Cost of equipment}}{\text{Estimated yearly cash inflow}}$$

Using the compact laser as an example, the medical office usually refers six patients per month to the podiatrist, but can now treat these patients. The cost of the compact laser is $44,000. The medical office will charge $360 for each treatment procedure, resulting in a revenue of $25,920 annually ($360 × 6 patients per month × 12 months each year). Using the payback period formula, we can calculate the number of years it would take to recover the cost of the compact laser:

$$1.74 \text{ years} = \frac{\$44,000}{\$25,290}$$

In other words, the machine will have paid for itself in 1.74 years, or about 1 year and 9 months.

Such information presents a strong case for the capital expenditure and should be included on the CER form. For other purchases, depending on the life of the item, the payback period may be too long in duration. If a piece of equipment can only be expected to last a few years, a shorter payback period may be required. As a result, the

CITYWIDE SURGI-CENTER
CAPITAL EQUIPMENT REQUEST FORM

BUDGET YEAR:	DATE:
BUDGET DESCRIPTION:	REQUESTED BY:

DEPARTMENT NAME:	Replacement	Yes ☐		No ☐
ACCOUNT / CENTER:				
CER AMOUNT:	New Item	Yes ☐		No ☐
DESCRIPTION OF NEED:				
	Revenue Stream	Yes ☐		No ☐

CAPITAL EQUIPMENT DESCRIPTION AND JUSTIFICATION
List all other associated costs such as additional staffing, maintenance agreements, supplies, etc.

EFFECT ON OPERATIONS
List quality benefits, operational efficiencies, productivity improvements, other rationale

COMPLETE THIS SECTION FOR ALL EQUIPMENT REQUESTS

Quantity	Vendor	Model Number

SIGNATURE APPROVALS

Director: _____   Date: _____

Administrator: _____   Date: _____

FINANCE SCREENING AND PURCHASE AUTHORIZATION

PROJECT CATEGORY	Budget Amount	CER Amount	
Professional Fees			Date: _____
Staff Salaries			☐ Approved
Fringe Benefits			☐ Approved with Modification
Supplies			☐ Disapproved
Computer Support Services			
Training			Comments:
Installation			
Maintenance			
Depreciation			
Trade In (Amount)			
TOTAL PROJECT COST	$ -	$ -	

REVIEW AND APPROVAL

DIRECTOR OF PURCHASING	Date	CHIEF FINANCIAL OFFICER	Date
CHIEF OPERATING OFFICER	Date	FINANCE - RELEASE OF FUNDS	Date

A

Figure 8.3 A, Capital expenditure request (CER) form. B, Elements of the CER. From Abdelhak, M, Hanken, MA: Health information: management of a strategic resource, ed 5, St. Louis, Elsevier.

Continued

CAPITAL EQUIPMENT REQUEST (CER) INSTRUCTIONS	
Budget year	Planned date of purchase
Budget description	Complete name and specifications of item to be purchased
Date	Date CER form is prepared
Requested by	Manager's name who initiates request
Department name	Department submitting CER form
Account/center	Ledger to be charged for items purchased
CER amount	Total amount should reflect Quantity $\times$ Price, less Discount
Description of need	Explanation of why item is needed; consequences if not approved
Replacement	Note if replaces existing item
New item	Note if does not replace existing item
Revenue stream	Note if generates new revenue (include pro forma)
Description and justification	Document business case why item is needed and any ancillary costs associated with purchase
Effect on operations	Describe anticipated benefits
Quantity	Include number of items requested
Vendor	Include complete name, business address, and contact
Model number	Verify exact model number of item to be purchased
Signature approvals	Signature denotes support for project (does not approve purchase)

B

Figure 8.3, cont'd

health services administrator may have to consider a less expensive piece of equipment or even leasing the item.

Leasing allows a business to pay for a large purchase in installments, such as monthly, rather than as an initial lump sum. To continue the earlier example, the medical office may decide to lease the compact laser for a year and then purchase the equipment if it proves to be a positive contribution to the revenue stream. If the cost of the lease is $1350 per month, the cost to the medical office will be $16,200 annually ($1350 $\times$ 12). Although the monthly cost is higher than an outright purchase, leasing allows the medical office to upgrade the compact laser and prevent being stuck with an obsolete piece of equipment in the future. In many lease options, the medical office may have the option to purchase the equipment later instead of providing an upfront large sum of money.

Operational Budget

Unlike the capital expenditure budget, the **operational budget** includes the fixed expenditures for the daily, routine operations of the business. This is the amount used to plan for payroll, utility bills, the cost of office supplies, and travel to conferences and educational events for continuing education. The operational budget also includes

operational budget costs related to the operation of the department, such as payroll, utilities, and supplies.

ANNUAL OPERATIONAL BUDGET	FIRST QUARTER			SECOND QUARTER			THIRD QUARTER			FOURTH QUARTER			TOTAL	%
	JAN	FEB	MAR	APR	MAY	JUNE	JULY	AUG	SEPT	OCT	NOV	DEC		
INCOME														
Professional Fees	180,000.00	180,000.00	180,000.00	180,000.00	180,000.00	180,000.00	180,000.00	180,000.00	180,000.00	180,000.00	180,000.00	180,000.00	$2,160,000.00	99.92%
Other Revenue	500.00	500.00	500.00	500.00	500.00	500.00	500.00	500.00	500.00	500.00	500.00	500.00	6,000.00	0.28%
Patient Refunds	(150.00)	(150.00)	(150.00)	(150.00)	(150.00)	(150.00)	(150.00)	(150.00)	(150.00)	(150.00)	(150.00)	(150.00)	(1,800.00)	-0.08%
Refund Insurance Companies	(200.00)	(200.00)	(200.00)	(200.00)	(200.00)	(200.00)	(200.00)	(200.00)	(200.00)	(200.00)	(200.00)	(200.00)	(2,400.00)	-0.11%
	180,150.00	180,150.00	180,150.00	180,150.00	180,150.00	180,150.00	180,150.00	180,150.00	180,150.00	180,150.00	180,150.00	180,150.00	2,161,800.00	100.00%
EXPENSES														
Salaries-Physician Owners	131,987.00	37,323.00	37,323.00	37,323.00	37,323.00	37,323.00	37,323.00	37,323.00	37,323.00	37,323.00	37,323.00	37,323.00	542,540.00	25.10%
Payroll Taxes - Physician	11,284.89	3,191.12	3,191.12	3,191.12	3,191.12	3,191.12	3,191.12	3,191.12	3,191.12	3,191.12	3,191.12	3,191.12	46,387.17	2.15%
Insurance - Physician	3,125.45	2,415.05	2,415.05	2,415.05	2,415.05	2,415.05	2,415.05	2,415.05	2,415.05	2,415.05	2,415.05	2,415.05	29,691.03	1.37%
Dues, Memberships, License Fees	312.33	312.33	312.33	312.33	312.33	312.33	312.33	312.33	312.33	312.33	312.33	312.33	3,747.96	0.17%
Meetings & Travel - Physician	300.00	300.00	300.00	300.00	300.00	1,300.00	300.00	300.00	300.00	300.00	300.00	300.00	4,600.00	0.21%
Meals & Entertainment-Physician	250.00	250.00	250.00	250.00	250.00	250.00	250.00	250.00	250.00	250.00	250.00	250.00	3,000.00	0.14%
Salaries - Primary Care Providers	15,007.00	15,007.00	15,007.00	15,007.00	15,007.00	15,007.00	15,007.00	15,007.00	15,007.00	15,007.00	15,007.00	15,007.00	180,084.00	8.33%
Salaries - Medical Support	16,666.00	16,666.00	16,666.00	16,666.00	16,666.00	16,666.00	16,666.00	16,666.00	16,666.00	16,666.00	16,666.00	16,666.00	199,992.00	9.25%
Salaries - Administrative	8,894.00	8,894.00	8,894.00	8,894.00	8,894.00	8,894.00	8,894.00	8,894.00	8,894.00	8,894.00	8,894.00	8,894.00	106,728.00	4.94%
Payroll Taxes - Staff	5,073.66	3,032.17	3,032.17	3,032.17	3,032.17	3,032.17	3,032.17	3,032.17	3,032.17	3,032.17	3,032.17	3,032.17	38,427.53	1.78%
Insurance for Staff	1,744.00	1,744.00	1,744.00	1,744.00	1,744.00	1,744.00	1,744.00	1,744.00	1,744.00	1,744.00	1,744.00	1,744.00	20,928.00	0.97%
Pension & Retirement Benefits	5,175.31	5,175.31	5,175.31	5,175.31	5,175.31	5,175.31	5,175.31	5,175.31	5,175.31	5,175.31	5,175.31	5,175.31	62,103.72	2.87%
Meetings & Travel-Staff	225.00	225.00	225.00	225.00	225.00	225.00	225.00	225.00	225.00	225.00	225.00	225.00	2,700.00	0.12%
Supplies - Drugs & Medications	4,306.94	4,306.94	4,306.94	4,306.94	4,306.94	4,306.94	4,306.94	4,306.94	4,306.94	4,306.94	4,306.94	4,306.94	51,683.23	2.39%
Supplies - Medical	12,253.04	12,253.04	12,253.04	12,253.04	12,253.04	12,253.04	12,253.04	12,253.04	12,253.04	12,253.04	12,253.04	12,253.04	147,036.54	6.80%
Supplies - Office/Administrative	668.50	668.50	668.50	668.50	668.50	668.50	668.50	668.50	668.50	668.50	668.50	668.50	8,022.00	0.37%
Supplies - Housekeeping/Maintenance	69.50	69.50	69.50	69.50	69.50	69.50	69.50	69.50	69.50	69.50	69.50	69.50	834.00	0.04%
Supplies - IT/Software	1,531.00	1,531.00	1,531.00	1,531.00	1,531.00	1,531.00	1,531.00	1,531.00	1,531.00	1,531.00	1,531.00	1,531.00	18,372.00	0.85%
Laboratory Services	7,435.00	7,435.00	7,435.00	7,435.00	7,435.00	7,435.00	7,435.00	7,435.00	7,435.00	7,435.00	7,435.00	7,435.00	89,220.00	4.13%
Rent - Buildings	8,147.00	8,147.00	8,147.00	8,147.00	8,147.00	8,147.00	8,147.00	8,147.00	8,147.00	8,147.00	8,147.00	8,147.00	97,764.00	4.52%
Utilities	938.00	938.00	938.00	938.00	938.00	938.00	938.00	938.00	938.00	938.00	938.00	938.00	11,256.00	0.52%
Rent/Lease-Furniture & Equipment	16,622.83	16,622.83	16,622.83	16,622.83	16,622.83	16,622.83	16,622.83	16,622.83	16,622.83	16,622.83	16,622.83	16,622.83	199,474.00	9.23%
Equipment Maintenance Contracts	1,662.00	1,662.00	1,662.00	1,662.00	1,662.00	1,662.00	1,662.00	1,662.00	1,662.00	3,167.25	1,662.00	1,662.00	21,449.25	0.99%
Accounting Services	800.00	6,000.00	9,200.00	4,700.00	700.00	1,325.00	700.00	700.00	700.00	700.00	700.00	1,450.00	27,675.00	1.28%
Legal Services	1,076.00	1,076.00	1,076.00	1,076.00	1,076.00	1,076.00	1,076.00	1,076.00	1,076.00	1,076.00	1,076.00	1,076.00	12,912.00	0.60%
Employee Development & Training	215.00	215.00	215.00	215.00	215.00	215.00	215.00	215.00	215.00	215.00	215.00	215.00	2,580.00	0.12%
Employee Relations	100.00	100.00	100.00	100.00	100.00	100.00	100.00	100.00	100.00	100.00	2,000.00	100.00	3,100.00	0.14%
Uniforms & Laundry	183.00	183.00	183.00	183.00	183.00	183.00	183.00	183.00	183.00	183.00	183.00	183.00	2,196.00	0.10%
Telephone/Internet Access	333.58	333.58	333.58	333.58	333.58	333.58	333.58	333.58	333.58	333.58	333.58	333.58	4,002.96	0.19%
Postage & Shipping	448.33	448.33	448.33	448.33	448.33	448.33	448.33	448.33	448.33	448.33	448.33	448.33	5,380.00	0.25%
Books & Subscriptions	175.00	175.00	175.00	175.00	175.00	175.00	175.00	175.00	175.00	175.00	175.00	175.00	2,100.00	0.10%
Marketing	500.00	500.00	500.00	500.00	500.00	500.00	500.00	500.00	500.00	500.00	500.00	500.00	6,000.00	0.28%
	257,509.37	157,199.71	160,399.71	155,899.71	151,899.71	153,524.71	151,899.71	151,899.71	151,899.71	153,404.96	151,899.71	154,549.71	1,951,986.38	90.29%
NET INCOME	$ (77,359.37)	$ 22,950.29	$ 19,750.29	$ 24,250.29	$ 28,250.29	$ 26,625.29	$ 28,250.29	$ 28,250.29	$ 28,250.29	$ 26,745.04	$ 28,250.29	$ 25,600.29	$ 209,813.62	9.71%

Figure 8.4 Operational budget.

any equipment leasing costs or maintenance agreements. A sample operational budget is illustrated in Fig. 8.4.

Some of these expenditures are **fixed costs**, such as the medical office space lease, malpractice insurance, and telephone and Internet services. Fixed costs can be counted on to stay the same month to month. **Variable costs**, however, change depending on the level of activity or volume. For example, the cost of drugs or medical supplies depends on the type and the amount ordered of these items. As a result, the budgeted amounts for variable-cost items are estimated based on the prior year's activity levels, along with any expected changes for the coming year.

Looking at the sample operational budget in Fig. 8.4, notice that the year is broken into quarters of 3 months each. This particular medical office begins its **fiscal year** in January; however, other medical offices may choose to begin their fiscal year in any month. For example, if the medical office's fiscal year begins October 1 and ends on September 30, the first quarter would include the months of October through December, the second quarter would be from January through March, and so on.

Variance

The operational budget is usually created and approved a year ahead of time. During the fiscal year, the health services administrator monitors income and expense to report on any *variances* from the budget, usually on a monthly basis. A **variance** is the difference between the budgeted amount for income and expenses versus the actual amount. Variances can be positive, meaning the office took in more money, or spent less than budgeted. Negative variances mean the office spent more than budgeted, or did not earn as much. Even though some actual monthly expenditures may be above budgeted amounts (a negative variance), some months can be below the budgeted amounts (positive variance). These fluctuations in totals should still be close to the annual budget projection.

fixed costs expenses in the operational budget that do not change on a monthly basis.

variable costs expenses in the operational budget that change month to month based on the volume of activity.

fiscal year a year structured for accounting or tax purposes.

variance a deviation from the projected spending or earning in the budget.

As seen in the sample operational budget in Fig. 8.4, the payroll portion is usually the highest percentage of the costs. The budget includes not only the salaries and wages of the medical office's employees, but also the fringe benefits, which include payroll taxes, retirement contributions, vacation, holiday, and sick pay. Usually, fringe benefits account for 30% of an employee's salary.

Payroll projections in the operating budget must also account for staff raises in the month the new wage becomes effective. The budget may be planned assuming the average wage increase for each of the employees in the medical office will be 3%.

In the following example, Bernice earns $36,000 a year, so the annualized amount before a raise in pay would be $3000 per month ($36,000 ÷ 12 months). If Bernice is given a 3% raise beginning October 1, an additional $1080 (36,000 × 0.03) would be added to her annual salary—$37,080, which is then divided by 12 months. The new monthly pay amount is then $3090 for her beginning with the October 1 payroll. The health services administrator would adjust the budget for the payroll increase as follows:

Employee	Starting Annual Salary	August	September	Salary Increase	New Salary	October	November
Patricia	$24,000	$2000	$2000	2%	$24,480	$2040	$2040
Bernice	$36,000	$3000	$3000	3%	$37,080	$3090	$3090
Ruby	$42,000	$3500	$3500	2%	$42,840	$3640	$3640
Hector	$33,600	$2800	$2800	5%	$35,280	$2940	$2940
Monthly Payroll Total		$11,300	$11,300			$11,710	$11,710

LEARNING CHECKPOINT 8.2

Budgeting

1. The retail clinic pays $18 each month for a firm to remove, shred, and recycle its paper waste securely. In May, the cost per month will rise to $25 per month. Is this a fixed cost or a variable cost?

2. A new all-in-one printer/copier/scanner/fax machine will cost $10,900, but it is expected to save $300 a month in staff time. What is the payback period for the item?

3. Henri's salary (including benefits) is $31,200, and he received a "3" on his performance review, meaning his work "Meets Expectations." As a result, he will receive a 3% raise in May. Dixon makes the same amount per year, but her score of "1", "Meets and Frequently Exceeds Expectations," will earn her a 5% raise. What is the payroll budget for these two employees for May?

● CASE STUDY

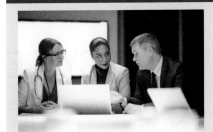

In the follow-up meeting with Dr. Lane and the staff, Brittney presented the following information:

- The cost of a basic echocardiogram machine is $250,000 and can be financed with the equipment provider for 7 years at 7.5% interest with a down payment of $15,000.

- The equipment vendor offers a lease program on echocardiogram machines. A medical office can lease the equipment for a term of 5 years, at which time they can buy the equipment for the current market value or lease an updated piece of equipment under a new deal. The terms for the echocardiogram are an initial payment of $20,000 with monthly payments of $3000. There is no general maintenance expense, with the vendor providing regular maintenance as part of the lease contract.
- The estimated annual maintenance cost if purchased is $2000 for service fees and replacement parts. The vendor offers a prepaid insurance plan for $2500 per year that covers all maintenance and replacement parts on the equipment and promises a same-day service call.
- The equipment will require that the medical office hire an echocardiogram technician with an estimated salary of $55,000 and an increased overall estimated staffing expense of $63,000 per year, including salary and benefits.
- Brittney estimates that 10 patients per week will need the echocardiogram services. If the office is open 50 weeks per year, that is an estimated 500 echocardiogram tests performed each year. The income expected from each test is $500, and the COGS for each test is $50.
- The purchase of equipment would be able to generate income immediately upon its purchase.

REVIEW QUESTIONS

1. What is the difference between long- and short-term liabilities?

2. In a health care facility, more than one revenue stream may be reported. What is a revenue stream, and why do you think a medical office would report separate revenue streams? Give an example of a revenue stream that you might find in a medical office.

3. Which accounting method reports cash as it comes in?

4. Which type of income reports revenue after COGS?

5. What are some questions that a health services administrator should ask before making a capital expenditure?

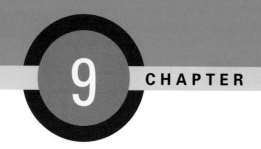

9 CHAPTER

REVENUE CYCLE

Nanette B. Sayles

CHAPTER OUTLINE

INTRODUCTION
HEALTH INSURANCE BASICS
  Cost Sharing
REIMBURSEMENT
  METHODOLOGIES
  Fee-for-Service
  Episode-of-Care Reimbursement
    *Medicare Prospective Payment
      System*
    *Resource-Based Relative Value
      Scale*
    *Hospital Outpatient
      Prospective Payment
      System*
    Ambulance Fee Schedule
    *Home Health Prospective
      Payment System*
  Managed Care

REVENUE CYCLE MANAGEMENT
  Front-End Processes
    Scheduling and Registration
    Insurance Verification
    Preauthorization
    Medical Necessity Coverage
      Advanced Beneficiary Notice
  Preparing for and Processing
    Claims
    Charge Capture
  Chargemaster
    Claims
      Claims Scrubber Software
  Coding
    *International Classification of
      Disease, Tenth Revision,
      Clinical Modification*

  *Healthcare Common
    Procedure Coding System*
  *Current Procedural
    Terminology*
  Clinical Documentation
  Billing/Claims Processing
  Postbilling Processes
    Payment Posting
    Denial Management
  Revenue Cycle Monitoring
    *Accounts Receivable (A/R)
      Days*
    Unbilled Accounts
    Clean Claims Rate
    Denials

VOCABULARY

advanced beneficiary notice (ABN)
allowable amount
Ambulatory Payment Classification
  (APC)
appeal
bundling
capitation
chargemaster
charges
claim
coinsurance
copayment (copay)
Current Procedural Terminology
  (CPT)
deductible
denial

fee-for-service
fee schedule
grouper
Healthcare Common Procedure
  Coding System (HCPCS)
International Classification of
  Disease, Tenth Revision, Clinical
  Modification (ICD-10-CM)
local coverage determination (LCD)
managed care
national coverage determination
  (NCD)
out-of-pocket limit
Outcomes and Assessment
  Information Set (OASIS)

outpatient prospective payment
  system (OPPS)
packaging
payer
preauthorization
premium
prospective payment system (PPS)
query
remittance advice (RA)
resource-based relative value scale
  (RBRVS)
revenue cycle
revenue cycle management
self-pay
subscriber

CHAPTER OBJECTIVES

After completing this chapter, the student should be able to do the following:

1. Recognize and use terms related to health
   insurance.
2. Summarize the different types of reimbursement
   methodologies used in health care.

3. Differentiate the processes in revenue cycle
   management.
4. Recommend metrics to be used to monitor the
   effectiveness of the revenue cycle.

INTRODUCTION

The **revenue cycle** is a set of functions associated with collecting revenue from a patient account. It starts when the patient makes an appointment, continues when the patient is seen by the health care provider, and ends when the health care facility receives reimbursement for the services provided. It is a complex and multistepped process that is subject to multiple laws and regulations, various coding systems, and health insurance and reimbursement procedures that involve many different staff members and health care providers. The objective of this chapter is to provide a general overview of reimbursement models, the revenue cycle process, and the role of the health services administrator in managing this process.

revenue cycle the processing of health information to obtain reimbursement for health care services provided.

● CASE STUDY

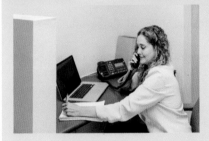

Great Valley Sleep Center offers diagnostic and treatment services to patients struggling with a variety of sleep disorders, such as sleep apnea, insomnia, narcolepsy, and restless leg syndrome. Sara, the health services administrator, knows that many patients reach the sleep center in an emotionally distressed state, and she is always ready to provide the highest level of customer service when interacting with patients and their families.

The patient on the phone has asked to talk to "someone in charge of insurance." He explains that his HMO has "lousy" coverage, and even though his family physician has referred him to Great Valley, he is skeptical that his insurance company will pay for an expensive sleep study. As you read the chapter, think about how insurance works and the steps in the revenue cycle that result in third-party payment. What should Sara tell the patient? How can she determine if the sleep study is covered by the patient's insurance coverage? What steps should she take if the study isn't covered?

HEALTH INSURANCE BASICS

Most medical care is paid by some type of health insurance, which may pay for all or some of the medical services provided. Health insurance is an agreement between an insurer and a consumer. An insurer is either a government or private organization that contracts with the health care consumer to pay either a portion or all of the medical expenses. The insurer is a third-party **payer**, who can be nongovernmental, such as Blue Cross and Blue Shield, or a government health care program, such as Medicare and Medicaid. A **subscriber** (sometimes referred to as an *insured* or *beneficiary* as a Medicaid recipient) is a consumer who purchases insurance from the insurer. Many employers provide health insurance for their employees as a benefit of employment; when insurance is purchased through an employer, it is known as *group insurance*. If it is purchased directly from the insurer, it is called *individual insurance*. To participate or be enrolled in a health insurance plan, the subscriber must make a payment (the **premium**) to keep the coverage active. Most subscribers will pay this premium monthly, but some may pay quarterly or even annually. Table 9.1 reviews terminology common to health insurance policies.

payer the entity responsible for most or all of a patient's bill to the provider.

subscriber the primary enrollee of an insurance policy (known as a beneficiary for Medicaid recipients).

premium a fixed amount paid to subscribe to an insurance policy.

Cost Sharing

Most health insurance companies have insurance policies that require sharing the patient's health care costs with the patient, called *cost-sharing charges*. A cost-sharing

TABLE 9.1

TERMINOLOGY COMMON TO HEALTH INSURANCE POLICIES

Term	Description
Benefit	The payment for specific health care services, or the health care services that are provided from an insurance policy or a managed care organization.
Beneficiary	One who receives benefits from an insurance policy or a managed care program, or one who is eligible to receive such benefits.
Benefit period	A period of time during which benefits are available for covered services, which varies among payers and policies.
Claim	The application to an insurance company for reimbursement of services rendered.
Coinsurance	A percentage of the amount owed to a provider for which the subscriber is responsible.
Copayment (copay)	A fixed amount paid by the patient (or the subscriber to the insurance policy) at the time of the health care service.
Coverage	The health conditions, diagnostic procedures, and therapeutic treatments for which the insurance policy will pay.
Deductible	A specified dollar amount for which the patient is personally responsible before the payer reimburses for any claims.
Exclusions	Medical conditions or risks not covered by an insurance policy; preexisting conditions and experimental therapy are common exclusions to standard policies.
Fiscal intermediary	An entity that administers the claims and reimbursements for a funding agency (i.e., an insurer or payer).
Guarantor	The person who is ultimately responsible for paying for health care services.
Insurance	A contract (policy) made with an insurer to assume the risk of paying some or all of the cost of providing health care services in return for the payment of a premium by or on behalf of the insured.
Out-of-pocket costs	Costs not covered by an insurer, which are in turn paid by the patient directly to the provider.
Payer	The individual or organization that is primarily responsible for the reimbursement for a particular health care service. Usually refers to the insurance company or third party.
Policy	Written contract detailing the coverage, benefits, exclusions, premiums, copays, deductibles, and other terms of the health plan.
Preexisting condition	A medical condition identified as having occurred before a patient obtained coverage within a health insurance plan.
Premium	Periodic payments to an insurance company made by the patient for coverage under a policy.
Primary care provider (PCP)	A physician or other provider designated by the patient to deliver primary care and refer the patient to other specialists as necessary.
Reimbursement	The amount of money that the health care facility receives from the party responsible for paying the bill.
Rider	An adjustment to a policy that increases or decreases coverage and benefits, corresponding to an increase or decrease in the cost to the insured.
Subscriber	A person who purchases insurance.
Third-party payer	An entity that pays a provider for part or all of a patient's health care services; often the patient's insurance company.

(From Davis N, LaCour M. *Foundations of health information management*, ed 4, St. Louis, 2015, Elsevier.)

TAKE AWAY •·········

Deductibles, copayments, and coinsurance are all cost-sharing measures.

○ **deductible** the amount of money a subscriber must pay for medical services before an insurer will pay claims.

charge is the amount the health care consumer has to pay for a medical item or service covered by the health insurance plan. Policies generally have three different types of cost-sharing charges: a *deductible, copayments,* and *coinsurance.* Not all health insurance plans include each of these three types of cost sharing. Premiums paid by the subscriber are not a type of cost-sharing charge.

Most policies require the subscriber to pay a **deductible,** which is a specified dollar amount a subscriber must pay before the health insurance company starts to pay for medical services. For example, if a subscriber has a deductible of $2000 and had a medical visit that costs $2600, the subscriber would be required to pay $2000 and the health insurance company would pay the remaining $600. The deductible amount is based on a calendar year, thus requiring the subscriber to pay another deductible starting January 1 beginning the next year. The deductible amount varies depending on the conditions of the policy, which may be based on the cost of the premium paid by the subscriber, whether the insurance plan is for an individual or a family, and, if provided by the employer, the size of the organization.

CURRENT TRENDS IN HEALTH CARE

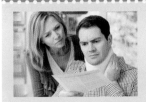

Due to the rising cost of health care, more health insurance plans are requiring deductibles and at higher amounts. In 2016 more than 83% of health insurance policies required deductibles with an average deductible of $1478, which is a 20% increase from 2011. Higher deductibles help to keep premiums lower, but require the subscriber to pay more out of pocket when medical services are needed.

Another method of cost sharing is a **copayment**, commonly called a *copay,* which is a flat amount paid to the health care provider at the time of service. A copay could be required for a provider visit, a laboratory test, an emergency room visit, or a surgical procedure. The copayment may vary depending on the type of service provided and if the health care provider is contracted (or considered in-network) with the health insurance company, or out-of-network. The in-network health care provider has contracted with the health insurance company to provide medical services at a predetermined rate, which provides overall cost savings and reduces the copayment of the subscriber. For example, a typical copayment for a routine visit to a primary care physician that is in-network would be $15 to $25, $30 to $50 for a specialist, $75 to $100 for an urgent care visit, and $200 to $300 for being treated in an emergency room. Copayments may also be required for prescription drugs, depending on the drug formulary adopted by the subscriber and whether the medication is a brand-name drug or a generic version. Depending on the individual health insurance plan, the copayment may contribute to the deductible, whereas other plans require the deductible to be met before the copayment applies.

Coinsurance is another method in which costs are shared between a health insurance company and the insured. Coinsurance is a percentage of the health care charges that the patient is responsible for paying; for example, the insurer pays 80%, and the patient is responsible for 20%. Like the copayment, the amount of coinsurance will depend on whether the health care provider being seen is in-network or out-of-network.

Considering there are so many different types of payments and cost-sharing methods, let's look at an example of a patient being seen by her in-network family physician. She has a $1500 annual deductible that must be met before her health insurance plan contributes and pays 80% coinsurance. Further, her copayment of $20 to see her family physician does not contribute to the deductible. At the end of her visit, she receives a bill for $2600. For this visit, she is responsible for paying $20 (copayment) + $1500 (deductible) + $220 [($2600 − $1500) × 20%], with a final payment of $1740. If she requires any additional medical visits this year, she will only be responsible for the copayment and 20% of the costs, as long as she sees an in-network health care provider, since she has already met her deductible for the year. At the beginning of the next fiscal or calendar year, she will be responsible for paying the $1500 deductible again.

Most health insurance policies have an annual **out-of-pocket limit**. Once the limit has been met through the payment of deductibles, copayments, and/or coinsurance, the health insurance company pays 100% of medical costs. In 2016, based on federal

copay (copayment) a fixed amount the insured owes to the provider at the time of service.

coinsurance a cost-sharing provision in which the health care consumer pays a percentage of the total health care cost.

out-of-pocket limit the most amount of money an individual will have to pay for covered medical services in a year.

guidelines, the maximum deductible amount was $6850 for an individual plan and $13,700 for a family plan. In general, the more an individual pays in premiums, the lower the out-of-pocket maximum is.

In the past, most policies had a lifetime maximum or limit, which is the total amount a health insurance company will pay for an insurer's health care costs during his or her life. Coverage ended once the lifetime maximum was met. Under the Affordable Care Act (ACA), however, health insurance policies with lifetime maximums are required to cover essential benefits, such as treatment for chronic diseases, visits to the physician's office, inpatient and outpatient hospital care, prescription drug coverage, pregnancy and childbirth, and mental health services.

LEARNING CHECKPOINT 9.1
Health Insurance Basics

1. The _____ is the person responsible for payment of health services.

   a. subscriber
   b. guarantor
   c. employer
   d. beneficiary

2. The charges for Moshe's magnetic resonance imaging (MRI) were $3199, and his policy stipulates a 10% coinsurance for this service. He has already met his deductible for the year. How much will Moshe have to pay out-of-pocket? _____

3. The processing of health information to obtain payment for health care services provided is called the _____.

   a. reimbursement cycle
   b. management of care
   c. billing cycle
   d. revenue cycle

4. Which feature of some health insurance policies was made illegal under the Affordable Care Act (ACA)?

   a. out-of-pocket maximums
   b. out-of-pocket minimums
   c. lifetime maximums
   d. lifetime minimums

5. Copayments and coinsurance are _____ for in-network providers than they are for out-of-network providers.

   a. higher
   b. lower

REIMBURSEMENT METHODOLOGIES

self-pay a reimbursement methodology in which a patient pays for his or her own health care services.

There are many ways health care providers and health care facilities get paid for their services. When payment comes directly from the patient, it is known as **self-pay**. However, most physician and health care facilities are compensated for providing medical services through reimbursements from a third-party payer. The services covered and the amount reimbursed depend on the patient's health insurance policy. There have been many models over the years to calculate health care provider reimbursement. The most common reimbursement models used are fee-for-service, episode-of-care reimbursement, and managed care.

Fee-for-Service

Fee-for-service (FFS) is the traditional model of health insurance where the health care provider receives payment for each service rendered. In an FFS reimbursement model, the insurer will either directly pay the health care provider or reimburse the patient after an insurance claim has been filed for each covered medical expense. The physician or other health care providers receive a payment for each service, such as an office visit, test, or procedure. Payments are issued only after the services are provided, and the insurer pays for part or all of the cost according to the contracted insurance policy and fee schedule.

A **fee schedule** is a list of each service that the insurer covers and the specific amount the provider charges for a specific service. **Charges** are the amount of money the health care provider submits for payment. The fee schedule is generally created by the health care provider and his or her staff, such as the health services administrator, based on the services they provide, the specialty, and the costs of providing the service.

Fee schedules may also be created by insurers because they usually do not pay what the provider charges but the "allowable amount." An **allowable amount,** or allowable charge, is the full amount the insurer will reimburse a provider that is in its network of providers for a covered service. The allowable amount is a predetermined rate rather than the actual charge based on the provider's fee schedule. For example, a patient sees an in-network provider that charges $150 for an outpatient office visit. However, the insurer's allowable amount is only $100 for the visit. The insurer will pay all or a portion of the $100—minus the patient's copayment and deductible—with the provider writing off the remaining $50 as contracted by being a participating provider. If the provider is out-of-network, the patient would be held responsible for the remaining amount not reimbursed by the insurer.

An insurer's allowable amount is based on the *usual, customary, and reasonable (UCR) rate,* which is calculated based on what providers in the geographical area usually charge for the same or similar medical service. The UCR rate is determined by three components. The *usual* is what the physician or other health care provider typically charges. The *customary* is based on what similar health care providers—same specialty, same experience—are charging in the geographic area. For example, the insurer will compare cardiologist fees in New York City to other cardiologists in the New York City area, not family physicians in Birmingham, Alabama. The third component is *reasonable.* The insurer will take into consideration the circumstances of the patient's care. The insurer then adjusts the payment based on the care required by the patient so they can provide reasonable reimbursement for the care provided.[1] The reimbursement may also be adjusted based on any contract that the health care provider has with the insurer and on any copayments and coinsurances that the patient's policy has.

Episode-of-Care Reimbursement

Unlike the FFS model, where medical services are not bundled and are reimbursed based on individual service provided, *episode-of-care reimbursement* models are used

---

TAKE AWAY

The most common reimbursement models used are fee-for-service, episode-of-care reimbursement, and managed care.

○ **fee-for-service** the traditional model of health insurance where the health care facility receives payment for each service rendered.

○ **fee schedule** list of each service that the insurer covers and the specific amount that they will reimburse a health care provider for that specific service.

○ **charges** the amount of money the health care provider submits for payment.

○ **allowable amount** the full amount the insurer will reimburse a provider that is in its network of providers for a covered service.

---

[1]Fordney, MT. *Insurance handbook for the medical office.* St. Louis, 2017, Elsevier.

to cover all services related to a condition or procedure with one lump sum or bundled payment based on the expected costs for clinically defined episodes of care. For example, a surgeon is paid a specified amount to provide preoperative care, to perform the surgical procedure, and to provide postoperative care. Although the FFS model is a dominant form of reimbursement, the episode-of-care reimbursement model is gaining popularity because of their strong incentives to reduce health care costs.

A type of episode-of-care reimbursement is a **prospective payment system (PPS)**, sometimes referred to as a *prospective payment bundle.* Prospective payment systems establish the amount of reimbursement that will be provided *before* the patient's care. Under a PPS, a health care provider will always receive the same payment for providing the same specific type of treatment. This contrasts with a retrospective payment system or bundle, such as the traditional FFS payment method, which pays each provider after services have been rendered.

Medicare Prospective Payment System

The Tax Equity and Fiscal Responsibility Act of 1982 required the establishment of PPSs for Medicare beneficiaries, with the system using diagnosis-related groups (DRGs). DRGs reimburse health care providers for inpatient care, like hospital stays. Since that time a number of other PPSs have been implemented for physician offices, hospital outpatient services, and many other health care facilities. In a PPS system, the reimbursement is not dependent on the actual costs of caring for the patient or the charges of the care, but rather on the predetermined amount for the diagnosis and/or procedure in the PPS system. For example, if a patient comes to the outpatient surgery center for an appendectomy, the payment remains the same regardless of how long it took to perform the procedure, how complicated it was, or how many supplies were used. Many of the Medicare PPS programs are discussed in this section.

prospective payment system (PPS) a reimbursement model that establishes the amount of payment before the patient's care based on the diagnosis or procedure.

CURRENT TRENDS IN HEALTH CARE

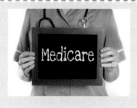

Understanding PPS programs is important because it is used by the Centers for Medicare and Medicaid Services (CMS), the largest third-party payer in the country. This means that a large percentage of a health care provider's patients are Medicare beneficiaries. Moreover, many private health insurers, including almost all health maintenance organizations (HMOs), utilize the same reimbursement methodologies as CMS.

Resource-Based Relative Value Scale

The **resource-based relative value scale (RBRVS)** is the system used to reimburse physicians for the care that they provide to Medicare patients. Using the RBRVS, procedures performed by a physician or other health care provider are assigned a relative value, which is adjusted by geographic region. This value is then multiplied by a fixed conversion factor, which may be adjusted annually, to determine the amount of payment.

Under the RBRVS, physician reimbursement is determined based on three components:
- *relative value unit (RVU)*
- *geographic practice cost index (GPCI)*
- *conversion factor (CF)*

Additionally, the RVU itself is made up of three different factors:
- *physician work (W):* the amount of time required of the physician as well as the level of difficulty of the patient's care. The more complex the patient's care, the higher the reimbursement.

resource-based relative value scale (RBRVS) the prospective payment system used for physician practices.

TABLE 9.2

EXAMPLES OF RELATIVE VALUE UNITS (RVUS) FOR DIFFERENT PROCEDURES

HCPCS Code	Procedure	Work RVU	PE RVU	MP RVU
90460	Immunization administration through 18 years of age via any route of administration, with counseling by physician or other qualified health care professional	0.17	0.53	0.00
69200	Removal of foreign body from external auditory canal; without general anesthesia	0.77	0.49	0.10
12032	Repair, intermediate, wounds of scalp, axillae, trunk and/or extremities (excluding hands and feet); 2.6–7.7 cm	2.52	2.70	0.38
70450	Computed tomography, head or brain; without contrast material	0.85	2.36	0.07
11011	Debridement including removal of foreign material at the site of an open fracture and/or an open dislocation (e.g., excisional debridement); skin, subcutaneous tissue, muscle fascia, and muscle	4.94	2.72	0.99

- *physician practice expense (PE):* the cost of running the physician's practice. The costs include salaries, office expenses, medical equipment, and other expenses.
- *malpractice insurance (MP):* the cost of purchasing professional liability insurance.

Medicare establishes the physician work, physician practice expense, and malpractice RVU for each Health Care Common Procedure Coding System (HCPCS) code, updated every October 1. Table 9.2 shows examples of three different procedures and the value associated with each part of the RVU. Note that the more labor-intensive and complicated the procedure, the higher the physician work (W) RVU factor is; the more resources required, the higher the practice expense (PE) RVU factor is; and the riskier a procedure is, the higher the malpractice (MP) RVU factor is.

The second factor for RBRVS reimbursement is geographic location. CMS recognizes that it costs more to live and work in some areas of the country than in others and there must be a cost-of-living adjustment. For example, the cost of housing and food is higher in California than in Mississippi, and so is the cost to pay employees and rent a building for a medical office. In turn, it is more expensive to provide care in California than it is in Mississippi, and reimbursement adjustments must be made to account for geographic variations in the costs of practicing medicine in different areas within the country. As a result, CMS assigns each health care provider a geographic adjustment to determine reimbursement amounts. This geographic practice cost index (GPCI) is not assigned specifically to individual states, but may be assigned based on cities or regions within the state, depending on the cost to do business in the different areas. For example, there is a GPCI for the city of Atlanta, Georgia, and separate one for the rest of the state of Georgia.

CMS assigns a health care provider a GPCI based on his or her location for each of the three components of the RVU. That is, a provider will have a separate GPCI factor for the work (W) RVU, the practice expense (PE) RVU, and the malpractice (MP) RVU. This adjustment is needed to accommodate the wide variation of costs across the country.

Finally, the last component of RBRVS is the conversion factor, which is a national figure that is used to convert the value of one RVU to dollars. When the conversion factor is higher, providers are paid more for services provided to Medicare patients. The conversion factor is adjusted annually by CMS. Thus the formula to calculate the reimbursement amount for any HCPCS code is:

$$[(W\ RVU \times W\ GPCI) + (PE\ RVU \times PE\ GPCI) + (MP\ RVU \times MP\ GPCI)] \times CF = Payment\ Amount$$

Table 9.3 shows how three physicians performing the same procedure in three different areas of the country will receive different payments from CMS.

TABLE 9.3

EXAMPLES OF RESOURCE-BASED RELATIVE VALUE SCALE PAYMENT CALCULATION FOR HCPCS CODE 69200 ACROSS DIFFERENT GEOGRAPHIC AREAS

Provider Location	RELATIVE VALUE UNIT (RVU)													
	W RVU	×	W GPCI	+	PE RVU	×	PE GPCI	+	MP RVU	×	MP GPCI	×	CF	=	Payment
Southern Maine	0.77	×	1.000	+	0.49	×	1.007	+	0.10	×	0.642	×	$35.8279	=	$47.57
San Francisco, CA	0.77	×	1.079	+	0.49	×	1.388	+	0.10	×	0.457	×	$35.8279	=	$55.77
Iowa	0.77	×	1.000	+	0.49	×	0.896	+	0.10	×	0.493	×	$35.8279		$45.08

outpatient prospective payment system (OPPS) the Medicare reimbursement system used to reimburse hospitals for outpatient services.

Ambulatory Payment Classification (APC) grouping of procedures and services that are provided to Medicare patients through the hospital outpatient prospective payment system.

grouper software used to convert diagnosis and procedure codes into Ambulatory Patient Classifications and other groupings.

packaging the inclusion of required minor services in a larger reimbursement grouping.

bundling payment for multiple procedures or services under one combination code.

Hospital Outpatient Prospective Payment System

Another type of PPS is the hospital **outpatient prospective payment system (OPPS)**, used to reimburse hospitals for outpatient services performed. These services include procedures, laboratory tests, and radiology services. The rate of reimbursement is based on **Ambulatory Payment Classifications (APCs)**, which group services that require similar care and similar costs together. The APC is assignment by software known as a **grouper** and uses Current Procedural Terminology (CPT) code(s) to assign the APC. If a patient has multiple services, such as a urinalysis and a chest x-ray, the patient can be assigned two or more APCs.

The OPPS utilizes both packaging and bundling methodology. **Packaging** occurs when a significant procedure requires minor services such as a laboratory test. The reimbursement for the procedure includes the minor services. **Bundling** assigns a code, when available, for an entire service rather than coding each test or procedure performed with that service separately. For example, there is a code for a complete blood count (CBC), which would be used rather than using individual codes for the hematocrit, hemoglobin, and other tests included in the CBC.

Ambulance Fee Schedule

The ambulance fee schedule is the Medicare PPS for ambulance services. As mentioned earlier in the chapter, a fee schedule is a list of services that are covered by an insurer and the amount the insurer will reimburse for ambulance transportation, which includes both ground ambulance and air ambulance services. To be eligible for reimbursement, the patient's condition must require ambulance transportation. The reimbursement amount is determined by a base rate established by CMS and includes mileage, supplies, and any additional services provided during the transportation.

Home Health Prospective Payment System

The *Home Health Prospective Payment System (HHPPS)* is the PPS used to reimburse home health agencies for the care they provide. Generally, the payment includes all supplies and services provided to patients in their home. Services covered by the HHPPS include intermittent skilled nursing, physical therapy, social services, and occupational therapy. For a patient to qualify for home health services, the patient must meet the following standards:

- Be homebound
- Require the services of a nurse or another skilled care provider
- Be under the care of a physician
- Receive the home care from an approved home health agency
- Receive care from a physician within the past 90 days of the date home care is started or within 30 days after the care is started and for the same reason home care is required.[2]

---

[2]Centers for Medicare and Medicaid Services. (2016). "Hospital outpatient prospective payment system." https://www.cms.gov/Outreach-and-Education/Medicare-Learning-Network-MLN/MLNProducts/downloads/HospitalOutpaysysfctsht.pdf

There are 20 patients in the physician's panel
No one received treatment in June

In July, 2 of the 20 patients receive treatment

All 20 patients come in for treatment

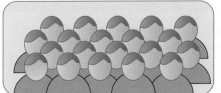 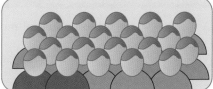 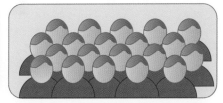

The payer pays $10 for each
patient this month.

The payer pays $10 for each patient in July,
regardless of whether they came in for a visit.

The rate does not change in August. The
payer pays a total of $200 for the panel.

Physician receives $200
with no expenses.

If each visit costs $12,
the physician receives
$176 in July.

Because the physician's expenses
outweigh his payment for August,
the physician loses $40 this month.

$10 × 20 patients   = $200
$12 × 2 patients seen = −$24
                              $176 net profit

$10 × 20 patients   = $200
− $12 × 20 patients seen = − $240
                                $40 net loss

Figure 9.1 Capitation scenarios with a pool of 20 patients. (From Davis N, LaCour M. *Foundations of health information management*, ed 4, St. Louis, 2015, Elsevier.)

The patient is assigned a home health resource group (HHRG) score based on the severity level of the patient's care and need, which determines the amount of reimbursement. The HHRG score is calculated based on a comprehensive assessment called the **Outcomes and Assessment Information Set (OASIS)**, which identifies data to be collected on each patient and assesses the services provided and the ability of the patient to care for himself or herself.

> ○ **Outcomes and Assessment Information Set (OASIS)** information collected on all Medicare home health patient care.

Managed Care

As discussed in Chapter 3, **managed care** is a type of health care whose focus is to control costs while maintaining quality of the care. One of the ways costs are controlled is to regulate the utilization of services through the use of primary care physicians (PCPs) as a gatekeeper. The PCP provides the majority of care for the patient. If the patient's condition warrants it, the PCP provides a referral to a specialist. The health care provider, in turn, is paid using a reimbursement methodology called **capitation**, which is a flat rate reimbursement the health care provider receives per patient for providing medical care. The PCP is paid the same rate regardless of the number of visits during a period of time, usually a month (Fig. 9.1).

> ○ **managed care** an insurance coverage and reimbursement structure that seeks to control costs by limiting the providers who can be seen by the patient and, in turn, discount payments to those providers.

> ○ **capitation** a flat rate reimbursement that a health care provider receives per patient for providing care.

■ **LEARNING CHECKPOINT 9.2**
■ **Reimbursement Methodologies**

1. Which reimbursement methodology establishes the payment amount before the patient receives medical services?

   a. fee-for-service
   b. self-pay
   c. episode-of-care reimbursement
   d. prospective payment system

Continued

2. A _____ is the amount of money the provider submits on a claim.

   a. UCR rate
   b. fee schedule
   c. charge
   d. DRG

3. Which is a component of the resource-based relative value scale (RBRVS)?

   a. malpractice costs
   b. geographical price differences
   c. the cost of running the physician's practice
   d. all of these

4. Which system groups services into Ambulatory Payment Classifications (APCs)?

   a. ambulance fee schedule
   b. outpatient prospective payment system (OPPS)
   c. resource-based relative value scale (RBRVS)
   d. Home Health Prospective Payment System (HHPPS)

5. _____ is a flat rate reimbursement that a health care provider receives per patient for providing medical care.

   a. fee-for-service
   b. capitation
   c. prospective payment
   d. UCR rate

REVENUE CYCLE MANAGEMENT

○ **revenue cycle management** the gathering of the administrative and clinical information required to obtain reimbursement for health care services provided.

Revenue cycle management is the gathering of the administrative and clinical information required to obtain reimbursement for health care services provided. It begins even before the patient visit and ends when the patient's account is paid in full. Some of the steps include scheduling and registration, insurance eligibility verification, coding and charge capture, processing claims, managing denials, and posting reimbursement received. The extent to which the medical practice and health care facility have a handle on these steps directly affects how much and how quickly they get paid.

Front-End Processes

Front-end processes cover scheduling and registration, insurance eligibility verification, obtaining preauthorizations, and addressing medical necessity coverage issues. All of these processes are performed before the patient receives services from the health care provider.

Scheduling and Registration

In most cases, the patient or referring physician calls to schedule the patient for health care services. The scheduling of the appointment begins the revenue cycle process, because information is collected during this initial contact with the medical office. Some services, such as a blood draw in a laboratory, do not generally require an appointment. Other services, such as mammograms and colonoscopies, must be scheduled.

Although the patient may be given paperwork to be completed before arriving at the health care facility, the registration process begins upon the patient's arrival at the health care facility. Information collected during patient registration includes demographics, employment status, and insurance information. The patient's identification must be verified by reviewing the patient's government-issued identification card, such as a driver's license, passport, or military ID card. A copy of the identification is made for the patient medical record. Additionally, the patient's insurance card is copied and included in the patient medical record. Having a record of the patient's insurance information is important because it includes the name of the health insurance company, the policy number and group number, the copays, coinsurance, and where to submit the claims. Chapter 4 discusses in more detail the process of scheduling and registering patients to ensure efficiency and proper workflow management.

Insurance Verification

Insurance verification is an important step in the patient registration process. A health insurance company will only pay for a patient's medical services if his or her health insurance policy is "active." This means that the patient has paid his or her premium for insurance coverage during a specific period and that the health insurance company will pay the health care provider for providing medical services to the patient or his or her dependent. If the health insurance is not active or the policy was cancelled due to lack of payment, then the insurance company will not process the claim and the health care provider will not be paid. Thus verification of patient insurance coverage must be verified each time the patient comes into the medical office or health care facility.

Insurance verification may be done by phone or electronically. Located on every insurance card is a contact phone number for the health insurance company, including numbers for specific departments like hospital admissions, referrals and preauthorizations, member services, and provider services. Verifying patient insurance coverage over the phone is time consuming. As a result, many health insurance companies provide electronic or online verification through a direct company website or by using an online clearinghouse. To use the provided clearinghouse service to verify insurance, the health care provider or health care facility must either subscribe to the clearinghouse or be a contracted provider with the health insurance company. Otherwise, verifying patient coverage information must be performed by phone.

Preauthorization

Preauthorization, sometimes called *prior authorization* or *precertification,* is the process of obtaining approval from the insurer for a service before the service is performed. Preauthorization is a determination of the medical necessity and appropriateness of treatment for certain covered services. This excludes any emergency procedures. Preauthorization may vary by health insurance policies, but it is generally required for high-cost services, such as magnetic resonance imaging, home health care, sleep studies, and specialty drugs. To obtain preauthorization, the insurer is contacted and provided with information about the recommended service and the patient's current diagnosis. A preauthorization is not a guarantee of benefits or payment. However, not receiving preauthorization could result in nonreimbursement of the provided service.

preauthorization the process of obtaining approval from the insurer for a service before the service is performed.

TAKE AWAY

A preauthorization is not a guarantee of benefits or payment.

A request for preauthorization may be done either by phone or by submitting a request form. The insurer will confirm the medical necessity of the requested medical care. This will help the insurer control costs and prevent any duplication of services, waste, and unnecessary medical procedures. Once approved by the insurer, an authorization number is provided. This number is submitted on the health care claim as proof that the service had prior approval. If the preauthorization has been denied, the patient, health care provider, or health care facility can appeal by providing the proper documentation to support the medical necessity of the requested medical care or service.

Preauthorization should be differentiated from *predetermination,* which is a voluntary request for review of treatment or services, usually considered not medically necessary, investigational, or cosmetic. Examples of reasons to request predetermination from an insurer are gastric bypass surgery for weight loss, breast reduction surgery, and dental implants. Similar to preauthorizations, predeterminations are done before medical services or care is provided to ensure coverage by the health insurance plan.

Medical Necessity Coverage

Insurers will only reimburse a health care provider for services that are deemed medically necessary. *Medical necessity* is a determination that services are required to diagnose and/or treat patients based on the specific needs of their disease or condition. Any service that is determined to be not medically necessary will be denied reimbursement.

Two tools to help determine the medical necessity of a service are national coverage determination and local coverage determination. **National coverage determinations (NCDs)** are guidelines and decisions that Medicare developed to determine whether or not a medical service is considered "reasonable and necessary" and, thus, will be covered and reimbursed on the national level. In the absence of an NCD, an item or service is covered at the discretion of the Medicare Administrative Contractor based on a local coverage determination (LCD). **Local coverage determinations (LCDs),** like NCDs, are guidelines to determine whether or not a service will be covered; however, they are for local use rather than for national use. All NCDs and LCD rules and decisions can be found on the Medicare Coverage Database.

Advanced Beneficiary Notice

An **advanced beneficiary notice (ABN),** also known as a *waiver of liability,* is a document sent by the health care provider notifying patients that Medicare will most likely not cover their treatment or service in a particular instance for certain reasons. The treatment or service in question may or may not normally be covered by Medicare, but, in this instance, the health care provider expects that Medicare will not find the care to be medically necessary and will therefore deny coverage. The health care provider must provide an ABN to the patient before providing services so that the patient can decide whether or not he or she wishes to assume responsibility for payment.

An ABN is not required for services that are not covered by Medicare. For example, Medicare does not generally pay for plastic surgery; therefore an ABN is not required for a patient having a liposuction unless it is deemed medically necessary.

Preparing for and Processing Claims

Preparing the health care claim continues during the patient's care as charges are captured. After the patient's care is completed, the charges are determined and codes are assigned during the processing of the health care claim. Once the health care claim is processed, it is submitted for reimbursement. These concepts are discussed further in this section.

national coverage determination (NCD) rules developed by the Centers for Medicare and Medicaid Services used to determine whether or not a service will be covered.

local coverage determination (LCD) rules developed by the Medicare Administrative Contractor used to determine whether or not a service will be covered within a local area.

advanced beneficiary notice (ABN) a written document notifying a Medicare patient that Medicare will not cover a service, usually because it is not determined to be medically necessary and the patient will be responsible for payment.

Charge Capture

During the patient's care, charges are entered into the patient account, which may include medications, supplies, and other charges for the patient's care. These charges may be entered using bar codes entered manually or determined through the electronic software system used by the health care facility. Charges should be entered immediately to the patient's account to prevent lost charges, which would result in loss of revenue to the medical office or health care facility.

Chargemaster

The **chargemaster** is a comprehensive list of all the services provided by the health care provider; the charges for those services; and the corresponding HCPCS (Healthcare Common Procedures Coding System), CPT (Current Procedural Terminology), or ICD-10-PCS (International Classification of Diseases, Tenth Revision, Procedure Coding System) codes.

> **chargemaster** a list of services provided, the charges, and the associated codes.

The uses of the chargemaster include:
- Collecting data to be included in an itemized statement
- Identifying charges and codes that go on the bill
- Monitoring statistics
- Providing data on cost of patient care[3]

It is important to keep the chargemaster current. This includes deleting services no longer provided, adding new services, and updating the codes. Failure to manage the chargemaster will result in problems in billing due to invalid codes, an inability to enter charges, and the submission of inaccurate claims.

Claims

Health care **claims** are the health care provider's request for reimbursement. Health care claims are generally submitted to the insurer or a health care clearinghouse, but may be submitted to the patient in the case of self-pay. The health care clearinghouse acts as an intermediary between the health care provider and the insurer. The health care provider submits health care claim data to the health care clearinghouse, which converts the data into the required format for submission. The health care clearinghouse would then submit the claim to the appropriate insurer for reimbursement to the health care provider.

> **claim** a statement of services sent to a health insurer for payment to the provider.

Claims Scrubber Software

Before a claim is submitted to an insurer, it should be reviewed by a claims scrubber software to ensure that it is a "clean" claim, meaning that it does not have any errors or omissions that would result in the insurer denying or underpaying the claim. The claims scrubber software checks the claims for errors such as:
- Invalid diagnosis or procedure codes
- Missing data
- Invalid data
- Improper formats

Any errors found must be corrected before submitting the claim to prevent a delay in reimbursement.

Coding

As discussed in Chapter 5, coding is assigning a universal numeric or alphanumeric number or code that represents a diagnosis, procedure, medical service, or equipment/supplies (Fig. 9.2). It is important to use these codes because the Health Insurance

---

[3]Pilato, J. Charging vs. coding: untangling the relationship for ICD-10. *J AHIMA* 2013;84(s):58–60.

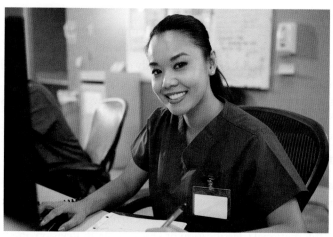

Figure 9.2 The medical coder assigns and verifies diagnostic, procedure, and other codes to a patient record.

TABLE 9.4		
SAMPLE CODES		
Coding System	**Diagnoses or Procedure**	**Sample Code**
ICD-10-CM	Gestational diabetes mellitus in pregnancy	O24.419
CPT	Pelvic exam and pap smear	88150
HCPCS – Level II	Annual women's exam visit	G0101

Portability and Accountability Act (HIPAA) mandates the specific code sets be used to submit diagnoses and procedures on health care claims. Diagnoses are reported using the coding system of the International Classification of Disease (ICD), Tenth Revision, Clinical Modification (ICD-10-CM). Outpatient procedures are reported on health care claims using the coding systems of Healthcare Common Procedure Coding System (HCPCS) and CPT. Table 9.4 shows some sample codes from each of these coding systems. In-patient procedures (and some outpatient ones) may use ICD-10-Procedure Coding System (PCS). The most common procedural coding system used in an outpatient facility will be ICD-10-CM and CPT.

International Classification of Disease, Tenth Revision, Clinical Modification

International Classification of Disease, Tenth Revision, Clinical Modification (ICD-10-CM) is a diagnosis coding system that is used for both inpatient and outpatient health care claims. It is based on the *International Classification of Disease, Tenth Edition* (ICD-10), which is published by the World Health Organization and is a statistical classification of diseases. The National Center for Health Statistics, a department within the Centers for Disease Control and Prevention, modified ICD-10 to assist in the classification of diseases in the health care setting in the United States.

ICD-10-CM was implemented on October 1, 2015, for all HIPAA-covered entities. ICD-10-CM is revised annually on October 1. The Official Guidelines for Coding and Reporting, the rules to follow when coding, is also revised on October 1 of each year. Clarifications of the rules and questions that coders have are published by the American Hospital Association in the *Coding Clinic for ICD-10-CM/PCS and/or HCPCS.*

The length of ICD-10-CM codes range from three to seven alphanumeric characters. To assign the code, the coder looks the diagnosis up in the alphabetical index, and then the code is confirmed in the tabular list. When coding outpatient services, the first code to be listed on the health care claim is known as the *first listed code*. The first listed code is the primary reason the patient sought health care services. Each health

International Classification of Disease, Tenth Revision, Clinical Modification (ICD-10-CM) diagnosis coding system used on health care claims.

care encounter should be coded at the level of complexity for that encounter as documented by the provider.

Healthcare Common Procedure Coding System

The **Healthcare Common Procedure Coding System (HCPCS)**, commonly pronounced as *"hic-pics,"* is a coding system developed specifically for Medicare recipients receiving outpatient services. It is divided into two levels:

- Level I: Current Procedural Terminology (CPT) system, discussed later.
- Level II: developed by CMS for codes not included in the CPT, such as durable medical equipment, medications, and supplies. The coding system begins with a single alphabetic character, and the remaining four characters are numeric.

Both Level I and Level II codes use modifiers to provide additional information about the services or procedure provided to ensure appropriate reimbursement. For example, modifiers may be used when performing a bilateral procedure, a reduced procedure, or a discontinued procedure.

> **Healthcare Common Procedure Coding System (HCPCS)** Coding system created by the Centers for Medicare and Medicaid Services for use in the hospital outpatient prospective payment system.

Current Procedural Terminology

Current Procedural Terminology (CPT) is a coding system that documents and reports medical, surgical, radiology, laboratory, anesthesiology, and evaluation and management (E/M) services. The CPT was first introduced in 1966 and is owned, maintained, and revised annually by the American Medical Association. All health care providers, health care facilities, and insurers use the CPT codes, and it is used solely for outpatient procedural health care claims. The CPT codes are five-digit numeric codes. Depending on the service provided, the code will be in one of three categories:

- Level I: These codes represent procedures that are consistent with contemporary medical practice and are widely performed. These procedures are commonly performed by health care providers, are approved by the Food and Drug Administration, and have shown clinical effectiveness.
- Level II: These codes are intended to facilitate the collection of information about the quality of care delivered by coding a number of services or test results that support performance measures. These performance measures have been agreed upon as contributing to good patient care.
- Level III: These codes represent temporary codes for new and emerging technologies. Unlike Level I codes, these procedures are not commonly performed by health care providers and are considered more experimental.

> **Current Procedural Terminology (CPT)** a coding system that documents and reports medical, surgical, radiology, laboratory, anesthesiology, and evaluation and management (E/M) services.

Clinical Documentation

The documentation in the patient's medical record must support the diagnosis and procedures coded and submitted on the health care claim. If the documentation is illogical, contradictory, or incomplete, it is the responsibility of the health services administrator or whoever is responsible for coding and submitting claims to query the health care provider.

A **query** is a tool used to ask the health care provider to clarify the current documentation or include missing information in the patient's medical record to ensure the correct codes are being submitted for reimbursement. The query should be in the form of a question to prevent any perceptions of leading the health care provider or to suggest an answer. In other words, the health services administrator should never tell the health care provider what to document or answer, but rather quote information in the health record and ask for clarification. Additionally, the amount of reimbursement should never be mentioned during the query. The query should only be concerned with clarifying or improving documentation and not increasing the reimbursement. Box 9.1 contains examples of appropriate and inappropriate queries.

> **query** a tool used to clarify the provider's documentation in the patient's medical record.

BOX 9.1	EXAMPLES OF APPROPRIATE QUERIES

EXAMPLES OF APPROPRIATELY WRITTEN QUERIES	EXAMPLES OF INAPPROPRIATE QUERIES
1. The chest x-ray indicates pneumonia, and the patient was placed on bronchodilators and antibiotics. If this is significant, please document this in the health record. 2. The history and physical states that the patient has type 1 diabetes mellitus; however, the discharge summary states that it is type 2. Please clarify the type of diabetes mellitus that the patient has.	1. Add pneumonia to the discharge summary. 2. If you add the atrial fibrillation, we can increase our reimbursement by $250.00. 3. Does the patient have hyperkalemia associated with the diabetes mellitus? Yes or No

Billing/Claims Processing

At the end of the patient's care, the medical chart is coded and any final charges are totaled. The health care claim is processed through the claims scrubber software, as described earlier. Once the health care claim is "clean," either it is submitted directly to the payer, such as Medicare and Blue Cross, or it is submitted to a health care clearinghouse.

According to the HIPAA Administrative Simplification Compliance Act (ASCA), health care claims for Medicare billing must be submitted electronically using the 837P (Professional) standard form. Under limited exceptions, Medicare will allow submission of paper health care claims from health care providers who meet the exceptions to the electronic submission requirements set forth in the ASCA. Examples of the exceptions are a medical practice that bills for Medicare reimbursement with fewer than 10 full-time employees or a medical practice that is experiencing an electrical or other disruption in communication that is beyond its control and expected to last more than 2 days. In these circumstances, health care claims may be submitted using the CMS-1500 paper form (Fig. 9.3). Regardless of how the health care claim is submitted, the following data must be provided:

- Patient identifying information
- Insurance information
- Diagnosis and procedure codes
- Charges
- Health care provider information
- Date(s) of service

Insurers have 30 days to submit reimbursement for a clean claim. Provided the claim is approved, the payer will submit reimbursement to the health care provider along with a *remittance advice,* which is discussed later.

Postbilling Processes

The revenue cycle continues when a health care claim is accepted or denied by a third-party payer. If the claim has been accepted, the third-party payer will reimburse some or all of the cost of the medical service. When there is more than one payer, "coordination of benefits" rules decide which insurer pays first. The "primary payer" pays what it owes on the claim first and then sends the rest to the "secondary payer" to pay. Additionally, patients may be billed for the coinsurance, deductible, or copay.

Payment Posting

remittance advice (RA) report that identifies the patient, the services that are being reimbursed, and the amount of the reimbursement.

The **remittance advice (RA)** is a list of all the claims submitted and all claims being reimbursed by the insurer, as well as any adjustments that need to be made to the payment (Fig. 9.4). Types of adjustments include denied claims, partial payments, any applied penalties, and additional or supplemental payments. The RA lists the itemized

HEALTH INSURANCE CLAIM FORM

APPROVED BY NATIONAL UNIFORM CLAIM COMMITTEE (NUCC) 02/12

| | PICA | | | | | | | | | PICA | |

1. MEDICARE ☐ (Medicare#) MEDICAID ☐ (Medicaid#) TRICARE ☐ (ID#/DoD#) CHAMPVA ☐ (Member ID#) GROUP HEALTH PLAN ☐ (ID#) FECA BLK LUNG ☐ (ID#) OTHER ☐ (ID#)   **1a. INSURED'S I.D. NUMBER**   (For Program in Item 1)

2. PATIENT'S NAME (Last Name, First Name, Middle Initial)

3. PATIENT'S BIRTH DATE MM ⎪ DD ⎪ YY   **SEX** M ☐ F ☐

4. INSURED'S NAME (Last Name, First Name, Middle Initial)

5. PATIENT'S ADDRESS (No., Street)

6. PATIENT RELATIONSHIP TO INSURED Self ☐ Spouse ☐ Child ☐ Other ☐

7. INSURED'S ADDRESS (No., Street)

CITY   STATE

8. RESERVED FOR NUCC USE

CITY   STATE

ZIP CODE   TELEPHONE (Include Area Code) (   )

ZIP CODE   TELEPHONE (Include Area Code) (   )

9. OTHER INSURED'S NAME (Last Name, First Name, Middle Initial)

10. IS PATIENT'S CONDITION RELATED TO:

11. INSURED'S POLICY GROUP OR FECA NUMBER

a. OTHER INSURED'S POLICY OR GROUP NUMBER

a. EMPLOYMENT? (Current or Previous) ☐ YES ☐ NO

a. INSURED'S DATE OF BIRTH MM ⎪ DD ⎪ YY   **SEX** M ☐ F ☐

b. RESERVED FOR NUCC USE

b. AUTO ACCIDENT? ☐ YES ☐ NO   PLACE (State)

b. OTHER CLAIM ID (Designated by NUCC)

c. RESERVED FOR NUCC USE

c. OTHER ACCIDENT? ☐ YES ☐ NO

c. INSURANCE PLAN NAME OR PROGRAM NAME

d. INSURANCE PLAN NAME OR PROGRAM NAME

10d. CLAIM CODES (Designated by NUCC)

d. IS THERE ANOTHER HEALTH BENEFIT PLAN? ☐ YES ☐ NO   *If yes*, complete items 9, 9a, and 9d.

READ BACK OF FORM BEFORE COMPLETING & SIGNING THIS FORM.
12. PATIENT'S OR AUTHORIZED PERSON'S SIGNATURE I authorize the release of any medical or other information necessary to process this claim. I also request payment of government benefits either to myself or to the party who accepts assignment below.

SIGNED _____   DATE _____

13. INSURED'S OR AUTHORIZED PERSON'S SIGNATURE I authorize payment of medical benefits to the undersigned physician or supplier for services described below.

SIGNED _____

14. DATE OF CURRENT ILLNESS, INJURY, or PREGNANCY (LMP) MM ⎪ DD ⎪ YY   QUAL. |

15. OTHER DATE QUAL. | MM ⎪ DD ⎪ YY

16. DATES PATIENT UNABLE TO WORK IN CURRENT OCCUPATION MM ⎪ DD ⎪ YY   FROM   TO   MM ⎪ DD ⎪ YY

17. NAME OF REFERRING PROVIDER OR OTHER SOURCE   17a. | 17b. NPI |

18. HOSPITALIZATION DATES RELATED TO CURRENT SERVICES MM ⎪ DD ⎪ YY   FROM   TO   MM ⎪ DD ⎪ YY

19. ADDITIONAL CLAIM INFORMATION (Designated by NUCC)

20. OUTSIDE LAB? ☐ YES ☐ NO $ CHARGES

21. DIAGNOSIS OR NATURE OF ILLNESS OR INJURY Relate A-L to service line below (24E)   ICD Ind. |

A. |____   B. |____   C. |____   D. |____
E. |____   F. |____   G. |____   H. |____
I. |____   J. |____   K. |____   L. |____

22. RESUBMISSION CODE   ORIGINAL REF. NO.

23. PRIOR AUTHORIZATION NUMBER

24. A. DATE(S) OF SERVICE						B. PLACE OF SERVICE	C. EMG	D. PROCEDURES, SERVICES, OR SUPPLIES (Explain Unusual Circumstances)		E. DIAGNOSIS POINTER	F. $ CHARGES	G. DAYS OR UNITS	H. EPSDT Family Plan	I. ID. QUAL.	J. RENDERING PROVIDER ID. #
From MM	DD	YY	To MM	DD	YY			CPT/HCPCS	MODIFIER						
1														NPI	
2														NPI	
3														NPI	
4														NPI	
5														NPI	
6														NPI	

25. FEDERAL TAX I.D. NUMBER   SSN ☐ EIN ☐

26. PATIENT'S ACCOUNT NO.

27. ACCEPT ASSIGNMENT? (For govt. claims, see back) ☐ YES ☐ NO

28. TOTAL CHARGE $

29. AMOUNT PAID $

30. Rsvd for NUCC Use

31. SIGNATURE OF PHYSICIAN OR SUPPLIER INCLUDING DEGREES OR CREDENTIALS (I certify that the statements on the reverse apply to this bill and are made a part thereof.)

SIGNED _____   DATE _____

32. SERVICE FACILITY LOCATION INFORMATION

a. NPI   b.

33. BILLING PROVIDER INFO & PH # (   )

a. NPI   b.

Figure 9.3 Paper CMS-1500 form.

(Right margin labels: CARRIER | PATIENT AND INSURED INFORMATION | PHYSICIAN OR SUPPLIER INFORMATION)

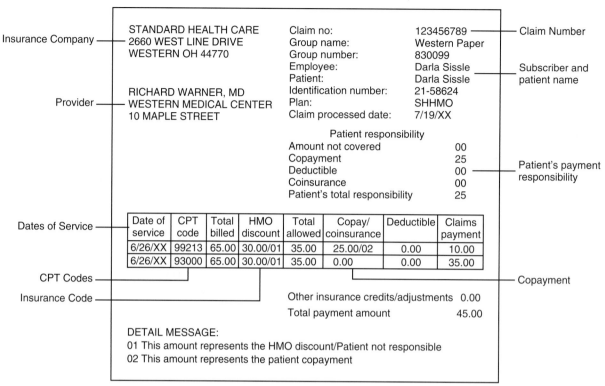

Figure 9.4 Sample remittance advice (RA). (From Bonewit-West K, et al. *Today's medical assistant: clinical & administrative procedures,* ed 3, St. Louis, 2015, Elsevier.

claims processing regarding the payments, deductibles and copayments, adjustments, denials, refunds, and any missing or incorrect data. The RA allows the health care provider to identify what claims have been paid and how much reimbursement was received. Once the RA is received, the reimbursement is posted or credited to the patient's account to show the receipt of the payment. In some situations, the RA may request that the health care claim be resubmitted with corrected information.

Denial Management

○ **denial** a decision by the insurer to not reimburse the health care provider for the service(s) billed.

In some cases, a health insurance claim may be denied by the insurer. **Denials** are decisions made by insurers to not reimburse some or all of the service(s) billed by the health care provider. The denial can be the result of many reasons, such as coding errors, services not covered by the insurance policy, or services that are deemed not medically necessary. There are three steps in denial management: tracking denials, determining what caused the denial, and improving processes to prevent denials from occurring in the future.

When a denial is received, the medical record and/or health care claim should be reviewed to determine if the health care facility agrees with the denial. To remedy a denial, the health care facility may merely need to check if numbers were not transposed (such as birth dates, billing codes, or patient identification numbers) or the correct sex of the patient was entered. If the health care facility agrees with the denial, no further action is required. However, the health care provider should track denials to identify problem areas that need improvement to prevent future denials and loss of revenue. If the health care facility disagrees with the denial, an appeal should be submitted.

○ **appeal** the request for an insurer to reconsider their decision to deny a health care claim.

An **appeal** is a formal request to the insurer to review its decision and, hopefully, to overturn the denial. An appeal is generally a letter to the third-party payer explaining why the health care facility disagrees with the decision. The letter should be written by the health care provider if the denial was based on the lack of medical necessity of the service or any other clinical issue. The health care provider's appeal should focus on the patient's condition(s) or diagnosis and explain why the service was medically necessary. If the denial was due to improper billing or an error in coding, the health services administrator or the medical biller or coder should write the letter. For a denial due to coding, the appeal should focus on documentation in the patient's medical record that supports the code submitted on the health care claim. The letter should also cite the coding rule that supports the claim and the submitted code. Fig. 9.5 shows an example of a denial letter.

Revenue Cycle Monitoring

Throughout the revenue cycle, there must be ongoing monitoring and review of the process to identify areas of concern and opportunities for improvement. Looking at specific metrics gives the health services administrator a picture of the health of the revenue cycle processes at the medical office. Furthermore, failure to identify problems may result in issues such as loss of revenue, increases in denials, and allegation of fraud.

Accounts Receivable (A/R) Days

The accounts receivable (A/R) report lists the number of days between the patient's date of service and the receipt of payment for services. If a patient is seen on

Birmingham Outpatient Services
1213 Main Street
Birmingham, Alabama 97865

March 23, 20XX

Department of Appeals
Trinity Insurance
203 Elm Street
St. Louis, Missouri 12345

Dear Appeals Coordinator:

I am writing in response to a coding error denial that was received by Birmingham Outpatient Services on Martha Jones for the date of services of February 18, 20XX. Ms. Jones had an XXX. The procedure code submitted was 45380. The denial letter states the code should be 45378. After review of the patient's medical record, we disagree with the change in code assignment. If you review the operative report, it specifically states that there was a biopsy performed. Please see the attached copy of the operative report. The relevant content has been highlighted for your convenience.

If you have any questions, please contact me at 555-555-5555 or by email at florence.wilson@birminghamoutpatient.org. Thank you for considering reversal of this denial.

Sincerely,

Florence Wilson

Florence Wilson, RHIA
Coding Supervisor

Figure 9.5 Sample denial letter.

September 1 and the A/R report lists a zero balance less than 2 weeks later, it reflects the submission of a clean claim that was paid promptly. When taken together, if the average A/R days of the medical office's patients are several months or longer, it indicates there is a problem with claims submission.

Unbilled Accounts

Unbilled accounts are accounts that have not yet been billed after a service was provided. Some medical offices are able to "drop the bill" the same day the patient was seen, but other offices are not as efficient and may have a lag time between when the service was provided and when the bill is sent. Generally, most medical facilities will seek to send out a bill within 1 to 2 weeks of a patient receiving services. If the billing process is taking longer than 2 weeks to submit, the health services administrator should do some investigation as to why bills are not being sent within a timely fashion. Are there enough coders and billers in the facility to keep up with the patient load? Do the coders and billers need training to increase their speed? Are providers not providing the needed documentation for accurate billing and coding? When there is a long lag time between services rendered and bills being dropped, there will also be a lag with reimbursements and a possible impact on the cash flow of the medical office.

Clean Claims Rate

Clean claims enable the health care provider to receive reimbursement quickly. The goal is for this number to be close to the number of claims submitted. For instance, if a medical office submits 300 claims in a month and 290 are clean, its rate of clean claims is 96.7%. A perfect month with no claims denied reflects a clean claims rate of 100%.

Denials

Similarly, the health services administrator should monitor the number of denials received to determine if the number is increasing or decreasing. The types of denials should also be monitored and tracked. Lastly, it is important to track the number of appealed denials that were overturned compared with all denials, keeping in mind that not all denials will be appealed.

● CASE STUDY

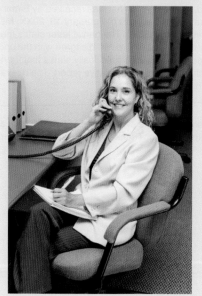

Sara tells the patient on the phone that she understands his concern about whether or not his insurance will cover a sleep study. She confirms that the facility has a referral from his PCP and that because of their expense, the office obtains preauthorization for all sleep studies. In fact, they submitted the preauthorization form when he made the appointment and have already received a preauthorization number, meaning that the facility is approved to provide the service. Sara stresses that this is not a guarantee that the service is covered, but that the HMO has confirmed the study is medically necessary.

LEARNING CHECKPOINT 9.3
Revenue Cycle Management

1. During the _____ process, administrative staff makes certain the patient's insurance is active.

   a. scheduling
   b. preauthorization
   c. verification
   d. coding

2. A _____ is a health care provider's request for reimbursement.

   a. claim
   b. appeal
   c. denial
   d. query

3. Which coding system is used solely for outpatient procedural health care claims?

   a. CPT
   b. HCPCS
   c. ICD-10-CM
   d. ICD-10-PCS

4. At the urgent care center, 910 of 1056 submitted claims are clean. What is the facility's clean claims rate?

   a. 86%
   b. 13.8%
   c. 910%
   d. 146%

REVIEW QUESTIONS

1. What features of health insurance plans attempt to share costs between the insurer and the subscriber?

2. Differentiate between the OPPS and the RBRVS.

3. Explain why documentation is so important to the revenue cycle.

4. Explain when a query is appropriate.

5. Who should write a denial letter?

6. How do A/R days indicate the effectiveness of a medical office's revenue cycle?

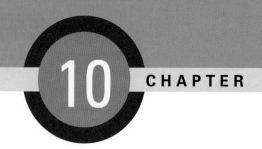

CHAPTER 10

QUALITY, PERFORMANCE IMPROVEMENT, AND RISK MANAGEMENT

Carol Colvin

CHAPTER OUTLINE

INTRODUCTION
QUALITY
  Measuring Quality
    Medicare Access and CHIP
      Reauthorization Act of 2015
      (MACRA)
    Healthcare Effectiveness Data
      and Information Set (HEDIS)
  Auditing
    Internal Audits
    External Audits

    Billing Audit
    Compliance Auditing
PERFORMANCE IMPROVEMENT
  Meetings
  Performance Improvement
    Methods
    Plan, Do, Check, and Act
      Method
    Lean Method
    Six Sigma Method
    Benchmarking Method

Performance Improvement Tools
  Data-Gathering Tools
  Data Presentation Tools
RISK MANAGEMENT
DISASTER MANAGEMENT
  Planning

VOCABULARY

Advanced Alternative Payment
  Model (APM)
audit
benchmarking
brainstorming
concurrent audit
decision matrix
epidemic
flowchart
graph
Healthcare Effectiveness Data and
  Information Set (HEDIS)

incident report
lean
Merit-based Incentive Payment
  System (MIPS)
outcome
performance improvement (PI)
Physician Quality Reporting System
  (PQRS)
pie chart
Plan, Do, Check, and Act (PDCA)
  method
potentially compensable event (PCE)

retrospective audit
risk management (RM)
sentinel event
Six Sigma
survey
table
unbilled charges
undocumented charges

CHAPTER OBJECTIVES

After completing this chapter, the student should be able to do the following:

1. Discuss the ways quality is monitored in the practice.
2. Understand the performance improvement methodologies used by health services professionals.
3. Distinguish data-gathering and data presentation tools and their uses.
4. Explain the function of risk management in health care.
5. Discuss the need for disaster management and the considerations in disaster planning.

INTRODUCTION

Quality control and risk management in a health care setting are critical requirements for any health care organization, and every staff member—from physicians to practitioners to support staff—plays an important role in maintaining and ensuring the delivery of quality health care.

This chapter discusses the way in which quality is defined and monitored in the health care setting. It also identifies tools for improving performance and introduces the function of the health services administrator in risk management and disaster management.

● CASE STUDY

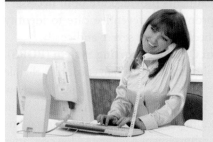

Margot Duque is the health services administrator at an ambulatory surgery center, and this week she is going to do some detective work. Once every 3 months, she sits down to review the documentation for all the surgical procedures performed at the clinic to make sure they are complete and free of errors that would cause delayed or rejected claims. As you read this chapter, think of the benefits of this process, called an *internal audit*. Why is auditing important? What can Margot do with the results?

QUALITY

Quality in a health care setting depends on many things and can be measured in many ways. Quality should focus on how health care is delivered, if it is patient centered, and if there is patient satisfaction. For example, patients judge the quality of health care based on their experiences with the facility and the provider, the results of the treatment, and the overall costs. Based on your own experiences, think of occurrences where you received less than quality health care services: perhaps you waited for hours to see a provider because of their scheduling error; your iodine allergy was not properly documented in your medical record, causing an adverse reaction during a procedure; or a claim with an incorrect procedure code was sent to your insurance carrier, resulting in a denial. In each of these cases, the actions or omissions of the health care team resulted in lower-quality care and, ultimately, dissatisfied patients.

High-quality care is not only central to maintaining and growing a patient base, but it is also essential to providing care that is both legally and ethically sound. The Institute of Medicine (IOM) defined what constitutes quality health care and identified six domains of quality:

- **Safe**: avoiding injuries to patients from the care that is intended to help them.
- **Effective**: providing services based on scientific knowledge to all who could benefit and refraining from providing services to those not likely to benefit.
- **Patient centered**: providing care that is respectful of and responsive to individual patient preferences, needs, and values and ensuring that patient values guide all clinical decisions.
- **Timely**: reducing waits and sometimes harmful delays for both those who receive and those who give care.
- **Efficient**: avoiding waste, including waste of equipment, supplies, ideas, and energy.

- **Equitable**: providing care that does not vary in quality because of personal characteristics such as gender, ethnicity, geographic location, and socioeconomic status.[1]

How do these examples fit into each of these domains? The patient who spent hours in the waiting room was not given timely care; the patient with the iodine allergy was not given safe care; and the billing error reflects inefficiency. The goal and responsibility of every health service administrator is to identify and monitor the practice's operations for quality and make improvements wherever possible.

Measuring Quality

Providing safe, effective, quality care is not only in the best interests of the practice, but also imperative to patients and insurance payers. As the entity paying for services, an insurance payer wants to ensure that the treatments provided are both necessary and effective, and it has a further interest in promoting preventive care to identify patients at risk for certain illnesses before they become more severe and costly.

One method to address this was the **Physician Quality Reporting System (PQRS)**, developed by the Centers for Medicare and Medicaid Services (CMS) to encourage eligible health care providers to report quality measures intended to improve care and show opportunities for improvement. When originally implemented in 2006, participation in the PQRS program was incentive based, with health care providers and organizations reportedly receiving a 1.5% increase in federal reimbursement payments. However, after the passage of the Affordable Care Act in 2010, CMS removed the incentive and instead financially penalized providers who did not report PQRS data by reducing payments.

○ **Physician Quality Reporting System (PQRS)** a Centers for Medicare and Medicaid reimbursement program that rewarded providers for collecting and reporting quality measures.

PQRS gave participating health care providers and health care organizations the opportunity to assess the quality of care they provide to their patients, helping to ensure that patients get the right care at the right time. By reporting on PQRS quality measures, individual eligible professionals and group practices could also quantify how often they met a particular quality metric. These PQRS measures were based on established best practices and clinical pathways developed by health care professionals and regulatory bodies. For example, the American Academy of Ophthalmology recommends that any patient over the age of 50 who has been previously diagnosed with age-related macular degeneration have a dilated macular examination performed. A health care provider or organization would track and report on how often they perform this test on the appropriate patient population.

○ **outcome** the result of a patient's treatment.

Despite an improvement in some patient **outcomes**, overall participation in PQRS was poor. Health care providers, especially single-physician and smaller practices, found the reporting structures and incentives difficult to understand, and annual changes made it hard to stay abreast of requirements. Additionally, because the processing time for reports was about 2 years, health care providers received no real-time feedback on their reporting process and were unable to correct errors or make any immediate changes.

Medicare Access and CHIP Reauthorization Act of 2015 (MACRA)

To improve upon the reporting system of the PQRS program and to minimize penalties for health care providers, Congress passed the Medicare Access and CHIP Reauthorization Act of 2015 (MACRA). MACRA repealed PQRS and the existing payment structure for health care providers and created the Quality Payment Program (QPP), establishing a new Medicare payment methodology for physician services and helping to improve data reporting and measuring of health care outcomes.

---

[1]Institute of Medicine (US) Committee on Quality of Health Care in America. (2001). *Crossing the quality chasm: a new health system for the 21st century.* Washington, DC: National Academies Press. Available from: https://www.ncbi.nlm.nih.gov/books/NBK222274/. doi: 10.17226/10027

The QPP allowed health care providers and organizations to choose how they wanted to participate in the program based on their practice size, specialty, location, and patient population. The QPP focused on moving the payment system to reward high-value, patient-centered care that accounts for diversity in health care delivery. To be eligible for QPP, the participant must bill more than $30,000 to Medicare; provide care to more than 100 Medicare patients per year; and be a physician, physician assistant, nurse practitioner, clinical nurse specialist, or certified registered nurse anesthetist.

The QPP has two distinct tracks: the **Merit-based Incentive Payment System (MIPS)** and the **Advanced Alternative Payment Model (APM)**. These seek to combine value-based services, electronic health record (EHR) technology incentives, and PQRS measures into a single program. For example, through MIPS, a health care practice collects quality data and information about how it uses technology during an observation period, which is then followed by discrete feedback from CMS. In MIPS, health care providers can earn a payment adjustment based on evidence-based and practice-specific quality data. Payments may increase, decrease, or stay the same depending on the amount of data submitted. Similarly, the APM program rewards practices that use EHR technology with much higher reimbursements and applies to a specific clinical condition, a care episode, or a population.

A large majority of health care providers will participate in the MIPS program. MIPS streamlines three currently independent programs—the PQRS program, the Value-Based Payment Modifier (VBM), and the Medicare Electronic Health Records (EHR) Incentive Program—into one program to ease the burden on health care providers. Later, a fourth component was added to promote ongoing improvement and innovation to clinical activities. The defined four performance categories for MIPS, linked by their connection to quality and value of patient care, are as follows:

- Quality—replaces current PQRS program
- Cost—replaces current VBM program
- Advancing Care Information—replaces Meaningful Use program
- Improvement activities (new component).

Successful participation in MIPS may require health care providers and organizations to enhance their staffing and information technology capabilities to ensure they support performance measurement, population health management, and feedback on quality and costs.

Merit-based Incentive Payment System (MIPS) a Centers for Medicare and Medicaid reimbursement program linking payments to the use of technology and the collection of quality data.

Advanced Alternative Payment Model (APM) a Centers for Medicare and Medicaid reimbursement program that rewards the use of technology during the care of certain clinical conditions and populations.

TAKE AWAY

Congress passed MACRA in 2015 to make improvements to the PQRS program, which tied quality data collection and reporting to Medicare reimbursements.

CURRENT TRENDS IN HEALTH CARE

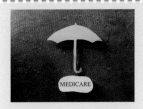

Researchers at the RAND Corporation estimate that MACRA and its value-based reimbursement models will decrease Medicare expenditures on physician services by $35 billion to $106 billion before the year 2030.

doi: 10.1377/hlthaff.2016.0559
Health Aff April 2017 vol. 36 no. 4 697-705

Healthcare Effectiveness Data and Information Set

Another set of performance measurements for health care and services is the **Healthcare Effectiveness Data and Information Set (HEDIS)**. Administered by the National Committee for Quality Assurance (NCQA), HEDIS provides a comparison tool for consumers to evaluate the quality of private and employer-based health care plans. Using a set of 81 measurements, HEDIS compares how well health plans performed across five domains:

- Effectiveness of Care
- Access/Availability of Care

Healthcare Effectiveness Data and Information Set (HEDIS) a performance measurement tool that allows comparison of health plans.

- Experience of Care
- Relative Resource Use
- Utilization and Risk-Adjusted Utilization

These measurements address a wide range of health issues, which are revised annually, and include:

- Adult BMI Assessment
- Lead Screening in Children
- Chlamydia Screening in Women
- Antidepressant Medication Management
- Annual Monitoring for Patients on Persistent Medications
- Avoidance of Antibiotic Treatment in Adults with Acute Bronchitis
- Flu Vaccinations for Adults Ages 18–64
- Prenatal and Postpartum Care
- Initiation and Engagement of Alcohol and Other Drug Dependence Treatment
- Call Answer Timeliness
- Antibiotic Utilization
- Use of First-Line Psychosocial Care for Children and Adolescents on Antipsychotics
- Health Plan Surveys

Data for HEDIS is collected directly from medical records and claims or via patient survey. Although HEDIS was originally intended to be used as a tool to compare health plans, the compiled data can be used by the insurers to identify areas for improvement.

Auditing

An old adage in management is "you get what you inspect, not what you expect." Any manager who wishes to ensure an operation is meeting quality standards must regularly monitor its processes and outputs. This inspection is done through an **audit**, which is an examination of the documents, procedures, and processes of an organization to evaluate how it is performing. More specifically, it is an independent activity by a person or team that presents objective findings and makes recommendations for corrective measures (Fig. 10.1). Audits in the health care setting provide a systematic way for organizations to evaluate, assess, and improve patient care. They measure performance against a standard or defined way of conducting business or providing patient care and provide feedback to the organization to let it know if it is doing the right things in the right ways.

Health care audits can produce valuable information for an organization. They can assure that the business is operating as it should, alert the organization that there are

○ **audit** an examination of the documents, procedures, and processes of an organization to ascertain how it is doing business.

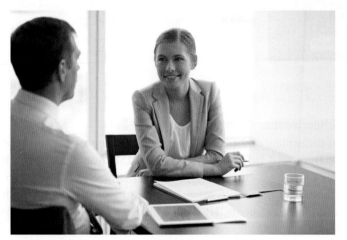

Figure 10.1 An auditor visits the health care facility to review its processes and make recommendations for improvement.

potential risks that need to be addressed, or provide accreditation and certification, as discussed earlier. The following types of audits can be conducted to collect information in a health care setting:

- Internal audits to confirm that internal controls are operating and effective.
- Medical reviews of the health care organization and affiliated networks to ensure that proper treatment is delivered based on patient information collected.
- Process reviews to provide technical assistance (financial and medical) in the development and expansion of new programs.
- Investigative audits to review health care beneficiary and provider information for fraud and abuse. The purpose of these audits is fraud prevention.
- Internal or external audits to evaluate current processes to modify those organizational policies or develop new ones.
- Mandated audits driven by executive leaders; local, state, or federal government bodies; the Health and Human Services Agency; or accrediting bodies.

Internal Audits

An internal audit helps a company ensure it has the proper controls, governance, and risk management processes in place. A robust internal audit function can find and correct deficiencies quickly and mitigate risks to minimize any legal or financial costs. For example, a medical office may perform an internal billing audit once each quarter to detect errors and provide opportunities for physician training to prevent coding and reimbursement issues.

Health care audits strengthen businesses and quality by uncovering inefficiencies and areas for improvement. Audits are often the driver of change in a health care system. When an audit flags a service, task, or process where resources are not maximized, an organization can address those areas and create new ways to operate.

Audits in health care assist in alerting management of errors taking place and allow for corrective actions to be taken. It is vitally important for the information from audits to be disseminated in a timely manner to the managerial stakeholders in the business. When errors are revealed, managers can take the information, determine the root causes, and enact reparative measures. These actions usually hold cost savings to the company in the form of reduction in errors, better provisions of services or billing that in turn reduces turnaround time for payment, and a reduction in legal expenses. On the other hand, health care organizations may find that the processes they have in place are effective and efficient, and only minimal, if any, improvements are needed.

External Audits

An *external audit* can be conducted in a similar manner to an internal audit, but is performed by an outside party or auditor. Examples of external auditors include accrediting and government agencies, such as The Joint Commission (TJC) and the Office of the Inspector General (OIG), respectively. Regardless of the type, the external auditor is independent of the organization that is being audited, and the objectives are to determine if an organization's processes and its documentation are in accordance with local, state, federal, and accrediting organization standards.

For example, TJC is an external auditor and is an independent, not-for-profit organization that accredits and certifies nearly 21,000 health care organizations and programs in the United States. TJC evaluates health care organizations to ensure they meet certain performance standards. One method of evaluation by TJC is performing onsite surveys, which focuses on continuous operational improvement in support of safe, high-quality care, treatment, and services. TJC's onsite survey includes activities such as:

- Survey-planning session.
- Opening conference and orientation to the organization.

TAKE AWAY ●·········

Audits can be done internally or externally. An *internal audit* is conducted by the organization, either by an employee of the organization or by consultants hired by the organization. An *external audit* can be conducted in a similar manner to an internal audit, but is performed by an outside party or auditor. Oftentimes, an internal audit will be performed before an external audit is.

TAKE AWAY ●·········

TJC performs onsite surveys of health care organizations to ensure they meet certain performance standards.

- Leadership session.
- Tracer methodology. The cornerstone of the TJC survey, the tracer methodology uses actual patients, residents, or individuals as the framework for assessing standards compliance.
  - Individual tracers follow the experience of care for individuals through the entire health care process.
  - System tracers evaluate the integration of related processes and the coordination and communication among disciplines and departments in those processes. The system tracers are specific time slots devoted to in-depth discussion and education regarding the use of data in performance improvement (as in core measure performance and the analysis of staffing), medication management, infection control, and other current topics of interest to the organization.
- Competence assessment process.
- Medical staff credentialing and privileging (hospitals only).
- Environment of care session, which includes a building tour.
- Exit conference, during which the survey team presents a written summary of the survey findings.

Billing Audit

One area commonly audited is the revenue cycle. Billing audits are conducted to verify that a health care organization's records are complete and in compliance with internal and external accrediting bodies and local, state, and federal government regulations. As discussed in Chapter 9, health care providers submit a claim to an insurance carrier for reimbursement, which the payer uses to review medical necessity and remit payment. The claim is the actual document representing the provider's request for reimbursement. Once charges have been submitted to insurance carriers for reimbursement, the claims are subject to audits. A billing audit is performed to determine if the services provided to a patient were medically necessary. The health care record must include a clinically documented diagnosis, which will substantiate the medical necessity of all services provided and submitted for reimbursement. The diagnoses documented must provide evidence for medical necessity for all procedures billed.

Billing audits can be done in one of two ways: concurrently or retrospectively. A **concurrent audit** is performed before the bill is generated and submitted to the insurance carrier. Concurrent audits may be done by either internal auditors or external auditors. If done externally by a clearinghouse, the audit will review claims before sending them to an insurance carrier for payment. A **retrospective audit** is performed after a bill has been submitted to the insurance carrier for payment. Similarly, retrospective audits may be performed internally or externally by a multitude of credentialing, licensing, or regulating agencies.

Billing audits compare medical records to bills submitted to insurance carriers and patients. In many instances, these audits pinpoint unbilled charges that represent unrecognized and lost income for the organization. **Unbilled charges** are services and/or procedures that have been performed by the health care providers or organization but were never billed to the insurer and/or the patient. When unbilled charges are found, the organization should consult the billing guidelines of the individual insurance carrier for a statute of limitations for submission of payment for those services. If the allotted time frame has not elapsed, the organization should submit the appropriate documentation along with explanation that the charges were omitted from the original bill in error. A standard protocol should be set for how the organization will account for unbilled charges if found after the time frame for submission. For instance, if an insurance carrier could have paid for the service but it was not submitted in a timely fashion, the charge would need to be documented as lost income. The root cause for

concurrent audit an audit performed before the bill is generated and submitted to the insurance carrier.

retrospective audit an audit performed after a bill has been submitted to the insurance carrier for payment.

unbilled charges services and/or procedures that have been performed by the health care providers or organization but were never billed to the insurer and/or the patient.

TAKE AWAY ●·········

Billing audits compare medical records to bills submitted to insurance carriers and patients.

the omission should be investigated, and corrective action should be put into place to prevent future occurrences and loss of revenue.

Billing audits may also uncover another type of error: **undocumented charges**. These are charges billed for services and/or procedures that were not documented in the patient's medical record. Billing of undocumented charges can happen due to an oversight in billing on a small scale, an employee error that would require additional training, or fraudulent behavior that should be addressed and eliminated immediately. Occurrences of undocumented charges must be corrected immediately, as it is seen as fraudulent billing practices and could lead to legal action or discipline by the OIG. When an instance of undocumented charges is found, the organization should investigate to find if it is an isolated incident or a pattern. The organization should take action to notify the appropriate insurance carrier that the incident occurred and submit necessary documentation so that a refund may be processed to return payment to the payer. Additionally, the health care organization should document the finding and the resolution for future audit purposes.

> ○ **undocumented charges** charges billed for services and/or procedures that were not documented in the patient's medical record.

Compliance Auditing

Compliance auditing is the independent assessment of whether a given organization follows guidelines issued by the applicable authorities in that business. Although an internal audit can be performed, more formal compliance audits are conducted by an individual or group of people representing an auditing organization. Compliance audits are typically carried out by assessing whether activities, transactions, and documentation comply with the guidelines issued by the authorities that govern the organization.

In health care, such compliance audits are conducted to ensure regulations and safeguards are in place to protect patients. When an external auditor reviews a health care organization, the focus is most often to review the information or documentation contained in medical records to determine if there has been fraudulent billing of patient care. If fraud or abuse is found to take place, the results could be heavy fines, loss of funding from insurance agencies, or loss of the ability to conduct business. As discussed earlier, being accredited by the TJC provides a health organization multiple benefits, such as:

- Fulfilling regulatory requirements in select states
- Providing deeming authority for Medicare certification
- Providing eligibility by insurers and other third parties for insurance reimbursement and participation in managed care plans or contract bidding

■ **LEARNING CHECKPOINT 10.1**

■ **Quality**

1. Which of CMS's quality reporting measures came first?

    a. Physician Quality Reporting System (PQRS)
    b. Quality Payment Program (QPP)
    c. Merit-based Incentive Payment System (MIPS)
    d. Advanced Alternative Payment Model (APM)

2. Who administers the Healthcare Effectiveness Data and Information Set (HEDIS)?

    a. the Centers for Medicare and Medicaid Services
    b. the National Committee for Quality Assurance (NCQA)

Continued

LEARNING CHECKPOINT 10.1—cont'd

Quality

c. The Joint Commission

d. The RAND Corporation

3. A TJC site survey is an example of an

   a. internal audit

   b. external audit

4. _____ charges are services and/or procedures that have been performed by the health care provider or organization but were never billed to the insurer and/or the patient.

   a. Unclaimed

   b. Undocumented

   c. Unbilled

   d. Retrospective

PERFORMANCE IMPROVEMENT[2]

○ **performance improvement (PI)** also known as *quality improvement (QI)* or *continuous quality improvement (CQI)*, refers to the process by which a facility reviews its services or products to ensure quality.

○ **sentinel event** an unanticipated event where death or serious injury occurs in a health care setting.

Performance improvement (PI), also known as *quality improvement* (QI), refers to the process by which an organization reviews its services or products to ensure quality. To be competitive in any marketplace, an organization should seek to improve its performance and not just simply meet a standard. PI can focus on one task or job in the overall organization or focus on a process that involves more than one department. Factors that would prompt a PI effort include changes in regulations, failure of a process to meet established standards, and sentinel events. A **sentinel event** is any unanticipated event in a health care setting resulting in death or serious physical or psychological injury to a patient or patients, not related to the natural course of the patient's illness. An example of a sentinel event is amputating the wrong limb.

The philosophy of PI is that by improving the process, the outcome, such as patient care, will ultimately be improved. The PI process begins with a formal policy on or statement of how the organization will conduct and document improvement efforts. Employees participate in teams to reach a solution to improve a process. The members of the team must be chosen for their expertise in the area being reviewed. Therefore teams are multidisciplinary and represent the active participants in the process, as well as the users of the process output. Thus a team working on improving patient registration data collection accuracy would likely include patient access staff, supervisors, medical assistants, patient financial service personnel, and clinical personnel.

Additionally, each team should have a sponsor, usually a management or administrative staff member, who can support the allocation of resources to the project, and a leader, who organizes and runs the meetings.

Meetings

When meetings are organized and managed effectively, they are an important method for bringing people and ideas together to improve performance. Meetings can be used

TAKE AWAY

PI teams are multidisciplinary and represent the active participants in the process as well as the users of the process output.

---

[2]The editors wish to acknowledge Nadinia Davis and Melissa LaCour, whose writing in *Fundamentals of Health Information Management* provides the basis for this section of the chapter.

to gather information from the people who are involved. Meetings are also used to inform and educate team members and to keep the team focused on the goal of improving the process.

In team meetings, the leader needs to foster a collaborative atmosphere. Meetings of individuals with disparate ideas and roles in the organization may result in contentious dialogue if ground rules and protocols are not clearly established. Further, individuals with strong personalities may monopolize the conversation. Therefore building a collegial team is very important to the success of the PI process.

In each PI meeting, there should be a facilitator. The team leader may also serve in this role, or another team member may be assigned the role of the team facilitator. The function of the facilitator is to keep the team focused on the goal and to ensure the team does not get sidetracked and deviate too far off course. Too much deviation or distraction in a meeting could impair the team's ability to accomplish its goal.

Performance Improvement Methods

An important tool in performance improvements is utilizing and developing a method, a framework or model that will support the way the team will conduct the project. The method not only helps the team document the PI process to support accreditation and certification standards, for example, but also provides a measure for the health care organization to monitor its efforts internally. There are a wide variety of PI methods, with many borrowed from other business industries but finding application in the health care setting. The following are some of the more commonly used methods in the health care setting.

Plan, Do, Check, and Act Method

One of the mostly commonly used methods in the health care setting for monitoring and improving performance is the **Plan, Do, Check, and Act (PDCA) method**, which was developed by Walter Shewhart. The PDCA method is easy to understand and follow (Table 10.1). The *Plan* phase consists of data collection and analysis to propose a solution for the identified problem. The *Do*, or implementation, phase tests the proposed solution. The *Check* phase monitors the effectiveness of the solution over time. The *Act* phase formalizes the changes that have proved effective in the Do and Check stages.

> ○ **Plan, Do, Check, and Act (PDCA) method** a performance improvement method with formalized steps for improving a process.

Lean Method

Although originally used in the manufacturing setting, specifically by Henry Ford in 1913 on the Model T automotive assembly line, the **lean** method has found application in health care settings. A somewhat less formal model than PDCA, the lean method,

> ○ **lean** a performance improvement philosophy that seeks to remove wastefulness from a process by constantly looking for ways to improve the way things are done.

TABLE 10.1			
PDCA METHOD			
Plan	**Do**	**Check**	**Act**
• Form a team • Identify the problem • Collect data • Discuss solutions • Concoct a plan • Project results	• Educate employees • Launch the new process • Collect data for analysis	• Analyze data • Check real results against planned/projected results • Adjust process as needed	• Change policy and establish new baseline

or "lean thinking," seeks to create value—which may be defined in this context as anything the customer would pay for—by reducing waste and wasteful activities. Lean thinking looks for ways to accomplish a task with less work and to reduce inefficiencies and thereby improve the process. Because the lean method assumes there are always ways to improve, it is a philosophy of continuous improvement. That is, the lean philosophy embraces a culture in which individuals in the organization are constantly looking for ways to improve the way things are done. This continuous improvement is expected of every member in the organization, not just managers or policy makers.

The lean PI philosophy has been adopted by health care organizations to improve many processes, including admission and discharge processes, patient scheduling, clinical processes, and coding and billing. For example, a common problem in many medical offices and health care organizations is patient wait time, or the amount of time before a patient is seen by a health care provider. Using the lean method, the team may start with monitoring a typical wait time over a certain period, such as a week or month(s). The team would set up a method to capture information related to the time each patient presents at check-in, time of recording of vital signs, time of first encounter with a health care provider, time of any key diagnostic or treatment activities, and time of departure. Using these data points trended over time and based on peak volume, as well as reason for visit, can help the PI team identify trends to alleviate wait times and improve timeliness of care to patients. Even though there are multiple, complex processes to accomplish and to provide patient care, the lean method's concept is that a waste of money, time, supplies, or goods will decrease value to both the health care organization and patients.

Six Sigma Method

Another PI method, originally developed by Motorola in 1986 but made famous by General Electric in 1995, is called the **Six Sigma** method. Six Sigma is a data-driven approach and methodology for eliminating defects (driving toward six standard deviations between the mean and the nearest specification limit) in any process, including patient care. Whereas the lean method can be thought of as a less structured approach used by an entire organization, Six Sigma is a highly regimented approach to PI, driven by specially trained individuals, called *Black Belts* and *Green Belts,* depending on their training and expertise, who guide others through a strict problem-solving method. Health care facilities that adopt this method of PI establish an organizational philosophy to systematically strive for performance improvement using an approach based on statistical analysis of performance.

Six Sigma uses different approaches to quality according to whether the facility is improving a current process or product—"DMAIC" for Define, Measure, Analyze, Improve, and Control—or creating a new process or product—"DMADV" for Define, Measure, Analyze, Design, and Verify. The basic steps for each approach are listed in Fig. 10.2.

Although a relatively new PI method to the health care industry, the Six Sigma method has been effectively used to reduce errors at any level of the patient care process, clinical or administrative.

Benchmarking Method

Benchmarking is a PI method used by one health care organization to compare performance of its processes with the same processes at another organization with noted superior performance. This method can also be used internally to compare current performance with a previous exemplary performance. By reviewing a process that is effective in another organization, the health services administrator may discover methods or processes that would improve his or her own facility and practices. Some

---

TAKE AWAY ●·········

The lean PI methodology focuses on removing wastefulness.

○ **Six Sigma** a performance improvement methodology that uses a regimented, formal structure to remove defects from a process.

○ **benchmarking** an improvement technique that compares one facility's process with that of another facility that has been noted to have superior performance.

DMAIC pronounced as "duh-may-ick"	DMADV pronounced as "duh-mad-vee" Also called DFSS – Design for Six Sigma
Used to improve existing process	Used to create a new process or product
Define the problem specifically	**Define** design goals
Measure the current process (collect data)	**Measure** and identify characteristics that are Critical To Quality (CTQ)
Analyze and investigate cause and effect relationships	**Analyze** for development and design
Improve the current process, pilot potential solutions	**Design** details
Control establish systems to monitor and maintain control of the new process	**Verify** the design, set up pilots

Figure 10.2 Two approaches for Six Sigma. (From Davis N, LaCour M. *Foundations of health information management*, ed 4, St. Louis, 2017, Elsevier.)

processes are better served by throwing out the old model or processes and starting with a best practice or a process that has been shown to be successful at another organization. The benchmarking method can provide the organization with new and better methods for accomplishing similar tasks. Additionally, benchmarking internally, against previous performance, allows the organization to compare previous practices to current ones.

Performance Improvement Tools

A wide variety of tools are used in the PI process. There are tools to organize the project and gather information, and other tools to present the information in a useful manner. Data-gathering tools help the team explore, or at least acknowledge, issues surrounding the process of concern. Organization and presentation tools make a statement about the information that is gathered. Two commonly used data-gathering tools—brainstorming and surveys—are discussed here, as well as several organization and presentation tools: bar graphs, line graphs, pie charts, decision matrices, and flowcharts. Table 10.2 contains a list of different PI tools and techniques.

Data-Gathering Tools

Brainstorming is a method in which a group of people discuss ideas, solutions, or related issues on a topic or situation. This is a data-gathering tool used to identify as many aspects, events, or issues surrounding a topic as possible. This method encourages the involvement of everyone in the group. All ideas are accepted, no matter how insignificant they may appear at the time. When brainstorming, the group should have a topic and a place to write down the ideas mentioned.

To begin the process, the team's facilitator or leader explains that the brainstorming tool is used to gather all ideas related to the issue—regardless of how unusual they may seem. For example, a PI team is organized to reduce the length of time that a patient waits to receive treatment at the medical practice. At the team's first meeting, the members brainstorm all of the possible factors that could have an impact on the patient's wait time. The team members are encouraged to mention anything that could affect this. Note that at this stage the members do not need to prove that the factors they mention actually affect the patient's wait time.

TAKE AWAY

Benchmarking is used to compare performance, either to another health care facility or to previous results from the same facility.

brainstorming a data-gathering quality improvement tool used to generate information related to a topic.

TAKE AWAY

Brainstorming is a tool for generating ideas.

TABLE 10.2

TOOLS AND TECHNIQUES FOR GATHERING AND PRESENTING DATA

Tool	Description	Example
Line graph	Shows data trends, usually over a period of time.	
Bar chart (or graph)	Compares categories of data during a single point in time.	
Pie chart	Displays the percentage each variable contributes to the whole.	
Pareto chart	Combination of bar and line chart that identifies the most common source of quality control problems. The left vertical axis indicates the frequency of an occurrence (the number of times something happened), and the right vertical axis indicates the percentage of time something occurred.	
Control chart	Displays variation in data points over time. A process is flawed when data points regularly stray outside the control limits.	
Scatter diagram	Displays relationships between variables, shows trends.	
Flowchart	Displays the process, identifies stakeholders, shows hand-offs in workflow.	

TABLE 10.2		
TOOLS AND TECHNIQUES FOR GATHERING AND PRESENTING DATA—cont'd		
Tool	**Description**	**Example**
Cause-and-effect (fishbone) chart	Displays multiple root causes of a problem and opportunities for improvement.	
Brainstorming	Rapidly generates multiple ideas, promotes buy-in of new ideas.	
Checklist	Controls data collection by reducing errors of omission	

Another commonly used data-gathering tool is a **survey**, which is a set of questions designed to gather information about a specific topic or issue. A survey can be used routinely to gather information from a group, or it can be designed as part of a PI team's efforts. Many health care organizations conduct a survey of patients after a visit to the practice. The purpose of the survey is to evaluate how the patient perceived the service and care, which can be used to measure patient satisfaction.

For example, in the previously mentioned patient waiting time example, the PI team could develop a survey to ask patients why they think it took so long to receive treatment. The questions on a survey can either be closed ended or open ended. Closed-ended questions can be answered with "Yes" or "No," or they have a limited set of possible answers (such as A, B, C, or all of the above). Closed-ended questions are often good for surveys, because they get higher response rates when users do not have to type so much. Also, answers to closed-ended questions can easily be analyzed statistically, which is commonly done with survey data. In contrast, open-ended questions are questions that allow users to give a free-form answer or answer in their own words. In open-ended questions, a richer and more qualitative response and data can be acquired. However, this method of questioning may sometimes be too broad and may not provide the necessary information to determine what improvements or changes need to be made. Table 10.3 provides an example of the same survey question asked in two different ways: open ended and closed ended.

survey a data-gathering tool for capturing the responses to queries; may be administered verbally or by written questionnaire; also refers to the activity of querying, as in "taking a survey."

Data Presentation Tools

Data organization and presentation tools are used to communicate information quickly to another person or group. Because PI is a team effort, it is important to organize information and display it so that the group can interpret or understand it quickly and accurately. Such data-presenting tools include graphs and tables. A **graph** is an illustration of data. A **table** organizes data in rows and columns. These visual tools can be quite persuasive, and positive information can be emphasized just as easily as negative information. For example, the number of cigarette-smoking freshmen on a college campus declined 40% between 2014 and 2018. However, overall smoking prevalence on the campus was virtually unchanged during that time. These data could be graphed in two different ways: the positive graph shows that the number of freshmen who smoke has decreased, and the negative graph shows that the total percentage of people who smoke remains unchanged. The positive data—the decrease in the number of

graph an illustration of the relationship between two or more variable quantities.

table a chart organized in rows and columns to organize data.

TABLE 10.3
SURVEY QUESTIONS

Open-Ended Questions	Closed-Ended Questions
How would you describe your visit to our waiting room?	Choose one of the following to describe the waiting room during your recent visit: a. Very clean b. Adequately clean c. Unclean d. Very dirty
How long did you wait in the waiting room before being called by a member of the clinical staff?	How long did you wait in the waiting room before being called by a member of the clinical staff? a. Less than 5 minutes b. 6–20 minutes c. 21–45 minutes d. Longer than 45 minutes

		Year				
		2014	2015	2016	2017	2018
Category	Number of freshmen who smoke	1299	1157	885	588	462
	Total freshmen	2095	2103	2099	2100	2098
	Percent of freshmen who smoke	62%	55%	42%	28%	22%
	Total smokers on campus	3247	3264	3254	3272	3269

A

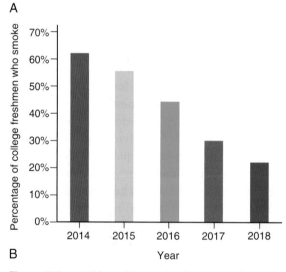

B

Figure 10.3 A, Table and B, graph of the same data. (From Davis N, LaCour M. *Foundations of health information management,* ed 4, St. Louis, 2017, Elsevier.)

TAKE AWAY ●··········

Data organization and presentation tools are used to communicate information quickly to another person or group.

freshmen who smoked from 2014 to 2018—can be plotted on a graph to show a positive trend in smoking cessation (Fig. 10.3). However, the graph can also provide a negative picture because the prevalence or overall number of people smoking on the campus remains about the same (Fig. 10.4).

Bar Graphs, Line Graphs, and Pie Charts

Bar and line graphs, also known as *charts*, relate information along the horizontal (*x* axis) and the vertical (*y* axis). In a bar graph, data are displayed for discrete elements, with one axis being used to represent the group or indicator and the other axis used to plot the data for the group. For example, Fig. 10.3 is a bar graph showing a category along the *x* axis that represents the years in which freshmen smoking was measured.

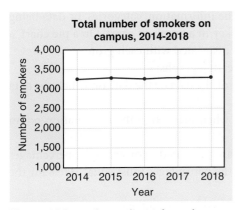

Figure 10.4 Total number of smokers on campus, 2014–2018.

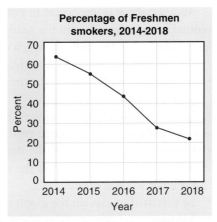

Figure 10.5 Line graph of percentage of freshmen who smoked, 2014–2018.

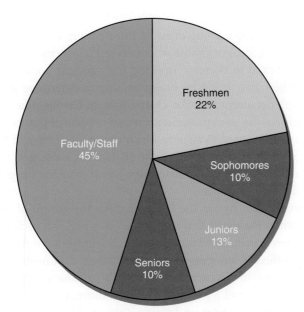

Figure 10.6 Pie chart of the percentages of different populations on campus who smoke. (From Davis N, LaCour M. *Foundations of health information management*, ed 4, St. Louis, 2017, Elsevier.)

The data plotted along the *y* axis indicate the percentage of freshmen who smoke for each year. Changing the bar graph to a line graph provides an illustration of the data points across a continuum and may display a percentage of people smoking over the course of the 5-year period. In Fig. 10.5, the bars have been replaced with points that are connected by lines. Line graphs are used to plot data over time. The line graph is an easy way to depict the trend of the same data as they are measured continuously, month to month or year to year.

A **pie chart** is a graphical illustration of information as it relates to a whole. For example, a pie chart can be used to illustrate the percentages of different populations on campus who smoke. When considering this type of chart, imagine a pie with individual pieces representing percentages. If the pie is cut into even slices, all of the pieces are equal. However, when the size of each piece represents the various smoking populations on campus, we can easily determine which group smokes the most based on sizes of the pieces (Fig. 10.6).

pie chart a graphical illustration of the percentage of data as it relates to a whole.

Additionally, it is important to note that the information, categories, or data being plotted is often described in the headings or key in a graph or chart. On a pie chart, a key might be used to indicate which color is associated with each group.

The following is a list of reminders for creating graphs:

- Include information about the time frame of the data or the date on which the data were collected.
- Make sure the graph is legible, especially when presenting the information on an overhead projector to a large group.
- Choose the best graph for the data that are presented—for example, percentages relate well on a pie chart, but the total of the percentages must equal 100% for the pie chart to be accurate.
- Be prepared to explain the graph if questioned by the audience.
- Software programs such as Microsoft Excel can simplify the creation of graphs, tables, and charts. These programs make it very easy to turn data into an easy-to-read presentation tool.

Decision Matrix

decision matrix a quality improvement tool used to narrow focus or choose between two or more related possible decisions.

A **decision matrix** can help a group organize information. This tool is used when the PI team must narrow its focus or choose among several categories or issues. For example, if a PI team is organized to decrease smoking for a patient population on a college campus, the members may begin by brainstorming to determine all the issues that influence a person's decision to smoke. Once the team has identified the factors that influence this decision, the team must decide which influential factors they can change. A decision matrix can be used to analyze which of the factors would cause a decrease in the number of smokers if removed. Table 10.4 shows a decision matrix in which each group of smokers is analyzed to determine which issue has the greatest influence on that group's decision to smoke.

First, note that the first row of the table identifies the groups of smokers and the first column identifies the issues that may influence a person's decision to smoke. To complete the decision matrix, the PI team analyzes each group according to the influences that the team identified. Team members can write their comments in the squares, or they can assign a value—in this case, 1 for least likely to influence the person to smoke, 2 for moderate influence, and 3 for most likely to influence the person to smoke. The final column on the right is a total, or decision, column. The influence with the highest rating or the influence that occurred in each of the categories would be the team's target. In this case, the first, and by far easiest, way to decrease smoking on campus would be to eliminate some of the smoking areas.

TAKE AWAY

The decision matrix weighs options to help the PI team make a choice.

Flowchart

flowchart a tool used to organize the steps involved in a process.

A **flowchart** is a tool used to organize the steps involved in a process. The flowchart provides an illustration of how a process works within the facility. It provides a sequence of movements or actions of people or things involved in a complex system or activity. Flowcharts help the team streamline a process and eliminate unnecessary steps. Flowcharts

TABLE 10.4						
DECISION MATRIX						
	Freshmen	**Sophomores**	**Juniors**	**Seniors**	**Faculty/Staff**	**Total**
Commercials	2	2	2	2	1	9
Smoking areas	3	3	3	3	3	15
Peer pressure	3	3	2	2	1	11

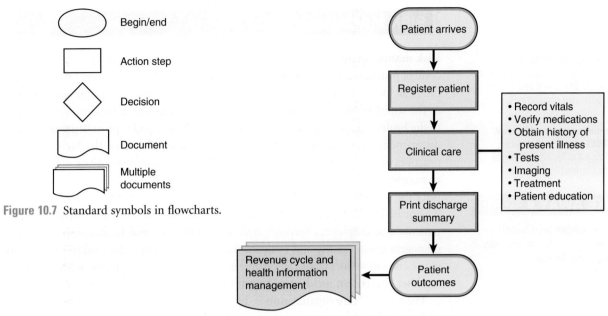

Figure 10.7 Standard symbols in flowcharts.

Figure 10.8 Patient admittance flowchart.

utilize standard symbols that are defined by the American National Standards Institute so that created flowcharts adhere to standardized symbols for universal understanding (Fig. 10.7).

Using a flowchart has a variety of benefits. It helps clarify complex processes and identifies unnecessary steps in a process, such as delays, duplicate work, added expense, and any breakdowns in communication. Flowcharts also help team members gain a shared understanding of the process and use this knowledge to collect data, identify problems, focus discussions, and identify resources. Oftentimes, flowcharts are utilized in the health care setting for medical processes or medical decision making. For example, Fig. 10.8 shows an example of a flowchart for patient admittance. By outlining the process for patient admissions by use of a flowchart, the admission process will be streamlined to improve timeliness and reduce staff stress.

◾ LEARNING CHECKPOINT 10.2
Performance Improvement

1. A(n) _____ is any unanticipated event in a health care setting resulting in death or serious physical or psychological injury to a patient or patients, not related to the natural course of the patient's illness.

2. The _____ PI methodology focuses on removing wastefulness.

3. _____ is a PI method used by the health care organization to compare performance of its processes with the same processes at another organization or with its own previous results.

4. A(n) _____ is a data presentation tool that illustrates workflow.

5. A(n) _____ is used when the PI team must narrow its focus or choose among several categories or issues.

RISK MANAGEMENT

risk management (RM) the coordination of efforts within a facility to prevent and control inadvertent occurrences.

potentially compensable event (PCE) an event that could cause the facility a financial loss or lead to litigation.

TAKE AWAY

Risk management monitors the operation for potentially compensable events (PCEs).

incident report an administrative discovery tool used by the health care organization to obtain information about a potentially-compensable event.

Risk management (RM) is the coordination of efforts within a facility to prevent and control **potentially compensable events (PCEs)**. A PCE is any event that could cause a financial loss or lead to litigation. Risk management is a TJC requirement and often one of the stipulations required by the insurance company that provides insurance coverage to the health care organization. Depending on the size and type of organization, the RM department may contain an attorney who is an employee of the facility. For smaller practices and organizations, RM may simply be the responsibility of one of the leaders or managers in the health care organization's administration. Whoever the risk manager is for the organization, the RM department or staff member must actively monitor PCEs, lead or be involved in the safety committee, and work to ensure a safe environment for patients and employees through training, education, and facility improvements. Risk managers must identify and evaluate risks as a means to reduce injury to patients, staff members, and visitors within an organization. Risk managers work proactively and reactively to either prevent an incident or to minimize the damages after an event.

Every health care organization is different and faces unique challenges; thus, RM may vary, as well as management solutions. Risk managers should develop a risk assessment plan that outlines the challenges faced by the health care organization that may include:
- Patient safety
- Mandatory federal regulations
- Potential medical errors
- Existing and future policy
- Legislation affecting the field of health care

An important function for risk managers is ensuring compliancy with documentation. The health record serves as evidence of patient-related events that occur within the facility. The patient health record includes documentation of the facts of an incident as they are related to the care of the patient. For example, if a patient is administered the wrong medication, the documentation in the patient's record would indicate the time and date of the occurrence. It would also document the medication and dosage given and any actions taken to remedy the situation.

This type of documentation in the health record is different from an **incident report**, which is completed when there is an inadvertent occurrence (Fig. 10.9). An incident report is an administrative discovery tool used by the health care organization to obtain information about the incident. The incident report is not a part of the patient's health record, nor is it mentioned in any documentation. Incident reports should be completed immediately by the supervisor, person involved, or a designee. The incident report is used to perform an investigation into the facts surrounding the incident. Facts discovered or reported after the incident can significantly affect an organization's ability to defend, prevent, or determine the cause of the incident or the liability of the parties in an incident. Examples of inadvertent occurrences that may be reported on an incident report are listed in Box 10.1.

BOX 10.1   EXAMPLES OF INADVERTENT OCCURRENCES

- An employee falls in the hallway on a slippery floor, injuring his knee.
- A visitor entering the elevator is struck by the door as it closes.
- A missing patient is found on the roof of the health care facility.

- A patient falls off the exam table; assessment of the patient found on the floor of the room reveals a broken arm.
- A nurse injures her back during transport of a large, uncooperative patient.

Incident Report

Evergreen Health

DATE OF REPORT:_____

REPORTED BY:_____

TITLE / ROLE: _____

INCIDENT INFORMATION

INCIDENT TYPE: _____

DATE OF INCIDENT:_____   TIME OF INCIDENT: _____

LOCATION OF INCIDENT: _____

DESCRIPTION OF OCCURRENCE:

POSSIBLE CAUSES OF INCIDENT:

DESCRIPTION OF INJURIES:

FIRST AID ADMINISTERED:

NAME(S) AND CONTACT INFORMATION OF PEOPLE INVOLVED:

1. _____

2. _____

3. _____

WITNESS(ES) AND CONTACT INFORMATION

1. _____

2. _____

3. _____

Supervisor name: _____

Supervisor signature: _____   Date: _____

Figure 10.9 Incident report.

The incident report should contain the following information:

- Name and contact information of the person involved
- Time, date, and location of the incident
- Description of occurrence
- Events that may have caused the incident
- Description of injuries
- First aid or treatment administered

Review of documentation by staff members may also identify a PCE. As a result, the medical record is used in risk management to gather facts surrounding an occurrence and sometimes support or defend a legal claim should the incident require litigation. It is also used in quality improvement activities to provide information to prevent future occurrences.

DISASTER MANAGEMENT

Another important function of risk management is disaster planning and management. Disaster management refers to actions taken to prevent or respond to such events and to recover the normal services of the facility as quickly as possible. Although unpleasant to think about, the reality is that catastrophic events can and do occur. Hurricanes, earthquakes, blizzards, forest fires, and other natural disasters are all possibilities in various regions of the country. Events like fire or flood may affect a single building. Terrorist and bioterrorist attacks by state-based and nonstate actors are possible anywhere. Additionally, public health outbreaks, such as influenza **epidemics**, can potentially overwhelm heath care systems. Health services administrators must evaluate and plan for each of these threats and take measures to prepare the staff and the facility in case of such an event.

epidemic a disease afflicting a community at the same time.

Planning

In disaster planning, health care organizations must take measures to secure their patient records. As discussed in Chapter 5, medical records are vital to providing efficient, quality patient care. Paper records must be kept in an area safe from the elements even in the case of a disaster, such as behind a fireproof door or in storage units that provide protection against moisture and fire. Ultimately, however, paper records are vulnerable to damage from the elements. For example, in the aftermath of Hurricane Katrina in 2005, area hospitals lost thousands of medical records during the flooding, and more were lost to mold in the ensuing weeks. This began a national effort by health information management professionals to transition to EHR technology, in which medical information is stored digitally. Practices using computer-based records should back up their information off-site daily.

TJC and other accrediting agencies require health care facilities to develop and maintain a disaster plan. Regardless of the types of disasters, the preparation can be quite similar because they often use the same types of resources. The disaster plan documents how the organization's resources will be utilized in the case of an emergency. It specifies what equipment and supplies are needed and divides the practice's staff into teams, designating a *chief* or *coordinator* to oversee the plan's execution.

Disaster planning may include having a planning committee with representatives from various departments. For example, a planning committee in a physician's office might include a member of the administrative staff, a medical assistant, a member of the nursing staff, a provider, a member of the laboratory staff, and an individual from patient reception. The committee may designate some individuals to other leadership positions. For example, it may name a safety officer to monitor safety protocols or a logistics officer to oversee supplies, equipment, and communications.

TAKE AWAY

TJC and other accrediting agencies require health care facilities to develop and maintain a disaster plan.

The disaster plan should also identify and maintain a list of community resources. This includes health departments at various levels of government, local hospitals and other providers, and nonprofit organizations, like the American Red Cross. The committee should update this list regularly.

The disaster plan itself dictates specific procedures in the event of a disaster. Each person is given assignments and responsibilities such as patient care or transportation or preparing the facility for evacuation. It designates an area of the building for the staff to gather for instructions and specifies routes of evacuation. The plan also documents how the facility will continue to operate if utilities become unavailable. For example, it lists a source of bottled water should the facility's water supply become contaminated or unavailable and the source of emergency electrical power should it become compromised. Such outages make surgical or invasive operations impossible; however, at the chief or coordinator's discretion, the health care organization may close and transfer its patients to another location.

LEARNING CHECKPOINT 10.3

Risk Management and Disaster Management

1. True or False. The incident report is part of the patient's medical record.

2. True or False. The person in charge of risk management at the facility should also be on the safety committee.

3. True or False. All facilities must have a disaster plan in place regardless of facility size.

4. True or False. The risk manager executes the disaster plan in the event of an emergency.

○ CASE STUDY

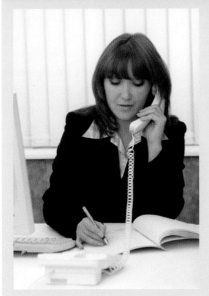

Margot reviewed all the medical records of patients at the surgical center for the past 3 months for errors that might cause delayed or denied claims. This is important not only to ensure the practice is being properly reimbursed but also to help her find and fix problems before they are identified by an external agency. The TJC has not been to her facility yet. But she knows that other surgery centers in the city have had site surveys recently, and compliance is essential for accreditation and reimbursement purposes.

Her internal audit showed that the practice was overall doing a good job with its recordkeeping. Unfortunately, the only issues she found were all from the records of one surgeon, Dr. Walsh, who joined the practice 6 months ago. On five occasions this quarter, Dr. Walsh neglected to sign his operative reports after transcription. This kind of omission would cause a claim to be rejected, resulting in lost revenue and a TJC standards violation. Margot decides to speak with Dr. Walsh about his relatively high frequency of incomplete records.

Continued

⬤ CASE STUDY—cont'd

Margot decides to create a visual aid to present her data to Dr. Walsh. She totals all the charting errors discovered during the internal audit from all the surgeons at the practice for the past 2 years, and she created the following table:

SURGEON	NUMBER OF CHARTING ERRORS	LOSS OF REVENUE
Dr. Patricia	1	$500
Dr. Daulis	0	$0
Dr. Graham	1	$500
Dr. Krashevsky	2	$1000
Dr. Walsh	11	$5500

The table indicates that Dr. Walsh is responsible for a significant number of charting errors identified during the internal audit. Margot then made a pie chart to show that he was responsible for nearly 75% of the errors and nearly 75% of the practice's lost revenue in the last 2 years, even though he had only been with the practice for 6 months.

Number of charting errors

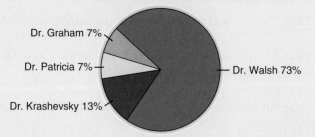

Margot braced herself for an uncomfortable conversation with Dr. Walsh, but hoped that her findings would convince him to be more careful with his recordkeeping and ultimately improve the surgery center's patient care and fiscal bottom line.

1. How can each of the six domains of quality improve patient care in an ambulatory care facility? Give an example for each domain.

2. At the retail clinic, you must reduce patient wait times. Using the PDCA method, what would you do in each step?

Match the data presentation tool with its use/description.

3. _____ Cause-and-effect (fishbone) chart

    A. Displays the percentage each variable contributes to the whole

4. _____ Line graph

    B. Displays relationships between variables, shows trends

5. _____ Bar chart (or graph)

    C. Displays the process, identifies stakeholders, shows hand-offs in workflow

6. _____ Pie chart

    D. Displays multiple root causes of a problem and opportunities for improvement

7. _____ Control chart

    E. Compares categories of data during a single point in time

8. _____ Scatter diagram

    F. Shows data trends, usually over a period of time

9. _____ Flowchart

    G. Displays variation in data points over time. A process is flawed when data points regularly stray outside the control limits.

10. How does the risk manager improve quality in the health care facility?

11. Discuss the need for disaster management and the considerations in disaster planning.

ETHICAL AND LEGAL CONCERNS

11 LEGAL ISSUES AND FRAUD IN HEALTH CARE
12 HEALTH INSURANCE PORTABILITY AND ACCOUNTABILITY ACT (HIPAA)
13 COMPLIANCE

CHAPTER 11

LEGAL ISSUES AND FRAUD IN HEALTH CARE

Deborah Proctor

CHAPTER OUTLINE

INTRODUCTION
OVERVIEW OF THE LAW
   Criminal Law
     Infractions
     Misdemeanor
     Felony
   Civil Law
     Tort Law
     Contract Law
   Administrative Law
CONSENT FOR TREATMENT
   Details Regarding Consent
MEDICAL LIABILITY AND
   MALPRACTICE
   Negligence
   Types of Damages
   Liability in a Health
     Care Facility

Liability, Malpractice, and
   Personal Injury Insurances
MEDICAL PROFESSIONAL
   LAWSUIT
   Interrogatories
   Depositions
   Subpoenas
   Inside the Courtroom
   Burden of Proof
   Verdict
   Statute of Limitations
   Mediation and Arbitration
LAWS AFFECTING THE HEALTH
   CARE FACILITY
   Patients' Bill of Rights
   Americans with Disabilities Act
   HITECH Act
   Compliance Reporting

Child Abuse Prevention and
   Treatment Act
Elder Abuse
Patient Self-Determination Act
Occupational Health and
   Safety Act
   Hazard Communication
   Ionizing Radiation
   Bloodborne Pathogens
Clinical Laboratory
   Improvement
   Amendments Act
HEALTH CARE FRAUD AND
   ABUSE
   Stark Law
   False Claims Act
   Sunshine Act
   Legal and Ethical Issues

VOCABULARY

abandonment
act
advance directive
arbitration
assault
battery
bloodborne pathogen
damages
defendant
deposition
emancipated minor

expert witness
guardian ad litem
implied contract
incompetent
informed consent
interrogatory
liable
libel
litigious
malpractice
materials safety data sheet (MSDS)

mediation
negligence
ordinance
plaintiff
respondeat superior
restitution
slander
statute
subpoena duces tecum
verdict

CHAPTER OBJECTIVES

After completing this chapter, the student should be able to do the following:

1. Compare criminal, civil, and contract law as they apply to the practicing health services administrator.
2. Explain the essential components of consent for treatment.
3. Define negligence and liability in a health care facility.
4. Describe the elements of a medical professional liability lawsuit.
5. Summarize pertinent laws that affect the health care facility.
6. Explain health care fraud and the laws designed to prevent it.

INTRODUCTION

litigious prone to engage in lawsuits.

Laws that affect health care facilities can be complex. In today's **litigious** society, health services administrators must take steps to protect themselves and their employers from lawsuits. Legal issues underlie many aspects of the provision of health care. Although the wording of laws and regulations is often long and complicated, health services administrators must be knowledgeable of the rules governing health care facilities and do everything possible to remain in compliance with the standards and regulations that oversee the medical industry.

CASE STUDY

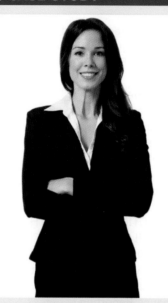

Carmen DeLotta is the new health services administrator for an urgent care facility in a suburb near where she lives. One of Carmen's first priorities at her new job is to make sure the facility complies with all laws that affect health care facilities, including the Health Insurance Portability and Accountability Act (HIPAA) and the Health Information Technology for Economic and Clinical Health Act (HITECH). She is knowledgeable about the importance of earning proper consent for treatment from patients, as well as the standards of patient care. Recently, she was subpoenaed to appear in court with medical records to testify about a patient who was seen for possible postoperative complications. The patient has brought a medical professional liability case against the surgeon who performed the procedure. Carmen is considered the custodian of medical records and will take them to court and answer questions about the information in them. As you read through this chapter, think about the interplay of law and medicine that happens every day in every medical setting. How does the health services administrator help providers follow the law?

OVERVIEW OF THE LAW

act the formal action of a legislative body; a decision or determination of a sovereign state, a legislative council, or a court of justice.

statute a law enacted by a state legislature.

ordinance authoritative decree or direction; law set forth by a governmental authority, specifically, municipal regulation.

Law is a custom or practice of a community. It is a rule of conduct or action prescribed or formally recognized as binding or enforceable by a controlling authority. The US Constitution is the supreme law of the United States. The rules established by the Constitution take priority over federal statutes, court opinions, and state constitutions. The state constitution is the supreme law within the boundaries of each state unless it conflicts with the US Constitution. States cannot pass laws that conflict with the US Constitution, nor can local governments pass laws that conflict with the state constitution.

A law enacted at the federal level, which must be passed by Congress, is called an **act**. **Statutes** are laws at the state level that have been enacted by state legislatures. Local governments create and enact **ordinances**. The two basic areas of law are criminal law and civil law, and both are important to understand in regard to health care.

Criminal Law

Criminal law governs violations of the law punishable as offenses against the state or the federal government. Such offenses involve the welfare and safety of the public as a whole rather than of one individual. There are many different types of crimes as defined by criminal law, but generally, crimes can be divided into four major categories:

- Personal crimes – "offenses against the person"
- Property crimes – "offenses against property"
- Inchoate crimes – "incomplete" crimes or crimes that were begun but not completed
- Statutory crimes – violation of a statute, rather than a common law

Many offenses constitute a personal crime, such as assault and battery. **Assault** is an intentional attempt to cause bodily harm to another. A threat to cause harm is an assault if it is combined with a physical action, such as a raised fist, so that the victim has a reason to assume there will be an assault. **Battery** is an intentional act of contact with another that causes harm or offends the individual being touched or injured. In health care, battery occurs when there is a violation of the patient's right to choose the treatments that affect his or her own body, such as when a treatment is performed without consent or against the patient's wishes. A health services administrator should become familiar with the different types of crimes under criminal law, especially in regard to health care and when managing staff.

In addition, criminal offenses are further classified into three general categories: infractions, misdemeanors, and felonies.

Infractions

An infraction, sometimes called a *petty offense,* is a violation of an administrative regulation, an ordinance, a municipal code, and, in some jurisdictions, a state or local rule. Infractions are often punishable by a fine and do not result in jail time. As a result, the offender does not have the right to a jury trial. The offender may hire an attorney, but the government does not have to appoint one. In some states, infractions are not considered violations of criminal law but of civil law. Examples of infractions are traffic violations, disturbing the peace, and fishing without a license.

Misdemeanor

A minor crime is called a *misdemeanor,* which is more serious than an infraction but less serious than a felony. Depending on the state and jurisdiction, misdemeanors may be further categorized into three classes: high or gross misdemeanors, ordinary misdemeanors, and petty misdemeanors. They are tried in the lowest local court such as municipal, police, or justice courts. Typical misdemeanors include petty theft, disturbing the peace, simple assault and battery, or drunk driving without injury to others. Punishment for misdemeanors can include payment of a fine; community service; **restitution**, which requires an offender to repay money or donate services to the victim or society; probation; and jail time. If convicted of a misdemeanor, individuals may spend up to a year in jail.

Felony

A felony is the most serious and major of violations of criminal law. Felonies often involve serious physical harm (or threat of harm), murder, rape, or burglary. Felonies also include offenses like white-collar crimes and fraud schemes, such as tax evasion, embezzlement, and identity theft. Many states divide felonies into subgroups or degrees, such as first degree, second degree, and third degree. A first-degree offense is generally the most serious. For federal felony offenses, each felony is assigned to one of 43 "offense levels," and each defendant is placed in one of six "criminal history categories." The category dictates the imposed sentence.

A felony charge can end with imprisonment for one or more years or even death for more serious crimes. An individual convicted of a felony may lose the right to vote; may not be employed in certain professions, such as teachers, social workers, and health care providers; are not allowed certain types of licenses, such as a medical license; and cannot buy or carry firearms.

assault an intentional attempt to cause bodily harm to another.

battery an intentional act of contact with another that causes harm or offends the individual being touched or injured.

restitution under criminal law, state programs that require an offender to repay money or donate services to the victim or society.

Civil Law

plaintiff the person or group bringing a case or legal action to civil court.

defendant a person required to answer in a legal action or suit; in criminal cases, the person accused of a crime.

Civil law is concerned with acts that are not criminal in nature but involve relationships with other individuals, organizations, or government agencies. In civil law, a party who seeks court intervention in a dispute is called a **plaintiff**. Conversely, the individual required to answer the legal action is called the **defendant**. Many types of civil law exist to address numerous issues. The three that most directly affect the medical profession are tort law, contract law, and administrative law.

Tort Law

Tort law provides a remedy for a person or group that has been harmed by the wrongful acts of others (Fig. 11.1). Tort law decides whether a person should be held liable for injury against another and what type of compensation the injured party is entitled to as a result of the injury. Four elements must be established in every tort action: (1) the plaintiff must establish that the defendant was under a legal duty to act in a particular fashion; (2) the plaintiff must demonstrate that the defendant, or *tortfeasor,* breached this duty by failing to conform his or her behavior accordingly; (3) the plaintiff must prove that the breach of the legal duty caused some injury or damage; and (4) the plaintiff must prove damages, the injury or loss suffered.

The three main types of torts are strict liability torts, intentional torts, and negligence (unintentional) torts. *Strict liability torts* are when a defendant places another person in danger, for example, based on the possession of a dangerous product, animal, or

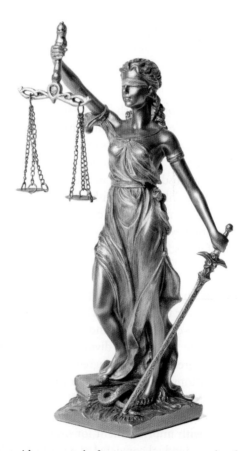

Figure 11.1 Tort law provides a remedy for a person or group that has been harmed by the wrongful acts of others. Statues representing Justice often depict her with scales to weigh the arguments of each side and a sword symbolizing authority. She is usually blindfolded to signify impartial judgment without prejudice.

weapon. The defendant is responsible for things that may go wrong even if the defendant did not intend for the wrong to occur. For example, if an individual has a Bengal tiger as a pet and the tiger accidently escapes and attacks another individual, the tiger's owner is liable for any damages. *Intentional torts* are acts that are intended to cause another person physical or nonphysical harm. There are many different types of intentional torts, such as assault and battery, false imprisonment, fraud, invasion of privacy, and conversion (theft). Defamation is another example of an intentional tort where a false statement, either written or spoken, harms a person's reputation; decreases the respect in which a person is held; or creates negative opinions toward another person. **Libel** (written) and **slander** (oral) are acts that fall into the category of defamation. A **negligence** *tort*, also called *unintentional tort*, occurs when an individual or party injures another party as a result of an action or inaction. Negligence torts are the most common types of torts and result from a breach of duty that causes harm to another party or a failure to act in a reasonable manner. Medical professional liability, or medical **malpractice**, is a common type of negligence tort. Medical malpractice occurs when a physician or health care provider fails to meet the standard of care as dictated by his or her profession or the medical industry. Medical malpractice is further discussed later in this chapter.

Contract Law

A contract is an agreement that creates an obligation. Contract law touches our lives practically every day, but we usually do not give much thought to its influences. If a person parks a car in a parking garage for a monthly fee and signs a contract for a year, even if the person begins parking elsewhere and refuses to pay the fee, the person may be liable for the fees for the duration of the entire contract. Further, if the person's vehicle is damaged while parked in the garage, the garage may be responsible for reimbursement, unless the contract states no responsibility for damages.

Contract law has many applications in health care. There may be written or oral (or verbal) contracts between the patient and the physician, health care provider, or health care facility. Written contracts may include an informed consent form, advance health care directive, and a Do Not Resuscitate lower. Although the patient may complete many forms before he or she is accepted by the provider, they often do not constitute a formal contract. Oral contracts also are valid in many states. An example of an oral contract is when the front office administrator in the health care facility makes an appointment for a new patient visit. Simply by scheduling that first appointment, the patient and provider are now in an oral contract for the provider to care for the patient and for the patient to comply with treatment protocols and payment of services. Box 11.1 lists the elements of a valid contract.

The provider–patient relationship is generally held by courts to be a contractual relationship that is the result of three steps:

- The provider invites an offer by establishing availability, such as by posting office hours.
- The patient accepts the appointment and makes an offer by arriving for or requesting treatment.
- The provider accepts the patient's offer by examining the patient and beginning treatment.

Before accepting a patient, the physician or health care provider is under no obligation to the patient and, thus, no contract exists. However, once the provider has accepted the patient, an **implied contract** exists. In this case, an implied contract assumes that the provider will treat the patient using reasonable standards of care and that the provider has a degree of knowledge, skill, and judgment that might be expected of any other provider in the same locality and specialty. It is extremely important that no express promise of a cure be made by a health care provider or staff member in the medical office because this would become a part of the contract.

libel A written remark that injures another's reputation or character.

slander a false spoken statement that injures another's reputation or character.

negligence the failure to behave in the manner of a reasonably prudent person acting under similar circumstances; it falls below the standards of conduct established by law for the protection of others against unreasonable risk of harm.

malpractice the failure of a physician to meet the standard of care as dictated by his or her profession or the medical industry.

implied contract a contract that lacks a written record or verbal agreement, but is assumed to exist.

BOX 11.1   WHAT CONSTITUTES A VALID CONTRACT?

A valid legal contract has four essential elements.

1. Mutual understanding and *agreement* on the intent of the contract.
2. The contract must involve something that is *legal*.

3. Both parties must be legally *competent*.
4. *Consideration* must be involved; consideration is an exchange of something of value (e.g., money) for the provider's time.

After the provider–patient relationship has been established, the provider is obligated to provide medical care to the patient until the care is no longer needed or the provider or patient terminates the contract. When a provider terminates the contract, the patient must be given notice of the provider's intentions so that the patient has sufficient time to secure another health care provider. The provider must write a letter of withdrawal of medical care from the patient, and it should be delivered by certified mail and return receipt requested. A copy of the letter and the return receipt should be included in the patient's medical record. Reasonable time should be allowed for the patient to secure other medical care, which is generally 15 to 30 days. During this time, the provider must continue providing emergency care and prescription refills.

In health care, the term **abandonment** means to discontinue medical care without proper notice after accepting a patient. Patient abandonment is considered a negligence tort. To protect the provider against a lawsuit for abandonment, the details of the circumstances under which the provider is withdrawing from the case should be included in the patient's medical record. To specify the withdrawal of care, a letter should be sent to the patient that includes a brief reason for withdrawal of care, such as missing appointments or failing to comply with treatment orders. The letter should also state the following:

- That professional care is being discontinued as of a particular date
- That the provider will supply copies of the patient's records to another provider on request
- That the patient should seek the medical services of another provider as soon as possible

The patient's responsibility in the physician–patient contract or agreement includes the liability of payment for received services and a willingness to follow the advice of the provider. A patient who wants to terminate the provider–patient relationship simply no longer seeks the provider for treatment. The patient does not have to inform the provider or the medical office; however, the office manager or provider should follow up with a confirmation letter, stating that the patient has ended the relationship.

A breach of contract occurs if there is a failure to perform any term of a contract, written or oral, without a legitimate legal excuse. For example, if a general surgeon performs an appendectomy on a patient but does not provide postoperative care, then a breach of contract exists.

Administrative Law

Administrative law involves regulations set forth by governmental agencies. For example, the Internal Revenue Service (IRS) has thousands of regulations and codes. The laws that allow the IRS to collect taxes and pursue restitution are administrative laws. Other examples of administrative laws that govern health care and the health care delivery system are the Health Insurance Portability and Accountability Act of 1996 (HIPAA), which helps regulate the electronic medical record, and the Occupational Safety and Health Administration (OSHA), which creates and enforces workplace safety regulations.

○ **abandonment** to withdraw protection or support; in medicine, to discontinue medical care without proper notice after accepting a patient.

LEARNING CHECKPOINT 11.1
Overview of the Law

1. Once the provider has accepted the patient, a(n) _____ contract exists.

2. An intentional act of contact with another that causes harm or offends the individual being touched or injured is called _____.

3. Tort law is a type of _____ law.

4. When a provider ceases a patient's medical care without proper notice, it is called _____.

CONSENT FOR TREATMENT

A provider must have consent to treat a patient, even though this consent usually is implied by the patient's appearance at the facility for treatment. This *implied consent* is sufficient for common or simple procedures generally understood to involve little risk. However, all heath care employees should ask the patient's permission to perform procedures, even noninvasive ones such as taking vital signs. You can achieve this by using expressed consent. *Expressed consent,* sometimes known as *general consent,* is consent given after the patient is asked a question, such as "Can I ask you some questions about your medical history?" If the patient replies "Yes," you have been given expressed consent to perform that procedure.

When more complex procedures are involved, the provider must obtain the patient's **informed consent**, which is the voluntary agreement, usually written, for treatment after being informed of the procedure's purpose, methods, benefits, and risks (Fig. 11.2). A provider who fails to secure consent could be charged with the crime of battery. A case for battery can be established if an individual is physically harmed or injured or if an illness occurs because of the contact. Battery may also occur if there is no physical harm but an act is considered offensive or insulting to the victim, such as touching a person without consent. If the patient refuses to consent to treatment and the treatment is performed anyway, the patient can then sue for battery.

informed consent voluntary agreement, usually written, for treatment after being informed of its purpose, methods, procedures, benefits, and risks.

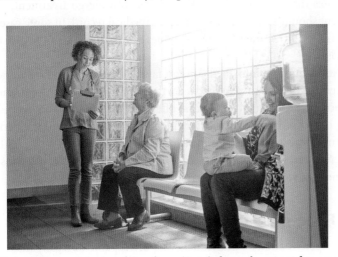

Figure 11.2 A medical assistant explains the written informed consent form to a patient.

Informed consent involves a full explanation of the plan for treatment, including the potential for complications, risks, and side effects. Informed consent is not satisfied merely by having the patient sign a form. A discussion must occur during which the provider gives the patient or the patient's legal representative enough information to decide whether the patient will undergo the treatment or seek an alternative. No other member of the medical staff, such as the health services administrator, may legally provide the information for the patient about informed consent. It is the provider's responsibility to make sure that each patient understands the treatment or procedure and answers all questions satisfactorily before the patient signs a consent form. However, the health services administrator can serve as a witness to the patient signing the document.

According to the American Medical Association, the provider's discussion with the patient about informed consent should include the following elements:

- Patient's diagnosis, if known
- Nature and purpose of the proposed treatment or procedure
- Risks and benefits of the proposed treatment or procedure
- Alternative treatments or procedures, regardless of the cost or the extent to which the treatment options are covered by health insurance
- Risks and benefits of the alternative treatment(s) or procedure(s)
- Risks and benefits of not receiving or undergoing a treatment or procedure

The discussion should be fully documented in the patient's medical record, along with a copy of the signed consent form. Treatment may not exceed the scope of the consent that the patient has given. Often consent forms are lengthy and mention excessive possibilities and complications. Some language may attempt to be all inclusive—for example, "included, but not limited to"—when risks are listed. It is wise to have an attorney review the forms used for informed consent—those that are too broad or too specific may cause the provider to be vulnerable to a medical professional liability case.

Patients cannot be forced to undergo any type of medical treatment or care. The ultimate decision about care must be left to the patient or the legal guardian. Although health care providers should disclose as much information as possible to help the patient make a sound, informed decision, the patient should never be persuaded to act in any manner or accept any treatment with which he or she does not agree.

After consideration, the patient either consents to the proposed treatment and signs a consent form or refuses to consent to the treatment. Should the patient decide not to undergo treatment the provider feels is necessary, the patient should sign an informed refusal of treatment form. This should be a statement similar to the informed consent, but it indicates that the patient has elected not to undergo treatment. Once signed, this document should be added to the patient's medical record. In some cases, a provider may discontinue all treatment if a patient does not participate in the care the provider recommends.

Each state has its own informed consent laws. Some states and insurance programs require a certain period to pass between the signing of the consent and the actual medical procedure. For instance, Medicaid often requires a 30-day waiting period between the signing of an informed consent form for a tubal ligation and the performance of the procedure. Health services administrators should become familiar with the laws in their respective states that apply to their particular health care facility. Most of the laws can be found easily by an Internet search.

Details Regarding Consent

Mentally competent adults—individuals who are capable of legally making their own decisions—can give consent to medical procedures. However, if the procedure is unlawful, the consent is invalid. For example, a provider cannot prescribe medical marijuana for a patient who gives consent for the treatment unless it is legal to do so in that state. Consent is also invalid if it is given by a person who is unauthorized to do so or if it is obtained by misrepresentation or fraud. For example, an adult child cannot give consent for a parent's treatment unless that parent has been declared **incompetent**, meaning that the individual is not able to manage his or her affairs due to a mental deficiency.

If a person is confused and unable to understand informed consent, a court of law would need to declare the person mentally incompetent and appoint a guardian to give consent for treatment. If this is the case, the only medical care that can be given without the guardian's consent is emergency treatment. The patient's ability to give informed consent can also be compromised if he or she is receiving pain medication or under the influence of alcohol or drugs. If the patient is not able to pay attention to the details of the procedure, as well as the risks and the alternatives to treatment, then it is impossible for the patient to give "informed" consent.

Generally, when the patient is a minor, consent for surgery or treatment must be obtained from a parent, guardian, or **guardian ad litem** (a court-appointed guardian), except in an emergency that requires immediate treatment. If the parents are legally divorced or separated, consent should be obtained from the custodial parent. In the case of joint custody or the child is visiting the second parent, consent may be obtained from that parent because, in such a situation, that parent has temporary custody.

Consent is not required for minors in the following circumstances:
- When consent may be assumed, such as in a life-threatening situation
- When a court order has been issued, as in a situation in which parents withhold consent for a necessary treatment because of religious reasons

In many states, even if there are consent laws, providers can still treat minors for sexually transmitted infections (STIs), drug abuse, alcohol dependency, pregnancy, or providing contraceptive methods without parental consent.

An area of potential confusion regarding consent to treatment is the *mature minor doctrine*, which allows minors to give consent to medical procedures if they can show that they are mature enough to make a decision on their own. Although it is only recognized in a few states, the mature minor doctrine has been applied in cases where the minor is 16 years or older and demonstrates understanding of the consequences of the proposed medical treatment or procedure. However, under the mature minor doctrine, the minor is still under the legal custody of a parent(s) or guardian.

Another exception to the need for parental consent is if the individual is an **emancipated minor**. An emancipated minor is a minor who is legally discharged or separated from the care and responsibility of his or her parents. There are a number of ways that a minor may become legally emancipated. The most common way is when the minor reaches the age of majority, usually 18 years of age. Eligibility for emancipation varies depending on state laws; however, it can be sought by those younger than the age of majority who meet one or more of the following conditions:
- Married
- In the armed forces
- Living separately and apart from parents or a legal guardian
- Self-supporting

Unless state law declares otherwise, an emancipated minor has the right to consent to treatment and the right to complete patient confidentiality, even from his or her parents.

incompetent refers to a person who is not able to manage his or her affairs due to mental deficiency (lack of IQ, deterioration, illness, or psychosis) or sometimes physical disability; the individual cannot comprehend the complexities of a situation and therefore cannot provide informed consent.

guardian ad litem an individual who is assigned by the court to be legally responsible for protecting the well-being and interests of a ward, typically a minor or a person who has been declared legally incompetent.

emancipated minor a person under the age of majority (usually 18) who has been legally separated from his or her parents by the courts; is responsible for their own care.

LEARNING CHECKPOINT 11.2
Consent for Treatment

1. What is a guardian ad litem?

   a. an emancipated minor
   b. a grandparent
   c. a parent
   d. a guardian appointed by the court

2. If a provider treats a patient without consent, what is the crime?

   a. battery
   b. assault
   c. malfeasance
   d. malpractice

3. Who provides information to the patient about the procedure?

   a. the health services administrator
   b. the medical assistant
   c. patient access staff
   d. the provider

MEDICAL LIABILITY AND MALPRACTICE

damages Money that is awarded by a court to an individual who has been injured through the wrongful conduct of another party.

As discussed earlier, when a patient is injured as a result of a provider's negligence, the patient may initiate a malpractice lawsuit to recover financial **damages**. Medical professional liability, or medical malpractice, occurs when a physician or health care provider treats a patient in a way that does not meet the medical standard of care and, as a result, the patient suffers harm.

Negligence

Medical malpractice may result from negligence, which, as discussed earlier, is an inattention to one's duty or business, or the implication of a lack of necessary diligence or care. In medicine, negligence is defined as the performance of an act that falls below the standards of care or behavior established by law or the failure to perform an act that a reasonable and prudent provider would do in a similar situation.

> **TAKE AWAY**
>
> Negligence does not occur any time a provider makes an error, but rather when the provider's performance does not meet professional standards of care.

Negligence is not presumed, but it must be proven. Box 11.2 lists the "Four D's" of negligence.

The standard of care and conduct is not defined by law but is left to the determination of a judge or jury, often with the help of *expert witnesses*. **Expert witnesses** are members of the profession involved—in this case, medicine—and usually belong to a certifying or qualifying organization, against which the defendant's qualities may be compared. Professional negligence in medicine falls into one of three general classifications:

expert witness one who provides testimony to a court as an expert in a certain field or subject to verify facts presented by one or both sides in a lawsuit.

- *Malfeasance:* Intentionally doing something either legally or morally wrong. For example, a physician performs a surgery for higher insurance payment when the patient could be treated with nonsurgical methods such as medication.
- *Misfeasance:* Performing an act that is legal but not properly performed. For example, the surgeon performs abdominal surgery that is indicated and necessary, but does

---

BOX 11.2   THE FOUR D'S OF NEGLIGENCE

The American Medical Association's Committee on Medicolegal Problems has determined that patients must present evidence of four elements before negligence has been proven. These elements have become known as the "four D's of negligence":

1. *Duty:* Duty exists when the provider–patient relationship has been established. Providers have a duty to provide the most accurate diagnosis and care and the duty to inform patients of potential problems the provider observes.
2. *Dereliction:* Dereliction refers to the failure of a provider to perform his or her duty; there must be proof that the provider neglected the duty.
3. *Direct cause:* The patient must prove that the provider was aware of potential risks but did not inform the patient and, as a result, the patient was injured.
4. *Damages:* If negligence is proven, the patient can collect financial compensation, which might include payment for lost wages, medical expenses, and emotional distress.

If all four of these elements exist, the patient may obtain a judgment against the provider in a medical professional liability case.

---

not do it under sterile procedures and the patient dies from complications for an infection that could have been avoided.

- *Nonfeasance:* Failure to perform an act that should have been performed. For example, there are diagnostic indications that a patient has a tubal pregnancy but the physician opts not to perform laparoscopic surgery to remove the tube.

What if the patient makes his or her condition worse? Perhaps the patient does not take the medicine prescribed or refuses to schedule surgery as recommended by the physician. Is the provider responsible for the bad outcome? *Contributory negligence* exists when the patient contributes to his or her own condition, and it can lessen the damages that can be collected or even prevent them from being collected altogether.

Types of Damages

Five types of damages are common in tort cases: nominal, punitive, compensatory, general, and special damages. The patient must prove that harm occurred due to the actions or lack of action of the provider.

Nominal damages are small awards that are token compensations for the invasion of a legal right in which no actual injury was suffered. For instance, if an unauthorized medical facility employee accesses a patient's health record and is discovered but has not revealed any of the information in the record, the patient has not actually been harmed but may be awarded nominal damages in a lawsuit for the invasion of the patient's privacy.

Punitive damages are designed to punish the party who committed the wrong in such a way so as to deter repetition of the act; these are sometimes called *exemplary damages.* These damages were historically set so that the amounts would discourage intentional wrongdoing, misconduct, and outrageous behavior. The amount of damages awarded is based on the wealth of the defendant. A specific monetary figure—for example, $500,000—has been suggested as a limit on punitive damages; some believe that plaintiffs should be allowed to collect only up to three times the amount of compensatory damages. Some states have passed legislation that caps one or more of the categories of damages.

Compensatory damages are designed to compensate for any actual damages caused by the negligent person. They are intended to make the injured person "whole." Of course, nothing can substitute for the loss of an arm or a leg, for example, but compensatory damages help the patient or the family recover from the loss.

General damages include compensation for pain and suffering, for loss of a bodily member or faculty, for disfigurement, or for other similar direct losses or injuries. The loss or damage must be proven, but the monetary value or amount does not need to be.

Special damages are awarded for injuries or losses that are not a necessary consequence of the provider's negligent act or omission. These may include the loss of earnings or costs of travel. The loss or damage must be proven, as well as the monetary value or amount.

Take Learning to the Next Level ·····················

Some states allow juries to award punitive damages in medical malpractice and professional liability cases, whereas other states limit punitive damages or place caps on the amount that may be awarded. Why do you think this is a controversial topic? What are the arguments for and against punishing medical professionals with punitive damages?

Liability in a Health Care Facility

respondeat superior legal doctrine stating health care providers are responsible for the actions of employees acting within the scope of their employment duties.

Under the doctrine of **respondeat superior,** the health care providers are legally responsible for employees acting within the scope of their employment duties. *Respondeat superior* is a Latin term meaning "let the master answer." Regarding health care, this principle means that the physician or employer is legally responsible for the actions of his or her employees—including health services administrators—when they are performing duties as outlined in their job descriptions. For example, although the health services administrator is liable for his or her own actions, the injured party generally sues the physician or employer because the chance of collecting damages is greater and because they are ultimately responsible for the actions or inactions of their employees. However, all health care professionals, regardless of their financial worth, can be held liable for negligent acts. This fact illustrates the continuing importance of exercising extreme care in performing all duties in the health care environment. All health care professionals must act ethically, legally, and professionally according to the responsibilities associated with their position.

TAKE AWAY ●·········

All health care professionals, regardless of their financial worth, can be held liable for negligent acts.

Liability, Malpractice, and Personal Injury Insurances

There are several different types of insurances that individual providers and health care facilities typically purchase. Health services administrators may be involved in researching, selecting, or renewing these insurance policies for their employers. The types of insurance available are:

- *Liability insurance* protects the health care facility if there is an accident in the facility that causes bodily injury or property damage. For example, if a patient falls in the parking lot of the facility and suffers a broken arm, liability insurance will cover this injury and protect the facility from financial loss.
- *Medical malpractice insurance* protects the provider and/or health care facility if there is a judgment against them for medical negligence, malfeasance, or malpractice. The majority of states require that providers have some form of medical malpractice insurance to protect them from legal action and lawsuits. The provider can either choose individual coverage or be part of a policy that incorporates the medical

practice or health care facility where the provider is employed. The premiums for malpractice insurance are determined by the provider specialty, with the insurance rate based on the probability of medical malpractice occurring. For example, orthopedic surgeons have higher premiums—due to the nature of their specialty and the increased risk of patient complications—than a primary care provider. Additionally, malpractice insurance rates vary according to the location of the medical facility. For example, malpractice rates are higher in the Northeast than they are in the Midwest states.

- *Personal injury insurance* covers both bodily harm and nonphysical, noneconomic harm. Examples of nonphysical harm are defamation (libel and slander), discrimination, and invasion of privacy, all of which may cause psychological harm or damage to the individual's reputation.

LEARNING CHECKPOINT 11.3
Medical Liability or Malpractice

1. The physician's assistant (PA) at the retail clinic failed to recognize signs that Carey had Lyme disease. Carey sued once the disease progressed, and the jury awarded $100,000 in _____ damages to make up for lost wages.

2. The type of negligence committed by the PA is _____.

3. The discharge instructions state that the physician ordered the patient to report to an emergency department if she experienced shortness of breath. The patient committed _____ negligence.

MEDICAL PROFESSIONAL LAWSUIT

Medical professional liability suits are far from rare, and every provider faces the risk of being sued during his or her career. The health care administrator may be involved in preparing documents for court and scheduling or participating in depositions. Attorneys will also help prepare the defense of the provider and the medical staff. If a medical lawsuit occurs, all employees of the medical staff should be truthful and present an accurate and complete statement to the representing attorney.

Interrogatories

Before the trial, the provider may be asked to complete an **interrogatory**, which is a list of questions from one party to the other in the lawsuit. Answers to the interrogatory must be provided within a specified time, and the answers are considered to be given under oath. Only the parties named in the lawsuit may be questioned through interrogatories.

interrogatory a list of questions from one party to the other in the lawsuit.

Depositions

A **deposition** is an oral testimony of a party or witness in a civil or criminal proceeding taken before trial. A witness who is not a party to the lawsuit may be summoned by subpoena for a deposition. A deposition is taken in the presence of a court reporter and under oath. The transcribed deposition is sent to the witness for review with the right to request changes or corrections in the document before it goes into the record.

deposition an oral testimony of a party or witness in a civil or criminal proceeding taken before trial.

Depositions are a *discovery* tool, which is the pretrial disclosure of pertinent facts or documents by one or both parties to a legal action or proceeding. The patient's medical record is often part of discovery requests because the record includes all pertinent data about the patient's care, such as diagnostic reports, progress notes, surgical records, and any communication between the provider and patient. Many states have extensive discovery statutes that require each side to reveal to the other the facts that they "discover" while investigating the case.

Subpoenas

A subpoena is a document issued by a court that requires a person to be present at a specific time and place to testify as a witness in a lawsuit, either in a court proceeding or in a deposition. A **subpoena duces tecum** is a court order to produce specific documents or records. This type of subpoena does not require the person named in it to give testimony at a deposition or trial.

In medical practice, a *subpoena duces tecum* is typically ordered for patient records needed in a malpractice lawsuit. The health care facility may charge a fee for the time spent in compiling the records and for photocopying charges. This fee must be requested at the time the *subpoena duces tecum* is served, or it is considered to be waived. Original records should never be released under any circumstances. If an original record is demanded in the subpoena, it usually is taken to court or to mediation by the provider or an employee of the provider's office. Copies can be released in advance of the court date. Release only the information requested in the subpoena, and provide only information that originated in the provider's office. Do not provide records sent from previous or consulting providers. Those records must be subpoenaed separately.

Before responding to a subpoena, make sure it is valid. Although variances may occur from state to state, some general rules can be used to judge the validity of a subpoena:

- A subpoena issued in one state court generally is not valid in another state. Always verify the state in which the subpoena was issued.
- A subpoena issued by a federal court in one state generally is not valid in another state unless a federal statute authorizes nationwide service of process.
- Any duly authorized law officer may execute a valid subpoena anywhere in the same state. The officer notifies the issuing court once the subpoena has been served.
- Generally, the person or entity subpoenaed has 21 days to respond, but this period may vary depending on the state and court.
- A *subpoena duces tecum* should be filed no less than 15 days before a trial. One served less than 15 days before a trial should not be honored.

Read the subpoena carefully to determine exactly what records are requested. The provider should always be notified of subpoenas served to the medical facility. Never copy records required in a subpoena without bringing the matter to the attention of the provider. It is also advisable to keep a log of subpoenas served to the office, what records were involved, and the disposition of the request, including when the records were presented to the court. Always inform the provider about the subpoena; the provider may want to present the document to an attorney for review before any information is released.

Inside the Courtroom

Knowing the role of each person in a court of law can be helpful. The person or party bringing the lawsuit to court is referred to by different terms, depending on the type of case. In a criminal court, the government brings the case and is represented by a prosecutor. In civil court, the person or group bringing the case to court is called the *plaintiff* (or *complainant* in some court systems), and the opposite or opposing party is called the *defendant* or *tortfeasor*. A judge presides over the case, giving instructions concerning the law to the jury, if a jury is present. If no jury is present, the judge decides the verdict of the case; this is called a *bench trial*.

Burden of Proof

In a criminal case the burden of proof is on the prosecution, which must prove guilt beyond any reasonable doubt. Reasonable doubt is defined as the level of certainty a juror must have to find a defendant guilty of a crime. It is based on reason and common sense after careful and impartial consideration of all the evidence, or lack of evidence, in a case.

Conversely, civil cases must be proven by a preponderance of the evidence. This means that the greater weight of evidence must point to the defendant as being responsible for the act involved in the case.

Verdict

Once both sides have presented their case to the judge or jury, they usually are given the opportunity to present a final summation of their case. The jury then retires to consider the **verdict**, which is the jury's decision in the case. In a bench trial where there is no jury, the judge's decision is called a *finding*, not a verdict. A verdict can take minutes, hours, days, or weeks. After the jury reaches a decision (Fig. 11.3), the judge may enter it as a final verdict or may disregard it if the evidence does not support the jury's decision. The judge may also revise the verdict to comply with statutes, such as statutory limits on the amount of punitive damages. The final decision of the trial court is reflected in the judgment, signed by the judge.

verdict the finding or decision of a jury on a matter submitted to it in trial.

Statute of Limitations

A statute of limitations is a period after which a lawsuit cannot be filed. The statute of limitations for medical malpractice issues varies from state to state, ranging from 1 to 5 years. Most states have a separate deadline for minors in medical malpractice cases. To research the limitations for minors in your state, refer to the National Conference of State Legislatures at http://www.ncsl.org/research/financial-services-and-commerce/medical-liability-malpractice-statutes-of-limitation.aspx.

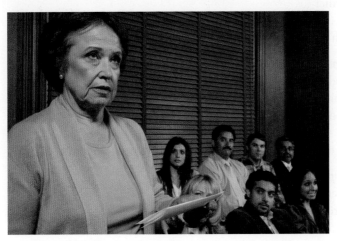

Figure 11.3 The jury foreperson announces the verdict.

The statute of limitations may be extended because of a delay in the discovery of an injury. For example, a patient has surgery to replace a heart valve, and the surgery appeared to be successful. One year later, the patient undergoes a routine echocardiogram, and the provider discovers that the valve was not implanted properly by the surgeon. Although it has been over a year since the surgery, the statute of limitations begins at the point of discovery of the injury; therefore the patient could now bring a lawsuit against the surgeon for the error.

Mediation and Arbitration

mediation a type of alternative dispute resolution involving the use of a neutral third party, called the mediator, to help those involved in a dispute come to a solution.

Before going to trial, the two parties may agree to Alternative Dispute Resolution (ADR), which refers to a variety of processes that help parties resolve disputes without a trial. *Mediation* and *arbitration* are two examples of ADR that share the goal of avoiding litigation in court. In **mediation**, a neutral third party, the mediator, helps those involved in a dispute come to an agreed-upon solution. The mediator facilitates the parties' decisions by helping them communicate and move through the more difficult parts of their differences in search of a compromise. Once the parties reach a solution, a final settlement agreement is signed. Successful mediation enables the parties to design and retain control of the process at all times and, ideally, come to a solution that meet both parties' needs.

arbitration a type of alternative dispute resolution that provides parties to a controversy with a choice other than going to court for resolution of a problem.

Arbitration is an alternative to trial in which a third party, an arbitrator, is chosen to hear evidence and make a decision about a case. The patient and the provider both have the opportunity to agree on who will arbitrate the case so that one side is not favored over the other. The arbitrator renders a legally binding decision based on highly specific rules.

Many providers and attorneys see mediation and arbitration as an effective way to solve the crisis of litigation in this country. Court battles can take years and can be extremely expensive, and much of the money reverts to the attorneys rather than the victors in the lawsuit.

LEARNING CHECKPOINT 11.4
Medical Professional Lawsuit

1. During which stage of trial is a deposition given?

   a. arbitration
   b. discovery
   c. mediation
   d. verdict

2. Which type of trial does not use a jury?

   a. bench trial
   b. mediation
   c. arbitration
   d. all of these

3. What order demands that medical records are brought to court?

   a. *subpoena duces tecum*
   b. interrogatory
   c. burden of proof
   d. all of these

LAWS AFFECTING THE HEALTH CARE FACILITY

Patients' Bill of Rights

The Consumer Bill of Rights and Responsibilities, more commonly known as the Patients' Bill of Rights, outlines the relationship patients should have with their health insurance companies and health care providers. The Patients' Bill of Rights was designed to strengthen confidence in the health care system, to encourage the development of quality provider–patient relationships, and to clarify that health care consumers also have a responsibility to participate in their own health care.

Most health care facilities have adopted a Patients' Bill of Rights that is a condensed version of the entire bill (Box 11.3). This information is typically shared with patients when they are admitted to health care facilities, or it may be posted in a prominent place in the facility. The health care facilities' policies and procedures should incorporate the provisions of the Patients' Bill of Rights. For health services administrators, every interaction with a patient should have the Patients' Bill of Rights in mind. For example, the health services administrator should explain procedures to patients and ensure they understand.

Americans With Disabilities Act

In 1990, President George H. W. Bush signed the Americans with Disabilities Act (ADA) into law with the intent of eliminating discrimination against individuals with disabilities.

TAKE AWAY

The ADA intends to eliminate discrimination against individuals with disabilities.

BOX 11.3   PATIENTS' BILL OF RIGHTS

I. INFORMATION DISCLOSURE
You have a right to receive accurate and easily understood information about your health plan, health care professionals, and health care facilities. If you speak another language, have a physical or mental disability, or just don't understand something, assistance will be provided so you can make informed health care decisions.

II. CHOICE OF PROVIDERS AND PLANS
You have the right to a choice of health care providers that is sufficient to provide you with access to appropriate high-quality health care.

III. ACCESS TO EMERGENCY SERVICES
If you have severe pain, an injury, or a sudden illness that convinces you your health is in serious jeopardy, you have the right to receive screening and stabilization emergency services whenever and wherever needed, without prior authorization or financial penalty.

IV. PARTICIPATION IN TREATMENT DECISIONS
You have the right to know all your treatment options and to participate in decisions about your care. Parents, guardians, family members, or other individuals whom you designate can represent you if you cannot make your own decisions.

V. RESPECT AND NONDISCRIMINATION
You have a right to considerate, respectful, and nondiscriminatory care from your doctors, health plan representatives, and other health care providers.

VI. CONFIDENTIALITY OF HEALTH INFORMATION
You have the right to talk in confidence with health care providers and to have your health care information protected. You also have the right to review and copy your own medical record and request that your provider amend your record if it is not accurate, relevant, or complete.

VII. COMPLAINTS AND APPEALS
You have the right to a fair, fast, and objective review of any complaint you have against your health plan, doctors, hospitals, or other health care personnel. This includes complaints about waiting times, operating hours, the conduct of health care personnel, and the adequacy of health care facilities.

VIII. CONSUMER RESPONSIBILITIES
In a health care system that protects consumer rights, it is reasonable to expect and encourage consumers to assume reasonable responsibilities. Greater individual involvement by consumers in their care increases the likelihood of achieving the best outcomes and helps support a quality-improvement, cost-conscious environment.

The act addressed many areas in which a person might experience discrimination, including telecommunications, housing, public transportation, air carrier access, voting accessibility, education, and rehabilitation.

In 2008, Congress passed the ADA Amendments (ADAA) Act to broaden the definition of disability. Per the ADAA Act, the definition of "disability" should be interpreted broadly to include any individual with a physical or mental impairment that substantially limits one or more of his or her major life activities; the individual has a record of such an impairment; or is thought to have an impairment. All individuals meeting this broad definition of disability should be provided the rights outlined in the ADAA Act.

For the public accommodations requirement, the ADAA Act requires that all new construction and building modifications must be accessible to individuals with disabilities. For existing facilities, barriers that make services inaccessible must be removed, if possible. Health care facilities fall under the category of public accommodations that must comply with specific requirements related to architectural standards for new and altered buildings.

Individuals with disabilities must be able to enter and exit the facility without difficulty. This means that individuals in wheelchairs need a ramp to enter and exit the building. They also must be able to navigate throughout the facility without major barriers. The law requires that public medical facilities must allow persons with disabilities to easily and safely:

- Reach door handles for opening and closing
- Enter and exit buildings
- Move through doors and hallways
- Use drinking fountains, phones, and restrooms (Fig. 11.4)
- Move from floor to floor (elevators are required for multilevel buildings)
- Do everything nondisabled persons can do in a public place
- Have access to communication devices if they have a problem with vision, hearing, reading, or comprehension

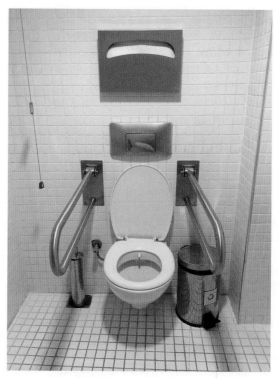

Figure 11.4 The Americans with Disabilities Act mandates that persons with disabilities have the same access to public facilities, such as restrooms.

HITECH Act

As discussed in Chapter 3, the Health Information Technology for Economic and Clinical Health Act (HITECH) was signed into law in 2009 to promote the adoption and meaningful use of health information technology. The HITECH Act allocated funds through the Medicare and Medicaid reimbursement systems as incentives for hospitals and providers who are "meaningful users" of electronic health record (EHR) systems.

Health care employees who do not comply with HITECH guidelines can be fined. The law encourages providers and health care entities to comply with HIPAA regulations or otherwise face stiff penalties for noncompliance. For example, according to this law, providers who do not adopt EHRs in their practices will be penalized in Medicare payments. Civil penalties can be as high as $250,000, with repeated violations costing up to $1.5 million. In addition, HITECH requires the Health and Human Services Department to conduct periodic audits of covered entities and business associates.

Compliance Reporting

The provider is charged with safeguarding and protecting patient confidences within the constraints of the law. But, depending on individual state laws, certain disclosures of patient information must be made. Frequently, the health services administrator is involved with the responsibility for compliance reporting and safeguarding patient information.

> **TAKE AWAY** •·········
>
> By law, the provider must report certain types of patient information, like births, deaths, injuries from violence, some diseases, and abuse.

Examples of mandatory reporting are occurrences of births and deaths. In some states, detailed information about stillbirths is required. Public health statutes also require compliance with reporting wounds from violence, such as gunshot wounds, knife injuries, or poisonings. Any death from accidental, suspicious, or unexplained causes must also be reported. In some states, occupational diseases and injuries must be reported within specific time limits.

Additionally, the federal government and every state monitors and tracks reportable diseases, such as STIs, anthrax, rabies, meningitis, and cancer. Individual states have their own list of reportable diseases. When a physician diagnosis a new case of syphilis, for example, the physician or a member of the medical team, such as the health services administrator, must report the case to the local or county health department (see Fig. 3.6). Depending on the disease, the reporting is done by either mandatory written report or mandatory report by telephone. Local health departments should be consulted for specific procedures and reporting protocols. The local or county health department will compile this data and report to the state health department, who will then report its statistics on new cases in the state to the Centers for Disease Control and Prevention, which tracks disease on a national scale.

The information gained from reporting allows the county or state to make informed decisions and laws about activities and the environment, such as animal control and immunization programs. County and state health departments may also periodically issue bulletins that are sent to health care providers with information about disease outbreaks and other statistics based on the reporting data.

Child Abuse Prevention and Treatment Act

The Child Abuse Prevention and Treatment Act (CAPTA), which was passed in 1974 and reauthorized in 2010, provides federal funding to individual states in support of preventing, investigating, and prosecuting child abuse. In addition, CAPTA sets forth a minimum definition of child abuse and neglect. Box 11.4 lists the signs of child abuse.

BOX 11.4   SIGNS OF CHILD ABUSE

OBVIOUS SIGNS
- Previously filed reports of physical or sexual abuse of the child
- Documented abuse of other family members
- Different stories between parents and child on how an accident happened
- Stories of incidents and injuries that are suspicious
- Injuries blamed on other family members
- Repeated visits to the emergency department for injuries

EXAMINATION FINDINGS
- Trauma to the nervous system
- Internal abdominal pain
- Discolorations/bruising on the buttocks, back, and abdomen

- Elbow, wrist, and shoulder dislocations

CHANGES IN CHILD BEHAVIOR
- Too eager to please the parent
- Overly passive and too compliant
- Aggressive and demanding
- Parenting the parent (role reversal)
- Delays in the normal growth and development patterns
- Erratic school attendance

PHYSICAL INDICATORS
- Poor hygiene
- Malnutrition
- Obvious dental neglect
- Neglected well-baby procedures (e.g., immunizations)

CURRENT TRENDS IN HEALTH CARE

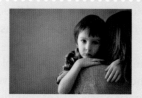

Child abuse is a leading cause of death among children younger than 5 years of age, and every state has statutes that require specific professionals and persons to report suspected child abuse and neglect to appropriate agencies, such as child protective services, a law enforcement agency, or a state's toll-free child abuse reporting hotline. The website, www.childwelfare.gov, lists each state's toll-free number for specific agencies designated to receive and investigate reports of suspected child abuse and neglect.

The professionals mandated by law to report cases of suspected child abuse include:
- Social workers
- Teachers, principals, and other school personnel
- Physicians, nurses, and other health care workers
- Counselors, therapists, and other mental health professionals
- Child care providers
- Medical examiners or coroners
- Law enforcement officers

Several states include commercial film or photograph processors, probation and parole officers, and members of the clergy. Additionally, many states require any person who suspects child abuse or neglect to report, regardless of profession.

When suspected abuse of a child is reported, the individual must provide his or her name; however, this is considered confidential information and is not given to the child's parent or guardian, nor is it given to the investigating officer. The individual making the report also is protected under the law from any liability for reporting suspicions of child abuse.

If the health services administrator or any other staff member suspects that a child is a victim of abuse, he or she should immediately consult with the physician or health care provider. In most states, the reporting can be done separately to the authorities. However, laws may vary, so state and local reporting protocols should be outlined in the office procedures manual. The report should be made as soon as evidence is discovered that gives the provider "cause to believe" that abuse, neglect, or exploitation has occurred. Even if the evidence is uncertain, the provider should report it and allow the government to investigate and determine what action to take to protect the child. However, it is essential to make every attempt to ensure that the report is legitimate and accurate because it could lead to the child being removed from the home and placed in foster care.

Elder Abuse

Another legal issue is recognizing and reporting elder abuse. In general, elder abuse is an act by a caregiver or any other person that causes harm or a serious risk of harm to a vulnerable adult and is considered intentional or negligent. Elder abuse occurs at all social, racial, and economic levels. The abuse may be physical, mental, sexual, material, or financial. It may involve neglect or failure to provide adequate care, including self-neglect when aging people are unable or refuse to care for themselves.

Abuse of elderly people by their caregivers may be difficult to identify. The aging victim could feel embarrassed, guilty, or afraid to report the abuse. Indications that a patient may be a victim of elder abuse are:

- Poor general appearance and poor hygiene
- Pattern of changing doctors and frequent emergency department visits
- Skin lesions, signs of dehydration, bruises (signs of new and old bruising together), abrasions, welts, burns, or pressure sores
- Recurrent injuries caused by accidents
- Signs of malnutrition and weight loss without related illness
- Any injury that does not fit the given history

If abuse is suspected, the caregiver and elderly adult should be interviewed separately by the appropriate staff member, which may be the provider, nurse, or health services administrator, before reporting. All 50 states have passed some form of elder abuse prevention laws that require reporting of suspected elder abuse. For more information, check the "State Resources" section of the National Center on Elder Abuse website (https://ncea.acl.gov/resources/state.html).

Patient Self-Determination Act

The Patient Self-Determination Act of 1990 brought the term *advance directives* to the forefront of medical care. This act requires health care facilities to develop and maintain written procedures that ensure that all adult patients receive information about advance directives and medical durable powers of attorney. **Advance directives** are legal documents that allow individuals to make decisions about end-of-life care issues. They are a way for patients to communicate their wishes to family, friends, and health care professionals about what type of care they would like to receive—or not receive—when their medical condition is terminal. Advance directives specify which treatments the patient wants if he or she is dying or permanently unconscious (Fig. 11.5).

advance directive documentation that details the types and limits of care in the event that a patient is unable to communicate his or her wishes.

Before completing an advance directive, patients should consider the following questions:

- What are your values about death and dying?
- Would you want treatment to extend life by any means in any situation?
- If you are suffering from a terminal illness, would you want lifesaving measures taken?

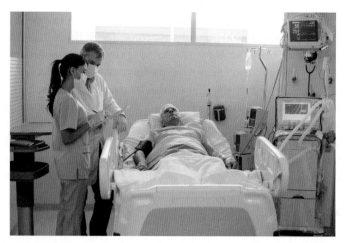

Figure 11.5 An advance directive indicates the patient's wishes for care in the event he or she is unable to communicate.

Patients can exert their right to accept or refuse treatment when they complete an advance directive form. Forms may be provided by health care facilities, hospitals, or long-term care facilities; they can also be accessed online. Advance directive forms ask patients to make decisions about a number of different treatment options. Patients completing these forms may need assistance from medical personnel to understand the ramifications of each option.

- The use of cardiopulmonary resuscitation or a defibrillator; this means the heart has stopped and needs to be artificially stimulated with drugs and machines.
- Whether a mechanical ventilator or respirator should be used if breathing complications occur; this means the patient would need to have an airway put in place or be intubated.
- Decide if, when, and for how long artificial feeding should be done; tube feeding supplies the body with nutrients and fluids intravenously or via a tube in the stomach.
- Determine if, when, and for how long renal dialysis should be done to remove waste materials from the blood if the kidneys stop functioning.
- Antibiotics or antiviral medications can be used to treat infections. Many debilitated individuals develop pneumonia near the end of life. Should infections be treated aggressively, or should they be allowed to run their course?
- Make decisions about palliative care that are used to keep individuals comfortable and manage pain; these may include being allowed to die at home, taking pain medications, and avoiding invasive tests or treatments.
- Organ and tissue donations can be specified in a living will; if organs are removed for donation, the individual is kept on life-sustaining treatment temporarily until the procedure is complete.
- Donating the body for scientific study to a local medical school or university can be specified in the living will.

When completing an advance directive, the patient may also identify a medical durable power of attorney or a health care proxy. This is someone who is trusted to make health decisions for the patient if he or she is unable to do so. The patient may choose a spouse, another family member, a friend, or a member of a faith community. This person can be a different person from the one chosen to be the executor of a will. The American Bar Association recommends the following when choosing a medical durable power of attorney:

- Meets your state's requirements for a health care agent
- Is not your doctor or a part of your medical care team
- Is willing and able to discuss medical care and end-of-life issues with you

TAKE AWAY ●·········

A medical durable power of attorney or a health care proxy makes health decisions for the patient if he or she is unable to do so.

- Can be trusted to make decisions that follow your wishes and values
- Can be trusted to be your advocate if there are disagreements about your care

Advance directives need to be in writing. Each state has different forms and requirements for creating legal documents. In some states the title of an advance directive can be different, such as a living will or an advanced health care directive. Depending on the state, a form may need to be signed by a witness or notarized. A lawyer can assist with the process, but it is generally not necessary. Links to state-specific forms can be found on the website of the National Hospice and Palliative Care Organization (http://www.caringinfo.org/i4a/pages/index.cfm?pageid=3289). The American Bar Association also has a basic, easy-to-use advance directive form that can be used in most states. All adults should prepare an advance directive because unexpected end-of-life situations can happen at any age.

After completion of the form, the patient should share it with his or her health care provider. A copy should be given to all providers involved in the patient's care, and a copy should be included in the patient's medical record. An advance directive can be changed at any time. However, a new form must be created and witnessed as required by the state of residence, and revisions should be shared with family members and health care providers.

In most states, a Physicians Orders for Life Sustaining Treatment (POLST) form can also be completed to plan for the type of desired care if the patient has a medical emergency, such as respiratory or cardiac failure. Unlike advance directives, a POLST summarizes the patient's wishes in the form of medical orders. The POLST form provides explicit guidance to health care providers based on certain medical circumstances and on the patient's current medical condition. The POLST forms are created by the patient and physician to inform emergency care providers, such as emergency medical technicians and ambulance workers, what treatments the patient wants and want to be withheld in a medical emergency. The patient does not need to have an advance directive to have a POLST form. The POLST form must be signed by a physician.

Occupational Health and Safety Act

In 1970, Congress passed the Occupational Safety and Health (OSH) Act to reduce fatalities, illnesses, and injuries incurred at the workplace. This law set standards to protect employees from hazards at work and created the Occupational Safety and Health Administration (OSHA) to enforce those standards. Under the law, employees have a right to safe working conditions, a right to be informed of potential hazards, and a right to file a formal complaint against an employer for breaching these rights. Employers must record and report job-related injuries and illnesses.

It is essential for the health services administrator to ensure the facilities and each staff are compliant with OSHA standards. The health services administrator should review "A Guide to Compliance with OSHA Standards" (OSHA 3187-09R) as it relates to occupational health practices and occupational exposures and hazards.

TAKE AWAY •·········

The Occupational Safety and Health Administration (OSHA) creates and enforces standards to protect employees from hazards at work.

CURRENT TRENDS IN HEALTH CARE

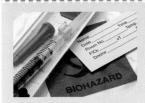

According to the Bureau of Labor Statistics, the health care industry had over 650,000 reported injuries and illnesses in 2010—the most of any industry and 150,000 more than manufacturing.

https://www.bls.gov/news.release/archives/osh_10202011.pdf#page=13

The OSHA safety standards cover all types of working environments, including many situations uncommon in health care, like ladder and machinery safety. Safety in case of a fire is a concern in nearly every work environment, including the medical office: the facility must have sufficient and marked exits in case of an evacuation. However, many hazards are particularly more prevalent in health care facilities than others, such as exposure to bloodborne pathogens, chemical exposures, and radiation. OSHA regulations specify measures to reduce exposure to each of these potential dangers and establish inspections and fines for noncompliance.

Hazard Communication

The OSH Act requires employers to inform their employees about hazardous materials in the workplace. This means that employees must have information on the kinds of hazards present in the facility and the ways in which they may be harmful. OSHA requires that each facility maintain a list of the hazardous chemicals stored in the office. For example, substances that can be dangerous, such as compressed gases, cleaning chemicals, and pharmaceuticals, must be properly labeled. In addition, the office must maintain a **materials safety data sheet (MSDS)** for each hazardous substance. The MSDS lists the physical properties of the hazardous substance, as well as its potential for harm, uses, proper storage, and responses to exposure. The MSDS may be kept in a binder or electronically. The health services administrator should also include employee training in handling chemicals, medical wastes, and any other hazards.

materials safety data sheet (MSDS) document stating the physical properties, use, and handling of a chemical substance.

Ionizing Radiation

In diagnostic imaging medical offices or in any ambulatory care setting with an x-ray machine, OSHA has several safeguards to protect employee health against excessive exposure to radiation. Each employer must survey the radiation hazards at the facility. This includes evaluating the materials and equipment on hand and the levels of radiation present. Exam areas must be restricted to limit employee exposure, and employees working in those areas must wear radiation monitors, such as personal dosimeters. In addition, OSHA specifies labels and signage in and around rooms and equipment where radiation is present, such as "Caution: X-Ray Radiation."

Bloodborne Pathogens

Concerns about the spread of hepatitis and HIV resulted in new OSHA regulations beginning in 1992 to emphasize precautions against **bloodborne pathogens**, or microorganisms in the blood that can cause diseases. Bloodborne pathogens may be transmitted in the workplace when a health care professional is accidentally stuck with a used or contaminated needle or other sharp instruments. Transmission may also occur when infectious material comes in contact with the eyes, nose, mouth, or broken skin. Any member of the medical staff, including housekeeping and the maintenance staff, are all at risk for exposure.

bloodborne pathogen microorganism in the blood that can cause disease.

OSHA's Bloodborne Pathogens standards require health care facilities to do the following to reduce exposure risk:
- List the organization's health care job classifications and tasks that risk exposure to bloodborne pathogens
- Create and have available an Exposure Control Plan that specifies measures to limit employee exposures to pathogens, to be reviewed and updated annually
- Provide employees with personal protective equipment (PPE), such as gloves, protective eyewear, masks, and gowns
- Provide handwashing facilities and training on proper handwashing
- Provide designated containers for the disposal of needles and other sharps
- Follow labeling guidelines when storing and transporting specimens

- Maintain the workplace in a clean and sanitary condition
- Vaccinate all employees for hepatitis B who may come into contact with the virus in their work.

Clinical Laboratory Improvement Amendments Act

As a way to regulate safety and accuracy in testing laboratories, in 1988, Congress enacted the Clinical Laboratory Improvement Amendments (CLIA) Act, which set forth regulations for diagnostic laboratories testing, established a regimen of on-site inspections, and issued certificates to compliant facilities. The CLIA regulations established quality standards for laboratory testing performed on specimens from humans, such as blood, body fluid, and tissue, for the purpose of diagnosis, prevention, or treatment of disease or assessment of health. This law regulated every test in every diagnostic laboratory throughout the United States, including those in physicians' offices, and ensured that the same test would yield the same results no matter where the testing was done.

However, some tests were "waived" from CLIA regulations. These tests included dipstick or tablet reagent urinalysis, fecal occult blood, ovulation tests, urine pregnancy tests, erythrocyte sedimentation rate, and hemoglobin testing. Additionally, hematocrit testing; blood glucose testing by Food and Drug Administration–cleared home-testing devices; and certain microscopic examinations performed personally by a physician, such as wet mounts, KOH preparations, pinworm examinations, fern test, postcoital examinations of vaginal or cervical mucus, and urine sediment examinations, were added as CLIA-waived laboratory tests. Even though a test is "waived," the physician office still needs the federal government's permission to perform it, even if the same or a similar test can be purchased over the counter at a pharmacy and performed by the patient at home.

> **TAKE AWAY** ●·········
>
> The CLIA regulations standardized laboratory testing.

▪ LEARNING CHECKPOINT 11.5
▪ Laws Affecting the Health Care Facility

1. Which set of laws protects disabled persons?

   a. ADA
   b. OSHA
   c. HITECH
   d. CLIA

2. Which physical findings may mean a patient is a victim of child abuse?

   a. scrape on knee
   b. bruise on the arm
   c. bruise on the back
   d. cut on the face

3. A(n) _____ makes health decisions for the patient if he or she is unable to do so.

   a. health care proxy
   b. provider
   c. adult child
   d. spouse

Continued

HEALTH CARE FRAUD AND ABUSE

Fraud may range from single individuals to entire institutions. Health care fraud is committed when a provider, consumer (patient), or company, such as an insurer or hospital, intentionally submits, or causes someone else to submit, false or misleading information with the intent to somehow profit from health care benefits payable, such as reimbursements, services, or pharmaceutical drugs. There are several examples of health care fraud, which will be discussed further, including:

- Knowingly submitting false statements for payment
- Knowingly seeking and/or accepting payment for referrals of items or services ("kickbacks")
- Billing for services that were not medically necessary
- Charging excessively for services or supplies
- Double-billing or filing duplicate claims for the same service
- Misusing codes on a claim, such as upcoding, which is billing at a higher level than the actual service provided, or unbundling codes, which is when the service is billed in steps rather than as one total procedure

Although it is more common for providers to commit health care fraud, patients may commit it by faking medical conditions to receive medications, falsifying medical claim information, or using someone else's insurance information to receive health care services.

Every state government and the federal government have laws against health care fraud. Regardless of the state law in place, federal health care fraud law will apply in most situations, which includes fraud committed against any health care benefits program, such as Medicare and Medicaid. Health care fraud is punishable by fines and/or prison time, which may be at the minimum 5 years in federal prison with fines ranging from $250,000 to more than $1 million, and even higher, depending upon the amount of money defrauded from the government.

Stark Law

The Stark Law is part of the Social Security Act and is commonly known as the "physician self-referral law." There are three components to the law:

1. Providers are prohibited from making referrals for certain designated health services (DHS) payable by Medicare to any facility or health care business that the provider or an immediate family member owns, has invested in, or receives payment from unless an exception applies. DHS include clinical laboratory; physical, occupational, or speech pathology; radiology; medical equipment and supplies; prosthetic devices; and prescription drugs.
2. Medicare or another third-party payer cannot be billed for those referred services.
3. It establishes a number of specific exceptions that do not pose a risk of provider abuse.

The Stark Law was passed to control provider conflicts of interest and to prevent using patient referrals for the provider's personal financial gain. It was originally enacted to prevent providers from ordering unncessary clinical laboratory tests as a way of increasing profits, but now covers an extensive list of testing and treatment facilities. However, providers can legally refer patients to testing facilities within a managed care organization.

False Claims Act

The False Claims Act (FCA) allows for recovery of money from anyone who knowingly submits a fraudulent claim for reimbursement of services to the government. Health services administrators must be very careful when billing any governmental body, such as Medicare and Medicaid, for provider services because any part of the claim that is fraudulent violates the FCA. Any false statement or document that supports a false claim can be considered breaking the FCA rules. If a provider or practice is convicted of submitting false claims, they can face fines of $5500 to $11,000 plus three times the government's damages for each claim under issue. Any individual can be held responsible if he or she is convicted of acting willfully, recklessly, or with deliberate ignorance when creating false claims. Those found responsible may even face criminal charges in extreme cases.

Sunshine Act

The Sunshine Act, or the Physician Payments Act, is designed to increase the transparency around the financial relationships between physicians, teaching hospitals, and manufacturers of pharmaceuticals, medical devices, and biologics. The law hopes to identify any questionable financial relationships between these parties and to help prevent inappropriate influence on research, education, and clinical decision making.

Manufacturers must submit annual reports to the Centers for Medicare and Medicaid Services (CMS) that then itemizes the payments and transfers of value made to health care providers. Some areas are acceptable under the law and do not require reporting, such as:

- A sponsoring manufacturer can provide food or drink to a large group of conference attendees.
- Small payments of less than $10 do not need to be reported except when the total annual value exceeds $100.
- Discounts and rebates for covered drugs or devices do not have to be reported.
- Manufacturers can donate supplies to patients who cannot afford them as long as the provider does not make money off the donation.
- Product samples, including coupons and vouchers, that can be given to patients do not have to be reported.
- Educational materials and items that directly benefit patients are excluded.
- Under certain circumstances manufacturers can pay a provider for speaking at a continuing education program.

Once the manufacture submits its annual report to CMS's Open Payments Program, which is the federal program that collects and compiles the data, the data are made available to physicians for review and to dispute any errors before the information is made public on the Open Payments website: https://openpaymentsdata.cms.gov/.

Legal and Ethical Issues

The primary objective of the health care profession is to render service and provide quality care to all individuals regardless of race, gender, sexual orientation, or

TAKE AWAY ●·········

Health care workers are bound by ethical standards to treat all patients with respect and to make ethical decisions based on principles rather than on personal beliefs and values.

socioeconomic status. The importance of respecting the confidentiality of information learned from or about patients in the course of providing patient care cannot be overemphasized. It is unethical to reveal patient confidences to anyone, including family members, a spouse, best friends, and other health care workers. Never mention patient names outside the place of employment even if the physician's specialty might reveal the patient's reason for consultation.

Regardless of the situation, health care workers are bound by ethical standards to treat all patients with respect and to make ethical decisions based on principles rather than personal beliefs and values. As a member of the health care team, the health services administrator is also responsible for reporting ethical infractions to supervisors and/or physician-employers. In addition, legal requirements may exist for the reporting of ethical issues to local or state authorities. An important role of each health care employee is to serve as the patient's advocate. In this role, it may be necessary to use legal means to protect the rights of patients in the practice.

● CASE STUDY

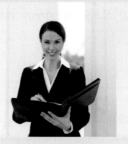

Even though none of the physicians at Carmen's urgent care center were being sued for malpractice, they did provide follow-up care, so it was important Carmen testify about the contents of the medical record. She explained to the court that the physicians in her clinic entered into a contract to treat the patient because they were open and available to offer treatment, the patient requested treatment, and the physician provided that treatment. She showed that the medical record documented the physician's discussion of informed consent with the patient: the patient was told of the diagnosis, proposed treatment, and risks of that treatment. The signed consent form was in the record, and Carmen herself was a witness to the patient's signature.

In medicine, the law works to protect both patients and providers. It is the duty of the health services administrator to make sure facility providers and staff understand and comply with policies and procedures.

▪ LEARNING CHECKPOINT 11.6
▪ Health Care Fraud and Abuse

1. The _____ was passed to control provider conflicts of interest and to prevent using patient referrals for the provider's personal financial gain.

2. The _____ shows relationships between physicians, hospitals, and manufacturers to help prevent inappropriate influence on research, education, and clinical decision making.

3. Filing duplicate claims for the same service is a violation of the _____ Act.

1. Compare criminal, civil, and contract law. What are their differences? Why is it important to understand their application in the health care environment?

2. What are the essential components of consent for treatment?

3. Describe negligence and liability.

4. What are the elements of a medical professional liability lawsuit?

5. Identify and explain a minimum of four laws that affect a health care facility.

6. How can ethical behavior influence patient care?

HEALTH INSURANCE PORTABILITY AND ACCOUNTABILITY ACT (HIPAA)

Carol Colvin

CHAPTER OUTLINE

INTRODUCTION
PORTABILITY
PRIVACY RULE

SECURITY RULE
ENFORCEMENT

Consequences of HIPAA
Noncompliance

VOCABULARY

administrative safeguards
business associate
civil money penalty (CMP)
covered entity
Health Insurance Portability and
    Accountability Act (HIPAA)

Notice of Privacy Practices (NPP)
Office for Civil Rights
physical safeguards
portability
privacy officer
Privacy Rule

protected health information (PHI)
Security Rule
technical safeguards

CHAPTER OBJECTIVES

After completing this chapter, the student should be able to do the following:

1. Explain the purpose and provisions of the Health Insurance Portability and Accountability Act (HIPAA).
2. List the provisions of the Privacy Rule and define protected health information (PHI).
3. List the guidelines of the Security Rule.
4. Discuss the enforcement of HIPAA regulations and penalties for noncompliance.

INTRODUCTION

As we have discussed in previous chapters, compliance is critical and must guide all aspects of health care. All employees in the health care organizations are bound by compliance regulations as established by the federal government to protect the interests and privacy of those that are serviced by the health care community. To help with providing guidelines and enforcement, in 1996, the United States federal government passed into law the **Health Insurance Portability and Accountability Act (HIPAA)**. Its primary goals are to make it easier for people to keep their health insurance by providing portability and continuity, protect the confidentiality and security of health care information, and help the health care industry control administrative costs. Additionally, HIPAA was designed with the following goals in mind:

- Reduce health care–related fraud and abuse
- Provide continuous health care coverage for Americans and their covered family members in instances when there is a loss or break in employment
- Standardize health care data and information submitted electronically, including for billing purposes
- Ensure protected, confidential handling of all protected health information
  HIPAA consists of five titles:
- Title I: Health Care Access, Portability, and Renewability
- Title II: Preventing Health Care Fraud and Abuse; Administrative Simplification; Medical Liability Reform
- Title III: Tax-related health provisions governing medical savings accounts
- Title IV: Application and enforcement of group health insurance requirements
- Title V: Revenue offset governing tax deductions for employers.

In regard to the role of the health services administrator managing a health care facility, Titles I and II will be discussed in detail, as they focus on the portability of health care and the privacy and security of health information.

○ **Health Insurance Portability and Accountability Act (HIPAA)** passed into law in 1996 by Congress and enforced in full in 2003, this regulation ensures equal access to certain health and human services and protects the privacy and security of health information.

CASE STUDY

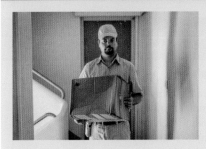

It was not a surprise when Dr. Estes announced his retirement, and in fact he had not worked full-time for a number of years. To stay sharp at the end of his career, he saw patients three days a week at the Drug Shoppe, a pharmacy with a retail clinic to treat minor ailments. When Dr. Estes decided to retire, the pharmacy's owner put the store up for sale, which was quickly bought by Black Mountain Medical, a nonprofit health system that provides community-based health care services in two states.

During the transition, Black Mountain attempted to deliver all the medical records for Dr. Estes' former patients to his apartment. However, when no one answered the door, the delivery driver left the cardboard box full of patient files in the hallway. As you read this chapter, what issues may occur with this treatment of medical records? What laws are in place to prohibit this type of action and protection patient information?

PORTABILITY

One of the primary provisions of HIPAA was to protect workers and their families during job transition or loss of work, or to maintain **portability** of health care insurance. Under Title I of HIPAA: Health Care Access, Portability, and Renewability, provisions

○ **portability** refers to the first guideline of HIPAA, which safeguards an American who is in transition between jobs by setting guidelines that health care insurance providers must follow and restricting exclusions from insurance coverage for certain reasons, such as preexisting conditions in certain situations.

are laid out where workers cannot be denied insurance coverage in a group plan due to a preexisting condition when they have had no significant break in insurance coverage after having been under a plan for 18 months or more. This guideline restricts group health plans from implementing eligibility rules or creating additional premiums for individuals based on health status, medical history, genetic information, or disability.

This section of HIPAA was intended to increase the number of Americans with health care insurance coverage by protecting the transferability of insurance during job transition. It also protected those who were seeking coverage under individual insurance plans when they were not eligible to be covered under a group, federal, or state plan.

PRIVACY RULE

Privacy Rule guidelines under HIPAA that give patients important privacy rights to their health care information, including who can access the information and to whom it can be released.

covered entity an entity that must comply with HIPAA regulations; this includes health care providers that transmit PHI electronically, health plans, and health care clearinghouses.

business associate a business that provides a service to a covered entity and uses PHI.

protected health information (PHI) the information protected under HIPAA regarding personal health care that must be transmitted, retained, and destroyed in the business of health care.

Under Title II, the **Privacy Rule** provides protection for the privacy of health information but does not interfere with patients' access to health care or the quality of health care delivery.

It governs the use of patient personal information by **covered entities**—any organizations that obtain and manage health information—in the way health information is held, stored, or transmitted. Covered entities include health care providers, health plans (insurers), and health care clearinghouses (Table 12.1). It also affects **business associates**—vendors who contract with covered entities and use health information in the course of providing a service. Some examples of business associates might be a transcription or translation service, accrediting agency, or software vendor. It stipulates who may access the information and under what conditions access is given. The Privacy Rule encompasses all modes of communication, including electronic data, paper documents, and oral communication (Fig. 12.1).

The Privacy Rule restricts or limits the use and disclosure of **protected health information (PHI)**, broadly defined as "individually identifiable health information." PHI is personally-identifiable information that includes the patient's medical history and health care. PHI includes many other common identifiers such as the examples in Box 12.1. It is important to note that identifying information alone would not be

TABLE 12.1	
COVERED ENTITIES	
Type	**Examples**
Health plan	• Dental insurance provider • Vision insurance provider • Health insurance provider • Employer group plan • Medicaid • Medicare • Military or veterans group plans
Clearinghouse	• Billing entity • Repricing company • Any business that facilitates or processes PHI
Provider	• Doctor • Dentist • Psychiatrist • Psychologist • Chiropractor • Pharmacy • Nursing home • Clinic

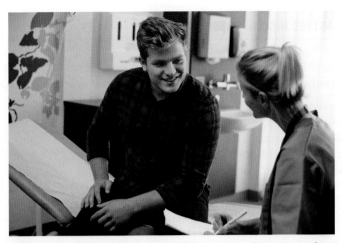

Figure 12.1 Health care professionals must be careful to protect the privacy of patients and their health information.

BOX 12.1	EXAMPLES OF PROTECTED HEALTH INFORMATION (PHI)
Name	Email address
Address	Social security number
Phone number	Account number
Geographic area	Unique patient numbers
Names of relatives	Dates (birth, death, admission,
Driver's license number	discharge)
Fax numbers	Photos
Ages	

designated as PHI, but it must be associated with the health information, such as on a laboratory report or hospital bill. These documents would contain a patient's name and/or other identifying information associated with the health data.

The Privacy Rule states that patients have the right to:

- Receive notices from the health care provider that inform of anticipated uses or disclosures of PHI
- Obtain a copy of personal health care information
- Request correction of information that is incomplete or incorrect
- Obtain an account of any PHI disclosures over the past 6 years

PHI may only be disclosed when authorized by the patient, except under certain circumstances (Box 12.2). Medical professionals may not give PHI to anyone unless the patient allows it, including to family members, friends, other doctors, and even insurance companies. If a patient objects to a disclosure to a family member, clinic staff are not allowed to discuss the patient's PHI with the family member. A provider may not send information about a patient's treatment to an insurer unless the patient signs a release allowing the provider to do so. The health services administrator should ensure that the health care facility has a process in place to obtain authorization to release PHI and that it has a policy that details the specific medical staff members authorized to use or disclose PHI and the purpose of the requested information. It should also require the patient's signature and the date of the request, as well as a statement of the patient's right to revoke the authorization.

When disclosing or using PHI, covered entities must only use or disclose the minimum amount of PHI necessary to meet the request or the intended purpose. Further, they

TAKE AWAY

Identifying information must be associated with the health information to be considered PHI.

TAKE AWAY

Health care professionals should limit access and use of PHI to the minimum amount necessary to do a task.

BOX 12.2   PERMITTED DISCLOSURES

Disclosures of PHI without patient authorization are permissible:

- During emergencies and disaster relief services
- For public health purposes as required by state and federal law
- To public agencies for health oversight activities (audits, civil, or criminal proceedings)

- To law enforcement officials
- To funeral directors or coroners
- To correctional institutions
- For medical research

---

should have limited access to only the PHI they need to fulfill their task or duties. For example, imagine a medical assistant sees her neighbor in the waiting room one afternoon. She doesn't get a chance to speak to her before she leaves, but decides to bring up her medical record to see why she was in the office today. This is a violation of patient privacy because the patient did not authorize the medical assistant to view her record and the medical assistant did not need the information to care for the patient. Box 12.3 lists several scenarios explaining the use and disclosure of PHI.

Remember that not all communication about a patient's health is PHI. In many cases, a patient is not identified by name; conversely, a patient may be identified, but nothing about his or her health is discussed. For instance, patients in a waiting room are commonly called by their first name, and, in hospitals, patient names are placed on charts outside of hospital rooms. Additionally, when data are aggregated for public health studies, no identifying information is attached to the health data. Thus PHI is health information that is linked to a specific individual.

BOX 12.3   PRIVACY AND SECURITY SCENARIOS

Scenario: A person breaks into a doctor's office at night and pries open the medical record file with a crowbar to gain confidential information about a patient. Can the privacy officer of the practice be prosecuted for this HIPAA violation?

Answer: No. HIPAA only requires that practices make a good-faith and reasonable effort to safeguard PHI. You might wish to safeguard highly sensitive information about high-profile patients offsite if it is not needed for day-to-day health care operations or treatment.

Scenario: Mr. Stabler is a physical therapy (PT) patient in your outpatient area. You receive a phone call from his grandson wanting to know how he is doing. What do you do?

Answer: Ask the grandson his name, then check the PHI Communication Resource form to see if the grandson is listed as an authorized person to receive

information. If not listed, you can give a general condition, but not specific PHI. You can direct him to someone listed on the PHI for specific information. If the patient requests "not to publish information" then you may not provide any information.

Scenario: Sarah is a physical therapist on the orthopedic floor. One day a fellow college classmate is admitted to the hospital. Sarah checks the chart and finds out that he was admitted with a diagnosis of cancer. When Sarah gets home, she calls all his friends to tell them he is in the hospital with cancer and to collect money for flowers. Do Sarah's actions violate HIPAA privacy?

Answer: Yes. Even though she might have had good intensions, she disclosed to a third party that the patient had been admitted. She also revealed PHI by disclosing the patient's diagnosis without his consent.

As required by HIPAA, the health services administrator must ensure that the medical office has a **Notice of Privacy Practices (NPP)**. The NPP is a document that communicates to patients their rights under HIPAA and includes the following information:

- The patient's right to the PHI and how to register any complaints
- How the covered entity may use and disclose PHI about the patient
- What the legal responsibilities of the covered entity in regard to the PHI are

The NPP must be written and in plain, simple language to ensure patient understanding. It must have an effective date, and any changes made to the NPP must be revised and distributed within 60 days. The health services administrator must ensure that every patient has signed it, with new patients completing the form no later than the first day of receiving medical services. If the notice is provided electronically, such as via email, the covered entity should request a return receipt for any kind of communication that the patient has received the notice. A sample NPP is shown in Fig. 12.2.

> **Notice of Privacy Practices (NPP)** document listing patients' rights as mandated by HIPAA.

LEARNING CHECKPOINT 12.1

Privacy Rule

1. What is a business associate?

2. Name five types of unique patient identifiers.

3. A covered entity must obtain an individual's written authorization for use of disclosure of protected health information in which scenario?

   a. A coder must review a patient's chart to code a recent hospital stay.
   b. A consulting physician needs to access a patient's record to inform his or her opinion.
   c. A hospital administrator needs to access patient data to create a report about how many patients were treated for diabetes in the last 6 months.
   d. None of the above.

SECURITY RULE

Health care facilities must take measures to ensure security of PHI and to prevent breaches of confidentiality. Under Title II, the HIPAA **Security Rule** provides guidelines for safeguarding how PHI is created, received, transmitted, or maintained. These nationwide security standards govern protection of PHI through administrative, physical, and technical safeguards (Table 12.2).

Administrative safeguards refer to the policies and procedures documented in writing that show how covered entities will comply with HIPAA. The administrative safeguards should include the covered entities' method for clearing or authorizing someone for access to PHI during the hiring process, modification of access during employment, and discontinuation of access upon termination. If the covered entity employs a third party for any service, it must determine what, if any, PHI is necessary for the services rendered and that the third party also has a plan in place to comply with HIPAA.

Administrative safeguards also require a plan for continuous training and education of employees (Fig. 12.3). Training creates a culture of compliance when it has demonstrated priority within a company. Training can be driven by internal audits that monitor HIPAA compliance in the business and identify areas where additional training and monitoring are needed. Additionally, most health care facilities may appoint a staff

> **Security Rule** guidelines under the HIPAA regulation that set the standards for the storage and transfer of electronic protected health information.

> **administrative safeguards** the policies and procedures documented in writing that show how a health care provider will comply with HIPAA.

Sample Notice of Privacy Practices

THIS NOTICE DESCRIBES HOW INFORMATION ABOUT YOU MAY BE USED AND DISCLOSED AND HOW YOU CAN GET ACCESS TO THIS INFORMATION. PLEASE REVIEW IT CAREFULLY.

Understanding Your Health Record/Information

Each time you visit a hospital, physician, or other health care provider, a record of your visit is made. Typically, this record contains your symptoms, examination and test results, diagnoses, treatment, and a plan for future care or treatment. This information, often referred to as your "health record" or "medical record," serves as a:
- Basis for planning your care and treatment
- Means of communication among the many health professionals who contribute to your care
- Legal document describing the care you received
- Means by which you or a third-party payer can verify that services billed actually were provided
- Tool in educating health professionals
- Source of data for medical research
- Source of information for public health officials charged with improving the health of the nation
- Source of data for facility planning and marketing
- Tool with which we can assess and continually work to improve the care we render and the outcomes we achieve
- Understanding what is in your record and how your health information is used helps you to:
- Ensure its accuracy
- Better understand who, what, when, where, and why others may access your health information
- Make more informed decisions when authorizing disclosure to others

Your Health Information Rights

Although your health record is the physical property of the health care practitioner or facility that compiled it, the information belongs to you. You have the right to:
- Request a restriction on certain uses and disclosures of your information as provided by 45 CFR 164.522
- Obtain a paper copy of the notice of information practices upon request
- Inspect and copy your health record as provided for in 45 CFR 164.524
- Amend your health record as provided in 45 CFR 164.526
- Obtain an accounting of disclosures of your health information as provided in 45 CFR 164.528
- Request communications of your health information by alternative means or at alternative locations
- Revoke your authorization to use or disclose health information except to the extent that action has already been taken

Our Responsibilities

This organization is required to:
- Maintain the privacy of your health information
- Provide you with a notice as to our legal duties and privacy practices with respect to information we collect and maintain about you
- Abide by the terms of this notice
- Notify you if we are unable to agree to a requested restriction
- Accommodate reasonable requests you may have to communicate health information by alternative means or at alternative locations

We reserve the right to change our practices and to make the new provisions effective for all protected health information we maintain. Should our information practices change, we will mail a revised notice to the address you have supplied us.

We will not use or disclose your health information without your authorization, except as described in this notice.

For More Information or to Report a Problem

If have questions and would like additional information, you may contact the Office of Civil Rights. Read more at the following website: http://www.hhs.gov/ocr/privacy/hipaa/complaints/index.html

If you believe your privacy rights have been violated, you can file a complaint with the Director of Health Information Management or with the Secretary of Health and Human Services. There will be no retaliation for filing a complaint.

Examples of Disclosures for Treatment, Payment, and Health Operations

We will use your health information for treatment. For example: Information obtained by a nurse, physician, or other member of your health care team will be recorded in your record and used to determine the course of treatment that should work best for you. Your physician will document in your record his or her expectations of the members of your health care team. Members of your health care team will then record the actions they took and their observations. In that way, the physician will know how you are responding to treatment.

We will also provide your physician or a subsequent health care provider with copies of various reports that should assist him or her in treating you once you are discharged from this hospital.

Figure 12.2 Notice of Privacy Practices (NPP).

We will use your health information for payment. For example: A bill may be sent to you or a third-party payer. The information on or accompanying the bill may include information that identifies you, as well as your diagnosis, procedures, and supplies used.

We will use your health information for regular health operations. For example: Members of the medical staff, the risk or quality improvement manager, or members of the quality improvement team may use information in your health record to assess the care and outcomes in your case and others like it. This information will then be used in an effort to continue improving the quality and effectiveness of the health care and service we provide.

Other Uses or Disclosures

Business associates: Some services in our organization are provided through contacts with business associates. Examples include physician services in the emergency department and radiology, certain laboratory tests, and a copy service we use when making copies of your health record. When these services are contracted, we may disclose your health information to our business associates so that they can perform the job we have asked them to do and bill you or your third-party payer for services rendered. So that your health information is protected, however, we require the business associate to safeguard your information appropriately.

Directory: Unless you notify us that you object, we will use your name, location in the facility, general condition, and religious affiliation for directory purposes. This information may be provided to members of the clergy and, except for religious affiliation, to other people who ask for you by name.

Notification: We may use or disclose information to notify or assist in notifying a family member, personal representative, or another person responsible for your care, location, and general condition.

Communication with family: Health professionals, using their best judgment, may disclose to a family member, other relative, close personal friend, or any other person you identify, health information relevant to that person's involvement in your care or payment related to your care.

Research: We may disclose information to researchers when their research has been approved by an institutional review board that has reviewed the research proposal and established protocols to ensure the privacy of your health information.

Funeral directors: We may disclose to funeral directors health information consistent with applicable law so they can carry out their duties.

Organ procurement organizations: Consistent with applicable law, for the purpose of tissue donation and transplant, we may disclose health information to organ procurement organizations or other entities engaged in the procurement, banking, or transplantation of organs.

Marketing: We may contact you to provide appointment reminders or information about treatment alternatives or other health-related benefits and services that may be of interest to you.

Fund-raising: We may contact you as part of a fund-raising effort.

Food and Drug Administration (FDA): We may disclose to the FDA health information relative to adverse events with respect to food, supplements, product and product defects, or post-marketing surveillance information to enable product recalls, repairs, or replacement.

Workers' compensation: We may disclose health information to the extent authorized by and to the extent necessary to comply with laws relating to workers' compensation or other similar programs established by law.

Public health: As required by law, we may disclose your health information to public health or legal authorities charged with preventing or controlling disease, injury, or disability.

Correctional institution: Should you be an inmate of a correctional institution, we may disclose to the institution or agents thereof health information necessary for your health and the health and safety of other individuals.

Law enforcement: We may disclose health information for law enforcement purposes as required by law or in response to a valid subpoena.

Federal law makes provision for your health information to be released to an appropriate health oversight agency, public health authority, or attorney, provided that a workforce member or business associate believes in good faith that we have engaged in unlawful conduct or have otherwise violated professional or clinical standards and are potentially endangering one or more patients, workers, or the public.

My signature below indicates that I have been provided with a copy of the notice of privacy practices.

_____   _____
Signature of patient or legal representative   Date

If signed by legal representative, relationship to patient: _____
Effective Date: _____

Distribution: Original to provider, copy to patient

Figure 12.2, cont'd

TABLE 12.2

THE SECURITY RULE'S ADMINISTRATIVE, PHYSICAL, AND TECHNICAL SAFEGUARDS

Safeguard	Examples
Administrative	• Staff training programs • Auditing and monitoring compliance with policies and procedures • Employee confidentiality agreements
Physical	• Controlling building access with photo-identification/swipe card system • Keeping offices and file cabinets containing PHI locked • Turning computer screens displaying PHI away from public view
Technical	• Tracking and auditing of all electronic systems for appropriate access and usage • Automatic log-off from an information system after a specified interval of time • Unique user identification with log-on and passwords

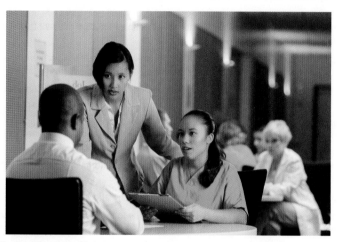

Figure 12.3 The health care administrator discusses protection of PHI during a training session, part of HIPAA's administrative safeguards.

> **privacy officer** an individual designated to enforce HIPAA compliance in the facility.

> **physical safeguards** guidelines to protect physical monitoring of protected health information.

member, such as the health services administrator, as a **privacy officer** who is responsible for training, performing internal audits, and the facility's security.

Physical safeguards are the second area covered by the HIPAA Security Rule and refer to the physical monitoring PHI. The HIPAA Security Rule defines these safeguards as "physical measures, policies, and procedures to protect a covered entity's electronic information systems and related buildings and equipment, from natural and environmental hazards, and unauthorized intrusion." This guideline requires that hardware and software used by covered entities be installed and removed properly to protect PHI. For example, healthcare organizations need to ensure that portable media—such as laptops or USB thumb drives—that contain PHI are secure and protected and monitor when they should be allowed to leave the facility. This rule also refers to physical information storage, such as files and records, and the control mechanisms in place to protect that data. Many health care facilities use a double-lock system—access to any PHI requires the ability to get through two locks, such as a locked room and a locked filing cabinet. This not only includes the storage of information, but also the destruction of information once it is no longer needed. Factors to consider when physically safeguarding PHI in the health care facility include:

- Keeping workstations with PHI out of high-traffic areas
- Having appropriate documentation of visitor sign-ins
- Restricting access to client data from third parties using facility equipment

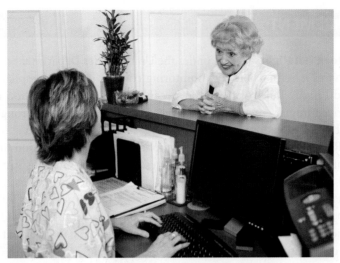

Figure 12.4 Many monitors in a medical setting can only be seen by the person sitting directly in front of the computer; the screen appears black to anyone else.

- Properly removing all client data from hardware or software before disposing of it
- Limiting employee access to areas where PHI is located
- Controlling and securing areas with PHI from third parties, such as janitorial services
- Verifying the training of third-party vendors
- Preventing the visibility of computer screens to unauthorized users (Fig. 12.4).

Technical safeguards are the final area and one of the most important aspects of the HIPAA Security Rule; this refers to the responsibility of the health care provider to monitor and safeguard PHI through all types of technology. With adoption of electronic health records (EHRs), every health care provider and covered entity should have a system for technical safeguards and a plan for internal monitoring to make sure that it is operational, effective, and sufficient in protecting data.

Technology includes all facets of the business using technical means of data storage and communication: emails, faxes, phones, and computer systems. Not only should data be secured at the point of use in the health care facility, but must also be secured and verified that they are received by the intended recipient. Use of a fax machine to send information to the wrong location is one of the greatest risk areas of inappropriate release of PHI. As discussed in Chapter 6, communication between health care providers and patients occurs more commonly using EHR or practice management software, which requires a user log on that leaves an audit trail (Fig. 6.8).

technical safeguards guidelines under HIPAA that safeguard protected health information through all mediums of technology.

TAKE AWAY

HIPAA established administrative, physical, and technical safeguards to protect patient information.

LEARNING CHECKPOINT 12.2
Security Rule

1. A(n) _____ is an individual designated to enforce HIPAA compliance in the facility.

2. None of the patient access staff have access to the progress note section of the patient's medical record. This is an example of a(n) _____ safeguard.

3. The housekeeping staff does not clean the file room, and they don't even have a key to get in. This is an example of a(n) _____ safeguard.

ENFORCEMENT

Office for Civil Rights the section of the US Department of Health and Human Services that is responsible for the enforcement of HIPAA regulations.

The **Office for Civil Rights** (OCR) under the United States Department of Health and Human Services is responsible for monitoring covered entities' compliance with the Security and Privacy Rules of the HIPAA regulation. Since its inception in 2003, the OCR has driven improvements in the privacy and security of PHI through corrective actions for HIPAA violations.

The OCR regulates HIPAA through compliance reviews, education and outreach initiatives, and complaint investigation and resolution. The OCR instituted a HIPAA Privacy and Security Rule Complaint Process through which it receives complaints of possible HIPAA violations and conducts the necessary follow-up actions. After receiving a complaint, the OCR will ask both the party filing the complaint and the one in suspected violation to present relevant information regarding the incident. During the review of a complaint, one of three actions may be taken:

- If a violation of the criminal provision of HIPAA is suspected, the complaint is referred to the Department of Justice for investigation.
- If a violation occurred, but was not in violation of the criminal provisions of HIPAA, the OCR will seek resolution through voluntary compliance, corrective action, and/or a resolution agreement.
- If no violation is uncovered, the complaint will be closed.

The majority of complaints filed with the Office for Civil Rights regarding HIPAA are resolved through voluntary compliance, corrective action, and/or a resolution agreement. Once resolution is reached, both entities are notified in writing of the findings and resolution.

CURRENT TRENDS IN HEALTH CARE

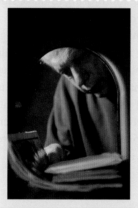

HIPAA violations are more common than you might think. For example, Walgreens Co., one of the United States' largest pharmacy chains, mailed free samples of Prozac capsules to patients who had an active prescription for the daily dosage of Prozac. This was an obvious violation of a patient's right to privacy because these patients received unsolicited medications with literature disclosing their name and medical condition to unauthorized persons—anyone who handled their mail.

Weber, G (2002). Avoiding a HIPAA nightmare. *The dermatologist*, 10(8), retrieved from http://www.the-dermatologist.com/article/707.

Consequences of HIPAA Noncompliance

After a covered entity is found to be noncompliant with HIPAA Privacy or Security Rules, most are given the opportunity to enter into voluntary compliance, corrective action, and/or a resolution agreement with the OCR. In some cases, covered entities who fail to abide by these resolutions force the OCR to levy **civil money penalties** (**CMPs**). CMPs are paid to the US Treasury and do not create any income for the entity that filed the complaint.

civil money penalty (CMP) fine levied on covered entities that violate HIPAA regulations.

CMPs are structured based on level of severity, as well as the intent of the violation. CMPs for HIPAA violations are also determined based on a tiered civil penalty structure, depending on the knowledge a covered entity had of the violation and the seriousness of the HIPAA violation. The OCR classifies violations into the following categories:

- Category 1 – A violation that the covered entity was unaware of and could not have realistically avoided had a reasonable amount of care had been taken to abide by HIPAA. Example: a health care employee forgets to log off her computer and leaves patient information on the screen where it is visible to others.
- Category 2 – A violation that the covered entity should have been aware of but could not have avoided even with a reasonable amount of care. The violation is done on purpose as a disregard of policies and procedures. Example: one employee uses another employee's password and accesses patient's medical information even though it is not a part of the first employee's job responsibility.
- Category 3 – This violation is done with malicious intent or "willful neglect" and with disregard of HIPAA standards but an attempt has been made to correct the violation. Example: a medical office failed to execute a business associate agreement before turning over thousands of patients' PHI to a potential business partner. The medical office required the business partner to return all PHI within 7 days.
- Category 4 – This violation is done with malicious intent or "willful neglect" and with disregard of HIPAA standards, where no attempt has been made to correct the violation. Example: selling PHI to malpractice lawyers or to the media or to people who will use this information to commit credit card fraud.

The amount of CMPs depends on the severity and category, as well as any prior history of violations by the covered entity, its financial condition, and the level of harm caused by the violation. If a violation is found, the CMP imposed will vary from $100 to $50,000 per violation per year the violation was allowed to persist. The maximum fine per violation category per year is $1,500,000.

In addition to civil penalties, HIPAA violation can result in criminal charges being filed against the covered entity responsible for a breach of PHI. Criminal penalties for HIPAA violations are divided into three separate tiers:

- Tier 1: Reasonable cause or no knowledge of violation
- Tier 2: Obtaining PHI under false pretenses
- Tier 3: Obtaining PHI for personal gain or with "willful intent"

Criminal penalties carry fines of up to $250,000 and potential imprisonment from 1 to 10 years in jail. In cases of criminal violations of HIPAA, the OCR would refer many of these cases to the state's attorney general to apply proper criminal penalties.

⬤ CASE STUDY

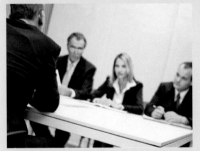

Dr. Estes' former patients' medical records were left in a hallway, unattended and accessible to anyone walking through the building. When he arrived home and discovered the box, Dr. Estes reported the event to the OCR.

The OCR investigated Black Mountain Medical for violating HIPAA's Privacy Rule because it failed to protect the PHI of many patients. Black Mountain Medical agreed to settle potential violations by paying a $30,000 fine. In addition, Black Mountain will adopt a corrective action plan to address deficiencies in its HIPAA compliance program.

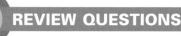

REVIEW QUESTIONS

1. When HIPAA was introduced to Congress, one of its primary goals was to increase the availability of health care to Americans, especially those in transition or between jobs. Which section of the HIPAA regulation is meant to ensure that workers are safeguarded when transitioning between jobs when it comes to the availability of health care insurance?

2. A superbill in the respiratory therapy center lists the patient's name and medical record number, and the CPT code is circled. Is this PHI? Why or why not?

3. Under the HIPAA Security Rule, what is the difference between physical and technical safeguards? Give examples of both.

4. What are the three tiers of HIPAA violations? Provide an example of each.

COMPLIANCE

Carol Colvin and Jaime Nguyen

CHAPTER OUTLINE

INTRODUCTION
COMPLIANCE PROGRAM
  Development
  The Office of Inspector
    General
  Compliance Plan
  Importance of Documentation

Implementation
Monitoring for Effectiveness
NONCOMPLIANCE
  False Claims Act
  Anti-Kickback Statute
  Physician Self-Referral Law
    (Stark Law)

OIG Audits and Actions
Disclosure
Resolution Process
  *Corporate Integrity
    Agreements*

VOCABULARY

action plan
compliance officer
compliance program
disclosure

Conditions for Coverage (CfC)
Conditions of Participation (CoP)
corporate integrity agreement (CIA)
exclusion

mandatory exclusion
Office of Inspector General (OIG)
permissive exclusion
stakeholder

CHAPTER OBJECTIVES

After completing this chapter, the student should be able to do the following:

1. Define a compliance program and understand its purpose.
2. Relate the role of the Office of the Inspector General (OIG).

3. List the elements of a compliance plan.
4. Describe the consequences of noncompliance.

INTRODUCTION

In the previous chapters, we have discussed some of the legal framework surrounding the delivery of health care. While providing medical services, situations may arise where noncompliance of laws and regulations occurs and fraud and abuse are uncovered in a health care organization, whether it is the result of intentional or unintentional actions. In some cases, noncompliance may be the result of misinterpretation of how a law or regulation applies to specific situations, which is an example of a nonintentional fraud or abuse. In other cases, some individuals may intentionally break the law and commit fraud for personal gain, such as a physician billing a health insurance company for a medical service that was never provided to the patient.

Not only is compliance important as a best practice to provide quality health care services to patients; it is also mandatory to legally and lawfully operate a health care practice. Health care compliance aids organizations and providers in avoiding trouble with government authorities. Thus all health care organizations and practices must incorporate a culture of compliance within their organization and among their staff. The health services administrator will play an important role in ensuring the health care organization maintains its compliancy. This chapter will discuss the role of compliance in health care and how to develop an effective compliance program.

● CASE STUDY

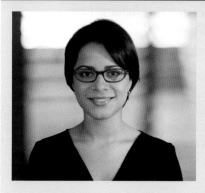

Carrie has been tasked with developing a compliance program for Community Health Care. Due to recent changes in health care regulations, the medical practice is no longer certain that its current policies and procedures are compliant. Carrie is instructed to select three staff members to be a part of her compliance committee and is given a timeline of 3 months to thoroughly review and identify any compliance issues and areas of risk. Once completed, the compliance committee will develop a compliance plan that will address any areas of risk, which will be presented to the board members of Community Health Care. When approved, Carrie and the compliance committee will implement the program and monitor its progress. She plans to assign sections of the compliance program management to individual team members. However, she is ultimately responsible for making sure that the practice discloses noncompliant areas, has a plan of action to correct those noncompliant areas, and is able to communicate and train all employees on the compliance plan.

Carrie begins by choosing three functional area leaders for the compliance committee to assist in her first step, which is to review current policies, procedures, and the daily activities of the practice. Each committee member is to document a written process for completing various tasks in his or her respective area and determine if those daily actions are compliant with current health care laws and regulations. Once completed, the committee will reconvene to discuss their findings.

COMPLIANCE PROGRAM

Ultimately, the purpose of health care compliance is to improve patient care. Health care compliance helps regulate both patients and health care providers and the relationship between the two parties. Patient care is improved when health care decisions are based upon appropriate and current clinical and legal standards of care, whereas noncompliance often results in patient errors and legal actions.

Every health care organization needs a compliance program. A **compliance program** is a set of internal policies and procedures put into place to help the health care organization comply with laws, regulations, and industry-accepted best practices. An effective compliance program can enhance the operation of an organization, improve quality of care, and reduce overall costs. It can also help identify problems upfront and allow the health care organization to correct them before they become systemic and costly. A compliance program must define appropriate conduct, train the health organization's staff, and then monitor adherence to the processes, policies, and procedures. The compliance program needs to address delivery of patient care; billing and reimbursement; managed care; Occupational Safety and Health Administration (OSHA), The Joint Commission (TJC), or other accreditation standards; and Health Insurance Portability and Accountability Act (HIPAA) privacy and security. Many of these compliance regulations and guidelines have already been discussed in previous chapters.

○ **compliance program** a set of internal policies and procedures put into place by an organization to help the organization comply with laws and industry-accepted best practices.

TAKE AWAY ●·········

An effective compliance program can enhance the operation of an organization, improve quality of care, and reduce overall costs.

CURRENT TRENDS IN HEALTH CARE

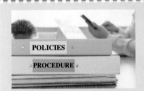

The Affordable Care Act (ACA) mandated that health care organizations with providers receiving Medicare and Medicaid payments are required to have a compliance program. Previously, many smaller facilities did not have staff solely dedicated to a compliance function, but instead tasked all employees with managing their daily routines in a compliant manner. However, due to increased scrutiny and penalties, it is becoming increasingly common for even the smallest medical practices to have a dedicated employee who functions as the compliance officer, such as the health services administrator. Another option for small medical practices is the contracting of a third party or legal counsel for internal compliance reviews at multiple points throughout the year.

Development

All health organizations need to develop their own compliance program based on the type of entity that they are and the type of service that they offer because they may be subject to additional or different laws and regulations than others. For example, clearinghouses, billing companies, small medical practices, nursing homes, and hospitals all need to tailor a compliance program to the type of services they provide.

Before the passage of the ACA in 2010, compliance programs were not mandatory by law or a requirement to receive reimbursements from federal health programs, such as Medicare and Medicaid. However, the requirement for an effective compliance program for health care organizations is transitioning from voluntary to mandatory, with the Patient Protection and Affordable Care Act requiring that health care providers applying to enroll as Medicare providers have a compliance program in place.

Although a compliance program is not a guarantee that fraud, waste, abuse, or inefficiency will not occur, the implementation of an effective compliance program will aid in better protecting the health care provider and organization from risk and may lead to several benefits for the organization, such as:

- Complying with federal guidelines and reducing the chances that an audit will be conducted
- Optimizing proper payment of claims and minimizing billing mistakes
- Avoiding conflicts with the self-referral and anti-kickback statutes.

The Office of Inspector General

One of the most important federal agencies that enforces compliance for health care organizations is the **Office of Inspector General (OIG)**. Under the division of the

○ **Office of Inspector General (OIG)** federal government office that prevents fraud and abuse in Department of Health and Human Services programs.

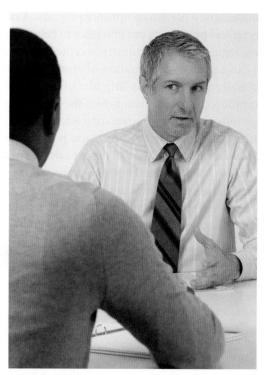

Figure 13.1 An auditor from an accrediting agency speaks to an employee during a site survey.

Department of Health and Human Services, the OIG monitors the department's federal health care program and those that benefit from those programs and protects these programs against fraud, abuse, and waste. A majority of the OIG's resources goes toward the oversight of Medicare and Medicaid.

Medicare and Medicaid are administered by the Centers for Medicare and Medicaid Services (CMS) and insure nearly 90 million people enrolled in these programs. CMS is the single largest payer for health care in the United States and accounted for more than 37% of the United States' health care spending, or $1.2 trillion, in 2015, according to the National Health Expenditure Data.[1] Federal spending on Medicare and Medicaid increased 8.9% in 2015 after growing 11% in 2014. The main factors in increased federal health care spending were the enrollment of newly eligible adults into Medicare due to the population aging and expanded health insurance availability made possible by the ACA.

In order for health care providers and health care suppliers to be eligible to receive payments or reimbursements for covered services provided by Medicare and Medicaid beneficiaries, they must be eligible, or "participate," in these programs. To participate, these providers and organizations must meet the standards of CMS' **Conditions of Participation (CoP)** or **Conditions for Coverage (CfC)**, depending on the type of participating entity. The CoPs are the health and safety requirements with which all hospitals, rehabilitation agencies, hospices, and most public health agencies must comply to participate in the Medicare and Medicaid programs, and CfCs include ambulatory surgical centers and skilled nursing facilities. Besides obtaining eligibility based on meeting federal requirements and guidelines, each health care organization must be either certified by a CMS-approved state agency or receive *deemed status* by obtaining accreditation from an accrediting body approved by CMS, such as TJC (Fig. 13.1).

Conditions of Participation (CoP) the terms that a facility or provider must follow to receive reimbursement from the Centers for Medicare and Medicaid Services.

Conditions for Coverage (CfC) the terms that a facility or provider must follow to receive reimbursement from the Centers for Medicare and Medicaid Services.

---

[1]https://www.cms.gov/research-statistics-data-and-systems/statistics-trends-and-reports/nationalhealthexpenddata/nhe-fact-sheet.html

Once participation is approved by CMS, the health care organization or provider must agree to accept assignment of claims for all services provided to Medicare and Medicaid beneficiaries. Additionally, providers must agree to Medicare- and Medicaid-allowed amounts as payment and not collect more than the allowed amounts for deductible and coinsurance from the beneficiary, which is based on the Medicare Physician Fee Schedule.

It is important for Medicare- and Medicaid-participating organizations and providers to remain compliant with the requirements of the CoPs and CfCs. Deficiencies in one or more of the conditions can result in denial of payment and may lead to exclusion from these federal programs if not corrected. Thus, to help ensure compliancy, the OIG encourages all health care organizations to develop a compliance program in order to internally monitor business operations and to ensure continuous compliance and efficiency in the use of federal and state funds. The OIG has published guidelines for each type of health care organization to develop internal monitors and controls to address statutes, regulations, and program requirements. Regardless of the type of health care organization or provider, the OIG lists fundamental elements that should be included in every compliance program (Box 13.1).

TAKE AWAY ●··········

Providers and organizations must meet CMS standards to receive payments for services to beneficiaries.

BOX 13.1   THE OIG'S SEVEN FUNDAMENTAL ELEMENTS OF A COMPLIANCE PROGRAM

1. Written policies and procedures.
   a. Create and write down the standards of conduct and other policies that make sense for the organization.
   b. Share them with everyone in the organization.
   c. Update policies periodically.
2. Compliance professional.
   a. Designate an individual to keep up with federal and state requirements and recommendations.
   b. Empower the individual with independence, authority, and a connection to people and information throughout the organization.
3. Effective training.
   a. Educate all employees.
   b. Ensure that they understand compliance program policies.
4. Effective communication.
   a. Facilitate communication between the compliance officer and all employees.
   b. Provide employees a way to report misconduct.
   c. Protect employees who report violations from retaliation.
   d. Comment boxes.

   e. Anonymous hotline.
   f. Open door policy.
5. Internal monitoring.
   a. Conduct audits—the heart of any effective compliance program.
   b. Use some kind of review to evaluate how the compliance plan is working.
   c. Good compliance programs identify problems from time to time.
   d. If no problems are identified, it could be a sign that what is being done is not effective.
   e. If a problem is detected, then the organization is in a position to do something about it.
6. Enforce your standards.
   a. It's not enough to develop, distribute, and educate employees about policies.
   b. Make sure that employees are following the policies.
   c. Take action when someone is not complying with procedures.
7. Promptly respond to issues.
   a. Look into reports of misconduct or other problems right away.
   b. Take steps to resolve the issues as quickly as possible.

Compliance Plan

An important component of a compliance program is the compliance plan. A compliance plan consists of written standards and procedures that include practice policy statements regarding patient care, personnel matters, and practice standards and procedures on complying with federal and state laws. A compliance plan should also include:

- **Standards of conduct.** Standards should be set in all areas. What is acceptable behavior, and what will not be tolerated? What activities drive compliant business operations, and what behaviors impede compliance? It should also be noted what associated disciplinary action will result from noncompliant behavior.

- **Assignment of compliance officer and a compliance committee.** Every plan needs a designated manager or leader for effectiveness and to guide success. The **compliance officer** is an individual whose role is to make sure the operations of an organization meet regulatory requirements. In a medical office, the health services administrator may be named the compliance officer. In larger health organizations, such as a hospital, the health services administrator may work alongside or underneath a chief compliance officer, who may be a lawyer or health care provider.

- **Development of compliance policies and procedures to standardize operational activities.** Each area of the business should have written policies and procedures that are guidelines for daily operation.

- **Benchmarks** for determining the effectiveness of the plan. For example, during the annual compliance training for all staff, the health services administrator may want to document staff knowledge by using pretests and posttests.

- **An anonymous system,** whether a hotline or online submission program, for reporting of suspected compliance violations without fear of retaliation.

- **New hire and annual education programs,** newsletters, and regulatory updates for all staff members, as well as specialized training for leadership and employees in high-risk positions.

- **Internal and external auditing** and monitoring programs. The health services administrator and other staff members in other departments should perform routine audits to identify any areas of risk in their respective departments and develop a method for dealing with these risk areas with *action plans,* when applicable. An **action plan** is a formal document listing goals and the people and resources needed to reach them within a certain time frame (Fig. 13.2).

compliance officer an individual whose role is to make sure the operations of an organization meet regulatory requirements.

action plan a formal document listing goals and the people and resources needed to reach it within a certain time frame.

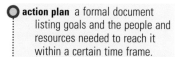

Action Area	Strategy	Task	Name and title of responsible person	Measurable	Timeline	Complete	
						Date	Init
Electronic Health Records (EHR)	Preventing security breaches of Protected Health Information (PHI)	Routine training of all staff and personnel	June Jones, Compliance Officer	Semi-annual training with 100% completion	Conduct training every 6 months	6/18	JJ
		Identify and limit access based on need only	Frank Stanley, Health Services Administrator	Compile list of staff with access and update monthly	List of staff access updated on 15th of every month	3/18	FS
						4/18	FS
						5/18	FS
						6/18	FS

Figure 13.2 Example of an action plan.

- **Organizational enforcement** of compliance-related issues. If a compliance issue or a violation has been identified, a process should be in place for prompt referral or disclosure to an appropriate government authority or law enforcement agency. It should also be assessed if the entire organization or specific departments need to be required to be retrained on compliance.
- **Screening mechanisms** to ensure eligibility of qualified employees, vendors, and contractor relationships. An important function of the compliance officer or the health services administrator is to ensure that all employees, medical staff, and independent contractors are not on the OIG's List of Excluded Individuals and Entities or the General Services Administration's List of Parties Debarred from Federal Programs, which will be discussed further later.
- **Annually updated** compliance plans that address areas of risk within specific departments or divisions. In addition, all employees should receive semiannual or annual training on how to perform their jobs in compliance with the standards of the practice and any applicable regulations.

Regardless of the type, every health organization should designate a compliance officer and compliance committee to develop, implement, and oversee the compliance program. The compliance committee should be composed of staff members from different departments who are responsible for compliance at the health organization, such as the compliance officer, a general counsel, a human resources representative, health care providers, and the health services administrator. The compliance committee should meet to review policies, procedures, annual compliance plans, and reports; perform risk assessments; and develop corrective and disciplinary actions. In addition, the committee would need to oversee internal and external audits and review the effectiveness of the compliance program.

Importance of Documentation

In Chapter 5, we discussed the importance of documentation in the health care setting, specifically regarding patient care, legal liability, reimbursement, administrative operations, and compliance. As part of a sound compliance structure, the organization and retention of information and documentation are of utmost importance. Even the strongest compliance plan will fail if the health care organization or practice is not able to document its business operations in a clear format for internal and external review.

> **TAKE AWAY** •·········
>
> Organized and safeguarded documentation is essential for compliance.

Proper documentation of patient medical records and claims is necessary in compliance for the following reasons:

- **Protect the programs.** Good documentation is important to protect federal health care programs, specifically Medicaid and Medicare. Accurate documentation ensures that federal health care programs pay the right amount to the right people for the right services.
- **Protect patients.** Good documentation is important to protect patients. It promotes patient safety and quality of care. Complete and accurate medical recordkeeping can help ensure that patients get the right care at the right time. For example, a surgical procedure for a patient may be delayed or not approved by the health insurer if the physician did not accurately document it in the patient's medical records.
- **Protect the provider.** Good documentation is important to protect the provider. It helps avoid liability and protects against allegations of fraud and abuse. If records do not justify items or services that were billed, the provider may have to pay that money back.

Timely, accurate, and complete documentation is important to patient care. This same documentation serves as a secondary function when a claim is submitted for payment as verification that the claim is accurate and that the necessary medical documentation supports it.

One of the most common areas where health care organizations experience compliance issues is in the documentation of diagnosis and treatment. The appropriate medical treatment for patients is heavily dependent on the physician's documentation, and it is also the basis for coding and billing determinations. A medical record documentation is used to validate:

- The site of the service
- The appropriateness of the services provided
- The accuracy of the billing
- The identity of the caregiver (service provider)

Health care organizations should develop a set plan and process for documentation and timing for the collection and review of documents. The health services administrator or compliance officer needs to be aware of federal, state, and local requirements for the statute of limitations, or the length of time that patient medical records should be stored and in what format (Table 5.2). As part of this plan for recordkeeping, a documented system for internal review to ensure compliance should be a part of the health care organization's compliance plan. Whether it be a random pull of files on a weekly basis or a systematic process for review of a specified number of files in a given time frame, a health care organization needs to have a plan in place and needs to follow that plan. Not only is the proper documentation by the physician and other health care providers necessary, but also auditing medical records and files and documenting findings are vital to maintaining compliance.

Implementation

After a compliance plan is developed, reviewed, and put into written policies and procedures, it must be implemented across the health care organization. An effective compliance program will involve all areas and levels of the business and will ensure that all employees are committed to being compliant. It must take into account tasks and processes in each area of the operation that affects the adherence to governing laws and regulations.

Employees and key **stakeholders**—any individuals with an interest in the process—must understand the importance of compliance in the areas addressed by the program. Thus, to effectively implement a compliance program, it must be communicated in a way that is understandable and relevant to the business and from the perspective of the employee reviewing the plan.

> **stakeholder** an individual with an interest in a work process or function.

There are six steps to implementing an effective compliance program:

1. **Foster a culture of compliance.** Committing financial resources is necessary to support an effective compliance program. If the organization invests in developing the necessary monitoring systems, training programs, and auditing processes, employees will take notice and buy into a culture of compliance.
2. **Support the compliance function with the right attitude.** Even more important than money and resources, the health care organization's attitude is critical to maintaining compliance. Compliance must be a part of the business' culture and not something thought of only once a year or during the compliance training. It must be incorporated in the daily operations of the health care organization. For example, maintaining compliance should be discussed at every staff meeting, and it should be kept in mind during every interaction with outside vendors, referring physicians, and patients. Additionally, celebrating employees who have effectively identified and resolved any compliance issues is an excellent way of displaying a positive attitude toward compliance.
3. **Create useful policies and procedures.** Policies should be specific to each job function and department in the health care organization. Review policies frequently

and make necessary updates as needed to keep the compliance plan relevant to the business and its daily activities. Confirm that every employee has received, reviewed, and understands the policies by conducting routine compliance training. Employees should be made aware of the policies by posting them in areas readily and easily accessible. A monthly newsletter can be created and distributed to all employees.

4. **Train often.** Training is an exercise; the more you do it, the better the outcome. Make training an essential function of every job in the health care organization. Be creative and generate compliance question-and-answer sessions or games to get everyone interested and involved. It is also important to be current by attending conferences and reading publications related to health care compliance.

5. **Promote communication.** Encourage communication and dialogue between employees and other stakeholders by staying visible and being approachable. Give staff frequent opportunities to express what is going right, as well as the areas for improvement. Develop and encourage employees to use an anonymous hotline or online system for reporting compliance issues. If an anonymous reporting system is used, develop a system to track and respond to complaints quickly and effectively. Review all incoming complaints, and investigate when necessary. This may require the designation of a compliance team to address these issues. In cases where compliance issues are found, take the appropriate corrective action. Provide feedback to employees regarding compliance issues that were identified and how they were resolved. Talk about a nonretaliation policy in staff meetings, and include it in all compliance policies and procedures.

6. **Conduct regular audits.** Identify risk areas, and audit and investigate any issues. Common health care risk areas include coding, contracts, and quality of patient care.

Monitoring for Effectiveness

After developing and implementing the compliance program, it is important to continually evaluate the program objectively to determine its effectiveness. When performing the evaluation, ask the following:

- Are benchmarks being met?
- Are the benchmarks effective in keeping the company in compliance?
- Are employees utilizing the anonymous reporting systems to address compliance issues?
- Are the corrective action plans in place sufficient to address the problems?

In a dynamic industry such as health care, compliance programs and the corresponding monitoring systems can quickly become outdated or obsolete. Thus, as regulations and laws change, the compliance program must reflect those changes. Processes and procedures may have to be updated for daily business activities to meet new requirements and to maintain compliance. An organization that can quickly interpret new regulations and laws, update the compliance program, communicate any new changes to all stakeholders, implement the compliance program, and monitor its effectiveness has an edge on its competitors.

For example, the health care organization should routinely audit claims submitted to health insurance companies. The audit should be preventative and proactive and should not be done when the insurer or federal government imposes an audit due to inaccurate billing. Depending on the health care organization and the type of services offered, it may be beneficial or necessary to retain an attorney who specializes in health care law to ensure compliance with certain laws or statutes.

LEARNING CHECKPOINT 13.1
Compliance Program

1. True or False. The OIG recommends an anonymous program for the reporting of compliance violations.

2. The _____ of a compliance plan describes acceptable and unacceptable behavior.

3. The _____ is an individual whose role is to make sure the operations of an organization meet regulatory requirements.

4. An _____ is a formal document listing goals and the people and resources needed to reach it within a certain time frame.

NONCOMPLIANCE

TAKE AWAY ●·········

The most important federal fraud and abuse laws that apply to health care providers and health care organizations are the False Claims Act (FCA), the Anti-Kickback Statute (AKS), and the Physician Self-Referral Law (Stark Law).

Chapter 12 discussed the legal and regulatory environment in health care in detail. With regard to compliance, the most important federal fraud and abuse laws that apply to health care providers and health care organizations are the False Claims Act (FCA), the Anti-Kickback Statute (AKS), and the Physician Self-Referral Law (Stark Law).

False Claims Act

The FCA is a federal law that makes it a crime for a health care provider or health care organization to knowingly make a false record or file a false claim regarding any federal health care program, such as Medicaid and Medicare, whether directly, through insurance, or otherwise, that is funded directly, in whole, or in part by the federal government or any state health care system. Examples of false claims include billing for services not provided, billing for the same service more than once, and making false statements to obtain payment for services.

Committing a violation of the FCA can be both a civil and a criminal act where significant fines, penalties, and even imprisonment may result. Physicians have gone to prison for submitting false health care claims. The OIG may also impose administrative civil monetary penalties for false or fraudulent claims.

Anti-Kickback Statute

The AKS is generally an anticorruption statute. It is a federal fraud and abuse statute that prohibits health care providers and health care organizations from conducting any business relationship or transaction intended to induce reward or patient referrals for services reimbursed by federal health care programs. For example, a physician or health services administrator may not receive money or any other kind of remuneration from a specialist in exchange for referring Medicare or Medicaid patients to that specialist. Penalties include sizable fines, imprisonment, and exclusion from participation in federal health care programs.

Physician Self-Referral Law (Stark Law)

The Physician Self-Referral Law, often called the *Stark Law,* is a "conflict of interest" law that prohibits physicians from referring patients to receive health services paid by federal health care programs where the physician or any immediate family member has a financial relationship, unless an exception applies. Exceptions to the Stark Law may be providing Medicare-covered preventative screening tests and immunization, eyeglasses and contact lenses, and implants and other prosthetics furnished in an ambulatory surgical center. Immediate family members are defined as spouse, natural or adoptive parents, children, siblings, stepsiblings, in-laws, grandparents, and grandchildren. Further, the Stark Law pertains only to a specific list of "designated health services," such as imaging studies, physical and occupational therapy, home health, durable medical equipment, and all inpatient and outpatient hospital services. For example, a physician receiving incentive pay for referring Medicare patients to a certain hospital would be in violation of the Stark Law. Penalties for physicians who violate the Stark Law include fines, as well as exclusion from participation in federal health care programs, which is discussed later. Fig. 13.3 is

ABC Health care LLC
ANNUAL CONFLICT OF INTEREST DISCLOSURE FORM
FOR LEADERSHIP and STAFF

Name (please print)   Department

Date   Title/Position at the organization

It is the policy of ABC Health care LLC to address how issues of actual, potential and perceived conflicts of interest involving trustees, officers, and employees of the Institute should be identified, disclosed and managed. This form is designed to identify and disclose known conflicts in an effort to properly manage them.

Please complete the following questions, and submit this form to the appropriate designated individual as noted on the last page of this form.

1. Are you or a member of your immediate family an officer, director, trustee, partner (general or limited), employee or regularly retained consultant of any company, firm or organization that presently has business dealings with the organization or which might reasonably be expected to have business dealings with the Institute in the coming year? _____Yes _____No
If yes, please list the name of the company, firm or organization, the position held, and the nature of the business which is currently being conducted with the Institute or which may reasonably be expected to be conducted with the Institute in the coming year:
_____
_____

2. Do you or does any member of your immediate family have a financial interest, direct or indirect, in a company, firm or organization which currently has business dealings with the organization or which may reasonably be expected to have such business dealings with the Institute in the coming year? _____Yes _____No
If yes, please list the name of the company, firm or organization, the nature of the interest and the name of the person holding the interest, and the nature of the business which is currently being conducted with the University or which may reasonably be expected to be conducted with the Institute in the coming year:
_____
_____

3. Do you or does any member of your immediate family have a financial or personal interest in an entity in which the organization has a financial or other vested interest? _____Yes _____No
If yes, please provide details below:
_____
_____

4. Have you or an immediate family member accepted gifts, gratuities, lodging, dining, or entertainment that might reasonably appear to influence your judgment or actions concerning the business of the organization? _____Yes _____No
If yes, please provide details below:
_____
_____

5. Do you have any other interest or role in a firm or organization, where that interest or relationship might reasonably be expected to create an impression or suspicion among the public having knowledge of your acts that you engaged in conduct in violation of your trust as a trustee, officer, faculty or staff member? _____Yes _____No
If yes, please provide details below:
_____
_____

Please add additional pages as needed.

Figure 13.3 Conflict of interest disclosure form.

Continued

ABC Health care LLC
ANNUAL CONFLICT OF INTEREST DISCLOSURE FORM
FOR LEADERSHIP and STAFF

If any material changes to the responses provided on the annual disclosure form occur before the next form is due, the trustee, officer or employee is required to update the information on this form in writing, and submit the update to the compliance officer or committee.

I have read ABC Health care LLC's Conflict of Interest Policy and understand that as an employee of the organization it is my obligation to act in a manner which promotes the best interests of the organization and to avoid conflict of interest when making decisions and taking actions on behalf of the organization.

My answers to this disclosure form are correctly stated to the best of my knowledge and belief. Should a possible conflict of interest arise in my responsibilities to the organization, I recognize that I have the obligation to notify, based on my position, the appropriate designated individual (compliance officer), and to abstain from any participation in the matter until the organization can determine whether a conflict exists and how that conflict shall be resolved. If any relevant changes occur in my affiliations, duties, or financial circumstances, I recognize that I have a continuing obligation to file an amended "Conflict of Interest Disclosure Form" with the appropriate designated personnel.

I understand that the information on this form is solely for use by ABC Health care LLC and is considered confidential information. Release of this information within the organization will be on a need-to-know basis only. Release to external parties will be only when required by law and/or Federal regulations.

Signature: _____   Date: _____

Figure 13.3, cont'd

an example of a form explaining a policy and asking for the employee to identify and disclose any potential conflicts of interest.

OIG Audits and Actions

In addition to providing recommendation on compliance, the OIG conducts audits of health care organizations and providers to ensure compliance with federal laws and health care regulations. The OIG investigates and evaluates organizations based on tips and information received from patients, current employees, former health care employees, and any other resources. After an investigation, the OIG will make decisions based on its findings. The result of the findings may lead to criminal, civil, and administrative penalties on individuals or organizations found guilty of any violation against federal law or health care statutes.

As discussed earlier, one of the penalties of committing fraud or abuse is **exclusion** from participation in federal health care programs. The OIG has the legal authority to exclude health care organizations and providers from receiving payments from federally funded health care programs, such as Medicare and Medicaid. Additionally, the OIG maintains a list of all currently excluded health care organizations and providers called the *List of Excluded Individuals and Entities (LEIE)*. Health care organizations and providers may be included in the LEIE by being convicted of the following types of criminal offenses:

- Medicare or Medicaid fraud, as well as any other offenses related to the delivery of items or services under Medicare or Medicaid
- Patient abuse or neglect
- Felony convictions for other health care–related fraud, theft, or other financial misconduct
- Felony convictions for unlawful manufacture, distribution, prescription, or dispensing of controlled substances

In addition, the OIG has discretion to exclude heath care providers and organizations on misdemeanor convictions related to health care fraud or in connection with the

exclusion disciplinary action that excludes a health care facility or provider from participating in any type of federal health care program.

unlawful manufacture, distribution, prescription, or dispensing of controlled substances; suspension, revocation, or surrender of a license to provide health care for reasons of professional competence, performance, or financial integrity; submission of false or fraudulent claims to a federal health care program; and engaging in unlawful kickback arrangements.

A health care organization that hires a health care provider on the LEIE and looks to receive payments from a federal health care program may be subject to penalties. If services are furnished by an excluded provider or health care organization, any federal health care payments received associated with the excluded provider or organization would have to be paid back. The facility would also need to show that it did not know and had no reason to know about the exclusion. For example, if a medical practice hires a physician who is on the exclusion list and he provides services that were paid for by Medicaid, the medical practice would be required to return the payment and justify to the OIG why the physician was employed with the practice.

Anyone can be excluded, from licensed clinicians to unlicensed personnel. Corporate entities and officers can also be excluded by the OIG. There are two types of OIG exclusions: mandatory and permissive exclusion. **Mandatory exclusions** are the result of:

- Conviction of program-related crime
- Conviction related to patient abuse or neglect
- Felony conviction related to a controlled substance
- Felony conviction related to health care fraud

A **permissive exclusion** can result from:

- Lying on an enrollment application
- Certain misdemeanors
- Loss of a state license to practice
- Failure to repay health education loans
- Failure to provide quality care

Being on the exclusion list has drastic results. The disciplinary action extensively narrows a health care provider's employment options with any health care organization that provides services to Medicare and Medicaid–eligible patients. While on exclusion, the health care provider is restricted to work in nonfederal health care payment settings, provide care to nonfederal health care beneficiaries, and/or seek nonpatient care employment opportunities.

The length of the exclusion for an entity varies, depending on the case and the basis for the exclusion, but the minimum period for a mandatory exclusion is 5 years. Individual exclusion is based on individual conviction or the part played in the actions causing the entity's exclusion. However, when the disciplinary action is administered, it is generally for a set period. Further, exclusions based on licensure action have an indefinite period.

After a health care provider or organization has completed the necessary terms of the exclusion, reinstatement is not automatic. At the end of the exclusion term, a provider must apply for reinstatement, with the OIG sending notice that reinstatement has been either granted or denied. However, before being reinstated, the OIG may conduct additional investigation, or it may require the contracting of a third party for auditing purposes to ensure that the proper safeguards are in place in terms of compliance with federal, state, and local laws and regulations for that health care provider or organization.

Disclosure

The OIG publishes a list on its website of all individuals and businesses that have received the disciplinary action of exclusion: https://oig.hhs.gov/exclusions/. This list

mandatory exclusion the result of conviction of a program-related crime, conviction related to patient abuse or neglect, felony conviction related to a controlled substance, or felony conviction related to health care fraud.

permissive exclusion the result of lying on an enrollment application, conviction of certain misdemeanors, the loss of a state license to practice, the failure to repay health education loans, or the failure to provide quality care.

TAKE AWAY ●·········

Routinely check the OIG website and the exclusion list for individuals and businesses that have received the disciplinary action of exclusion.

is published for the protection of health care providers to keep them from entering into employment contracts with organizations that are under exclusion and for the purpose of alerting the public of those individuals and organizations that have been found guilty of fraud and abuse of federal health care programs.

In monitoring the compliance program, the health services administrator, compliance officer, or a designated member of the compliance committee should routinely check the OIG website and the exclusion list. If it has been discovered that the health care organization has employed or done business with an excluded entity or provider, it is necessary for the organization to self-disclose the interaction or relationship to the OIG and take the necessary actions to correct the situation. In any compliance program, timely corrective action, including self-disclosure, is essential. In a **disclosure**, the organization works collaboratively with the government toward a resolution. Providers who voluntarily disclose noncompliant behavior are looked at more favorably and may receive reduced penalties compared with those being investigated due to the result of a complaint or reporting. Disclosing a problem voluntarily demonstrates a culture of compliance.

In addition to the self-disclosure, it is important for the organization to take corrective actions. Corrective actions would include refunding any payment from the federal health care program received as part of the unlawful rendering of service to the beneficiary. Moreover, if an organization keeps federal health care program payments it is not entitled to, it faces additional penalties under the False Claims Act and the Civil Monetary Penalties Law.

When noncompliance is discovered, steps must be taken to address the situation based on its severity:

1. Clarify the issue and confirm that it is a potential case of fraud. For instance, overpayments and unintentional errors can be reported to the health insurance company through the normal refund process.
2. In the case of more significant findings, consult with a health care attorney who has federal health care experience. The attorney would be helpful in confirming that there is, in fact, a violation and what the options are for reporting it.
3. Decide where and to whom to disclose the conduct. Disclosure to the local federal attorney's office may be appropriate depending on the conduct. When applicable, the OIG has a self-disclosure link on its website, and it should be used for reporting noncompliance when necessary.

Self-disclosure and self-reporting offer health care providers benefits that would not be available should an issue of fraud or abuse be discovered by a third party. This allows the provider or the health care organization to minimize the potential cost and prevent a full-scale audit. It may also allow the organization to negotiate a reduction in penalties and avoid being placed on the OIG exclusion list.

Resolution Process

Voluntarily disclosing noncompliant behavior is both necessary and beneficial to a health care organization. Thus the organization should have an established protocol for voluntary self-disclosure. When developing such a protocol, the health care organization must consider the following points:

- **Timing of a disclosure.** Think carefully to avoid disclosing prematurely. Rushed disclosure reporting may result in inaccurate results or the elimination of relevant data. Conversely, a lack of urgency in reporting could lead to the issue being reported by a third party instead, resulting in more stringent and severe disciplinary actions.
- **Full description of the conduct.** Incomplete submissions may be rejected and may delay the review process.

disclosure the voluntary self-reporting of an infraction.

TAKE AWAY •·········

Self-disclosure and self-reporting allow health care providers to minimize the potential cost and prevent a full-scale audit.

- **Prompt response to requests for additional information.** The OIG needs and expects the cooperation of the organization if it is to reach a resolution. All requests for information should be treated as urgent, requiring immediate attention.

Corporate Integrity Agreements

In the case a health care provider or organization has been found to be in violation of federal health care programs, sanctions and penalties for the misconduct may be required, as well as being placed on the OIG exclusion list, or the LEIE. In some cases, the OIG may allow the provider or organization to enter into a **corporate integrity agreement (CIA)** to reduce penalties and avoid being placed on the exclusion list. A CIA is an enforcement tool used by the OIG to strengthen its efforts to enforce federal health care statutes and actively address cases of fraud and abuse. A CIA is a settlement negotiation between the OIG, the federal and/or state government, and the health care provider or organization in violation. A CIA guides organizations through the implementation of an effective compliance program that will, for example, ensure proper billing practices, including submission of accurate and complete claims for payment to federal health care programs, appropriate arrangements with physicians, and improved quality of care for program beneficiaries.

> **corporate integrity agreement (CIA)** an enforcement tool used by the Office of the Inspector General (OIG) to promote compliance.

Since the mid-1990s, the OIG has entered into more than 1000 CIAs or similar agreements. In recent years, the OIG has expanded its reach and entered into CIAs with a number of different health care organizations and suppliers who have been in violation of federal health care laws, including pharmaceutical manufacturers, clinical laboratories, nursing homes, home health agencies, and durable medical equipment and pharmacy suppliers. The OIG posts all currently active CIAs on its website. The health services administrator or compliance officer should review new CIAs as part of a routine evaluation of the compliance program and risk assessment process.

Although labor intensive and often expensive to comply with, most health care providers and organizations would rather agree to the requirements of a CIA to reduce monetary penalties than to be placed on the OIG's exclusion list, which would make them ineligible to participate in federal health care programs. In return, the health care provider or organization commits to being compliant with federal health care guidelines and laws and the provisions to the CIA. Most CIAs are 5 years in duration.

Although the terms and conditions of these CIAs vary depending on the nature and extent of the fraudulent or abusive action, they have many similar elements. One of the most important requirements of a CIA is the implementation of a comprehensive compliance program modeled after the OIG's published guidelines, which was discussed earlier in the chapter and includes:

- Hiring a compliance officer/appointing a compliance committee
- Developing written standards and policies
- Implementing a comprehensive employee training program
- Retaining an independent review organization to conduct annual reviews
- Establishing a confidential disclosure program
- Restricting employment of ineligible persons
- Reporting overpayments, reportable events, and ongoing investigations/legal proceedings
- Providing an implementation report and annual reports to the OIG on the status of the entity's compliance activities

LEARNING CHECKPOINT 13.2
Noncompliance

1. A provider sees and treats a patient for routine foot care, but bills Medicare for "nail avulsion," a more complicated and more expensive procedure. This is a violation of the:

   a. False Claims Act
   b. Anti-Kickback Statute
   c. Stark Law
   d. Conditions of Participation

2. Oliver is an advance practice registered nurse (APRN) at a retail care clinic and sees many patients who complain of having a sore throat. Generally he can treat his patients with over-the-counter or prescribed medicine, but occasionally he must refer his patients to an ear, nose, and throat (ENT) specialist (an otolaryngologist). He always sends his patients to Dr. Nickerson, who gives Oliver $50 for any new referrals. This is a violation of the:

   a. False Claims Act
   b. Anti-Kickback Statute
   c. Stark Law
   d. Conditions of Participation

3. Which action could result in a mandatory exclusion?

   a. Failure to provide quality care
   b. Felony conviction related to health care fraud
   c. Loss of a state license to practice
   d. Failure to repay health education loans

CASE STUDY

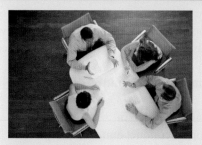

Carrie gathers the compliance committee back together after a month of observation and finds that, for the most part, the business is running compliantly. However, two main concerns have been identified. The first is that one of the services offered by the health care provider is not being coded correctly when it is submitted for payment. It has consistently been coded incorrectly as a service that will result in higher reimbursement. The second issue is that patient medical records are not being consistently documented by all the clinical staff. Some medical records are missing documentation. Carrie decides that these are the first two processes that she will suggest a written policy for, and then she will roll out training. She decides the company should self-disclose because the repercussions will be worse if fraud or abuse is discovered by a third party.

1. What is a compliance program, and why is it important?

2. What is the role of the OIG in compliance?

3. Who develops a compliance plan?

4. What are the potential consequences of compliance violations?

5. Why is it important to self-report or self-disclose when noncompliance has been identified in a company? What happens if the company does not self-disclose?

COMMUNICATION

14 BUSINESS COMMUNICATION AND PROFESSIONALISM
15 MARKETING

CHAPTER 14

BUSINESS COMMUNICATION AND PROFESSIONALISM

Meredith Robertson

CHAPTER OUTLINE

INTRODUCTION
PROFESSIONALISM
  Patient Respect
  Dependability
  Professional Team Collaboration
EFFECTIVE COMMUNICATION
  Communication Barriers
    Privacy
    Lack of Time
  Special Populations
    Elderly Patients
    Cultural Sensitivity and
      Competency
    Hard-to-Reach Populations
    Patients in Pain
  Verbal Communication
    Phone Etiquette
      Answering the Call
      Confirming Appointments
      Test Results

Billing
Closing the Call
Triage and Call Flow
  Management
  Patient Visit
Nonverbal Communication
Written Communication
  Email Etiquette
    Email or Phone Call
    Replying to Incoming Email
    Subject Line
    Message Content
    Closing and Signature
    Proofreading
    Carbon Copy and Blind
      Carbon Copy
    Reply to All
    Forwarding Emails
    Attachments

Professional and Formal
  Business Letters
  Business Address
  Date of Letter
  Recipient Address
  Greeting
  Main Body
  Closing
  Signature
  Form Letters
  Memorandums
  Heading
  Body or Content
  Formatting
  Distribution
  Meetings
  Agenda
  Minutes

VOCABULARY

agenda
blind carbon copy (bcc)
business letter
carbon copy (cc)
complementary and alternative
  medicine (CAM)

cultural competency
cultural sensitivity
hard-to-reach population
memorandums (memo)
minutes
needs assessment

nonverbal communication
patient-centered medical home
  model
professionalism
verbal communication
written communication

CHAPTER OBJECTIVES

After completing this chapter, the student should be able to do the following:

1. Distinguish professional behavior from nonprofessional behavior.
2. Understand barriers to communication, including patient privacy and time constraints, and techniques to overcome them.
3. Utilize verbal and nonverbal communication strategies in health care settings.
4. Understand the importance of respect for patients, especially those with special needs, such as the elderly, individuals with cultural diversity, hard-to-reach populations, and patients in pain.

5. Understand the importance of dependability and team collaboration on patient outcomes.
6. Utilize proper phone etiquette with patients and other health care professionals.
7. Communicate in writing through clear and concise emails, business letters, and memorandums.
8. Distinguish between business letters and memorandums and the different parts of each.
9. Describe what should be included in meeting agendas and minutes.

INTRODUCTION

Regardless of the type of business, successful professionals are usually those individuals who behave in certain ways. These professionals are most often honest, trustworthy, ethical, dependable, accountable, respectful, and show personal integrity in their work. Businesses who strive to maintain these values and foster these kinds of professionals tend to see "repeat customers" because they develop relationships with their clients and form bonds of trust.

Leaders in the health care field with these professional values are usually the colleagues you want to work with, the respectful employer you want to work for, or the reliable employee you want to hire. However, health care professionals must go further to ensure positive relationships with their unique customers—patients.

In this chapter, we will discuss behaviors and skills of successful health care professionals, specifically the importance of respect and dependability, and how to consistently display professionalism through effective communication. Not only are professionalism and good communication important to learn now; they are attributes and skills that can continually improve throughout one's career.

CASE STUDY

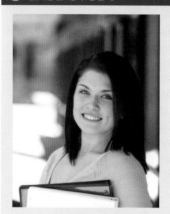

Zeina is the health services administrator for a dialysis center. The center has a new patient, Stella, who is elderly and does not understand English well. Several of the staff members are struggling to communicate with her. What can Zeina do to help her staff and Stella? What kind of training can Zeina provide to her staff to help them with other patients with communication challenges?

PROFESSIONALISM

> **professionalism** the skills, judgments, and behaviors that are expected in the workplace.

Professionalism is defined as the skills, judgments, and behaviors that are expected in the workplace. Health care professionals must be honest and show integrity in the work that they do. Each health care professional must be responsible for his or her own behavior and work products or outcomes. To be truly altruistic and to advocate for patients' care, health care professionals must be compassionate and show empathy and respect toward patients. In a health care setting, professionalism may include, but is not limited to:

- Adhering to patient safety guidelines
- Safeguarding patient privacy
- Ensuring continuous quality improvement
- Maintaining accurate and timely medical records
- Following professional rules of ethics
- Complying with billing practices
- Strengthening patient relationships through effective communication and timely follow-up

Patient Respect

Health care professionals must put the patients' needs and safety above all other priorities. This means that responsiveness to patients' needs supersedes self-interest. Health care professionals can show respect by responding to the patient as a person and not just as a case or a number—for example, "the coughing patient in room 12." Patients who are treated with respect are more engaged in their health care decisions and have higher patient satisfaction than those who are not. Further, patient health outcomes are improved when patients express their own thoughts, expectations, and concerns.

Dependability

When people follow through on promises and commitments, they become more trustworthy and dependable. The importance of dependability is the fostering of trust, which is directly applicable for developing a successful patient–provider relationship. Patients must be able to depend on their health care providers to give the advice and services needed to keep them healthy. All team members must understand that all of their actions affect the reputation of the business as being dependable. For example, simply returning a phone call when promised or completing tasks in a timely manner promotes trust in the patient relationship.

Professional Team Collaboration

The office environment also benefits from professionals who can similarly be trusted by their colleagues to be available when needed and are willing to accept responsibilities. Professionalism among peers is critical in today's health care setting. It is increasingly difficult for a single provider to have all the knowledge needed to treat a patient in the best manner possible. Without teamwork and respect, health care professionals cannot achieve desired results for their patients. When conflicts among team members arise, health care professionals should remember that, above all, the patient's health and needs should be the primary focus when working to resolve the conflict.

Collaboration from members of the health care team is also addressed in the Affordable Care Act, specifically in the Accountable Care Organizations (ACOs). As discussed in Chapter 3, the ACO is a model of patient care where groups of doctors, hospitals, and other health care providers voluntarily collaborate to give coordinated high-quality care to their Medicare patients. The goal of this coordinated care is to ensure that patients, especially the chronically ill, get the right care at the right time, while avoiding unnecessary duplication of services and thus preventing medical errors.

Another model of collaborative patient care is the **patient-centered medical home model (PCMH)**, which is a health care delivery model in which patient care is coordinated through the primary care physician. The objective of the PCMH model is to have a centralized setting that facilitates partnerships among individual patients, their physicians, and the patient's family, when appropriate. Patient care through the PCMH model is facilitated by registries, information technology, health information exchange, and other means to assure that patients get the appropriate care when and where they need and want it and in a culturally and linguistically appropriate manner. As a result, the PCMH model improves the quality and accuracy of information exchanged and thus optimizes resources and improves patient health outcomes. In addition, it aids in providing coordinated care and continuity of care to patients and reduces the likelihood of bias and provider fatigue, which ultimately will reduce patient adverse events.

Being a health care professional means treating other team members with respect and sensitivity. This improves overall team collaboration and the work environment, can reduce employee turnover, and increase job satisfaction. It should also be noted that professionalism is shown through one's ability to take constructive feedback from

TAKE AWAY ●·········

The patient's needs and safety are the top priority.

◯ **patient-centered medical home model** a health care delivery model in which patient care is coordinated through the primary care physician.

supervisors in a receptive and nondefensive manner. Recognizing one's limits and seeking help when needed are signs of a responsible employee, and, although this can be challenging, it does lead to improved patient care.

LEARNING CHECKPOINT 14.1
Professionalism

1. Which aspect of professionalism is the focus of the patient-centered medical home model?

    a. Sensitivity
    b. Respect
    c. Collaboration
    d. Dependability

2. Why is dependability an important professional behavior?

    a. It builds trust.
    b. It safeguards patient privacy.
    c. It helps improve safety.
    d. It improves collaboration.

EFFECTIVE COMMUNICATION

TAKE AWAY

Better communication leads to better care.

Better communication in patient care leads to better health outcomes and improved overall quality of care for patients, as well as increased patient satisfaction, greater patient safety, fewer medical errors, and fewer malpractice lawsuits. Being able to effectively communicate with patients, their families, and other health care professionals is critical because poor and ineffective communication can harm patients' lives. The inability to effectively communicate can lead to receiving inaccurate patient history, such as medication history, which can lead to drug allergies, drug interactions, toxicity, and other inappropriate therapeutic decisions. This contributes to patient confusion and frustration and nonadherence to treatment regimens, whereas good communication can increase the likelihood of patients adhering to medical recommendations, self-managing chronic conditions, and adopting preventative health behaviors.

All health care professionals need to assess their communication skills to better ensure that information regarding treatment and therapy, prevention, and health promotion are delivered effectively to patients, thus improving health outcomes (Fig. 14.1).

The Joint Commission, which is an independent organization responsible for the accreditation of more than 21,000 health care organizations and programs, has indicated that miscommunication is a significant driver of medical errors. Although The Joint Commission requires accredited organizations to use a standardized approach to communications, breakdowns in communication have been a leading contributing factor in unexpected events involving death or serious physical or psychological injury or the risk of death or injury. In addition to patient harm, poor communication has led to delays in treatment, inappropriate treatment, and increased length of stay in the hospital. Further, another study showed that poor team communication was the main cause for nearly 66% of all medical errors. The study also found that communication between health care professionals is further inhibited by stressful, high-task situations that can lead to breakdowns in effective communication, increasing the likelihood of medical errors.

Fortunately, effective communication skills can be learned and continuously improved through professional commitment and practice. Working environments where colleagues

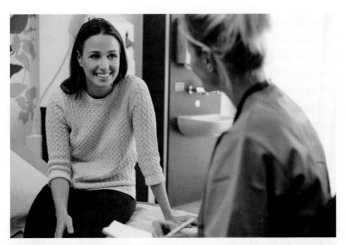

Figure 14.1 Effective communication leads to better patient outcomes.

BOX 14.1	EXAMPLES OF HEALTH CARE COMMUNICATION

- Explaining office protocol, insurance requirements, and patient financial responsibility
- Communicating with patient, families, and other health care professionals
- Seeking informed consent for procedures and/or information sharing
- Asking questions and listening for patient history and complaints

- Including the patient in decision making
- Explaining diagnosis, medication, and treatment regimens
- Delivering bad news
- Providing discharge instructions
- Making recommendations for health behavior changes, improved control of risk factors, and other patient education

effectively communicate improves the quality of working relationships and reduces staff turnover. In fact, researchers have found that there is a direct relationship between job satisfaction for health care professionals and their ability to show compassion and warmth to patients. Health care professionals are more satisfied in work environments where they feel supported, respected, and valued, with clearly defined job roles, and experience work equity and fair compensation. Furthermore, those who have effective communication skills are more likely to have successful careers. Box 14.1 lists examples of communication in health care.

Communication Barriers

Today's health care environment presents many challenges to effective communication with patients, their families, and even other health care professionals. Patients are experiencing shorter hospital stays, which creates more demand on ambulatory care services, providers, and resources.

We begin our discussion of communication barriers in the health care setting by first considering the beginning of the patient experience. Unlike with other businesses, patient clients arrive at the reception desk not because they *want to* be there, but because they *must* be there. They are immediately placed in a position with little control. They likely have more anxiety than other types of business "customers" because they have stress about loss of time, potential financial costs, and their overall future health. Patients

TAKE AWAY ●·········

Lack of privacy and inadequate time are two communication barriers in health care.

are too often greeted with orders, such as "give me your insurance identification," "sit over there," and "wait until we can see you." Patients will then be moved into an isolated room where they are asked to remove their clothing and await a stranger who will walk into the room at any minute. This situation may put patients at a point of high stress and anxiety and creates a communication barrier for health care professionals. It is the responsibility of the health care professional, including the health services manager, to help ease patients' concerns and make them as comfortable as possible during the patient visit.

Privacy

One of the most important communication barriers is privacy. If patients feel confident and trust that their information will be kept confidential, they are more likely to disclose more personal information, which will assist in accurate diagnosis and treatment planning. In addition to the Health Insurance Portability and Accountability Act (HIPAA) privacy provisions, discussed in Chapter 12, health care professionals are legally bound to keep confidential and not share, discuss, or disclose patient information with anyone, including family, friends, or another health care professional, without the consent of the patient.

Additionally, every effort should be made for health care professionals to speak with patients in a private space and to avoid discussions with colleagues or other patients in public areas, such as hallways, elevators, parking lots, and the waiting room (Fig. 14.2). A patient's comfort with the environment also makes it more likely that the patient will ask more questions about the diagnosis and treatment plan rather than avoiding perceived "embarrassing" or "stupid" questions. This improves patient education and understanding and makes patient medical adherence more likely.

Lack of Time

A lack of time with patients may be a significant communication barrier for health care professionals. Studies have shown that the amount of time spent with patients directly affects their satisfaction and experience. However, patients are often rushed when sharing their medical history with health care professionals, which may affect the accuracy of the medical diagnosis and treatment. Patients are also less likely to offer additional information, which may be important to aid in their diagnosis, if they feel the provider appears rushed and does not have time to listen.

Interruptions during a patient visit may deter from information gathering and damage the overall patient relationship. It also makes the patient feel disrespected and that his

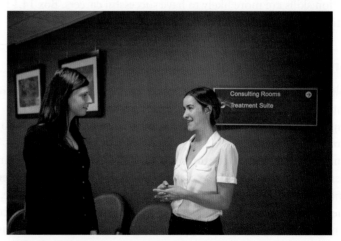

Figure 14.2 A health services manager offers to speak with a patient in a private consulting room.

or her visit and time are less important than other office business. Thus the physician–patient visits should be uninterrupted, unless there is an urgent situation that demands the physician's immediate attention.

The health services manager can focus on workplace processes and flow that improve efficiency and allow each patient adequate time for his or her visit. For ambulatory care facilities, such as physician offices, this can be done by the scheduling process and allocating sufficient time for each patient. Another strategy that saves time and promotes effective communication is being prepared—for example, reviewing the patient's intake and medical history before seeing the patient.

Special Populations

Working in health care means working with a diverse population of patients with unique communication challenges. Groups of different ages, races, ethnicities, socioeconomic status, and those with acute or chronic conditions will have special communication needs, and health care professionals must have the appropriate skills to meet these needs.

Elderly Patients

According to the US Department of Health and Human Services' Administration on Aging, the number of individuals age 65 or older is likely to double from 45.1 million in 2014 to about 98 million by 2060. Elderly patients have some of the most complicated health issues of all Americans, and many have comorbidities, or multiple chronic conditions. Older adults also require more visits to their health care providers compared with any other age group. As a result, it is important to understand the unique challenges that face elderly patients and how to best communicate critical health information with them.

Some of the earliest signs of aging in elderly patients are hearing and vision loss and impairment. The population 65 years old and over account for roughly 37% of all hearing-impaired individuals and 30% of all visually impaired individuals. In general, visual and hearing impairments can reduce physical, functional, emotional, and social well-being, such as isolation and depression. For the elderly population, this may lead to an additional decrease in independence in performing the activities of daily living, getting from place to place, or communicating with others.

Age-related hearing loss, or *presbycusis*, is the loss of hearing that gradually occurs as we age. Most hearing impairments for the elderly patient come from the inability to distinguish high-frequency sounds, which is what makes it difficult for them to tell differences between background sounds and conversation. Thus it helps communication if the health care professional faces the older patient so that the patient can use lip reading to understand what is being said. During the patient visit, it is also recommended to keep the conversation focused on a single topic to avoid overwhelming the patient with too much information.

Visual impairment is vision loss that cannot be corrected by glasses or contact lenses alone and is increasingly common in the elderly. Visual impairment, including blindness, has four main causes: cataracts, glaucoma, diabetic retinopathy, and age-related macular degeneration. Also common as a result of aging is the gradual loss of the eyes' ability to focus on nearby objects, called *presbyopia,* occurring most commonly by the mid-40s and worsening until around age 65. Additional visual impairments in the older population include reduced peripheral vision, reduced ability to distinguish some colors, and a sensitivity to bright glaring lights and surfaces that are highly reflective. Thus it may be difficult for older patients to read patient instructions and other printed materials. The health services manager should ensure that the medical office includes important

TAKE AWAY ●·········

Diverse patient demographics present unique communication challenges.

forms and patient education material in a larger type size, as well as any signage used in the office or waiting area.

Although many elderly patients may have others, such as family members, with them, always speak to the patient. Do not assume that the patient is incompetent. When scheduling appointments with older patients, you may want to allow extra time for the visit because, as mentioned earlier, they are more likely to have multiple health-related issues that need to be discussed with the health care provider. It is particularly important when working with older patients that the health care experience be unhurried. It may also be beneficial to some older patients to have appointments scheduled when the office is less busy. Take time to engage them in conversation, speaking slowly and clearly. Do not assume all older patients have hearing challenges. It is also best to avoid any slang or youth-oriented phrases. And, most important, treat elderly patients with the same respect that all patients deserve.

Cultural Sensitivity and Competency

Patients have varied ethnic, cultural, and socioeconomic backgrounds. These factors and characteristics often affect the reasons patients seek health care, and they may influence the relationship and interactions between the patient and health care providers. Therefore professional behavior in the health care setting includes not only showing compassion and respect to patients, but also being sensitive and aware of the cultural needs of the patient population. Unprofessional and unethical behavior that may lead to illegal actions, on the other hand, would include discrimination and harassment based on age, race, color, creed, religion, citizenship, sex, marital status, sexual orientation, disability, military status, and national origin.

Health care professionals must have **cultural sensitivity** to effectively advocate for their patients' health. Cultural sensitivity means having the understanding and knowledge of cultural characteristics, history, values, belief systems, and behaviors of the members of different ethnic groups. Further, **cultural competency** in the health care setting is the ability of providers and health care organizations to effectively deliver health care services that meet the social, cultural, and linguistic needs of patients. A culturally competent health care organization can help improve health outcomes and quality of care and can contribute to the elimination of health disparities for their patients.

In health care, effective intercultural communication can affect a patient's mental and physical health overall.[1] It is important to remember that some patients have their own cultural beliefs that may not always align with American cultural beliefs, including spiritual roles, use of medication and nutrition, how diseases are spread, and approaches to decision making. Make sure to talk to the patient about his or her values and beliefs and work to integrate those into the patient experience and treatment plan. When taking the medical history, ask patients if they are using any **complementary and alternative medicine (CAM)** as part of their health care plan. CAM generally includes natural products, such as herbs and nutritional supplements, and mind and body practices, such as hypnotherapy and acupuncture (Fig. 14.3). According to the National Institutes of Health, more than 30% of adults in the United States use health care approaches developed outside of Western or conventional medicine.

There are also several nonverbal communication strategies to be aware of when it comes to working with cultural differences. These are described further in the "Nonverbal Communication" section of this chapter.

cultural sensitivity knowledge and interpersonal skills that allow health care professionals to understand and work with individuals from diverse cultures.

cultural competency the ability of providers and health care organizations to effectively deliver health care services that meet the social, cultural, and linguistic needs of patients.

complementary and alternative medicine (CAM) health and wellness therapies used along with (and complementary to) conventional medicine, focusing on the "whole person," including the physical, mental, and spiritual health of the individual.

---

[1]Voelker, R. Speaking the languages of medicine and culture. *JAMA.* 1995;273(21):1639–1641. doi:10.1001/jama.1995.03520450007003.

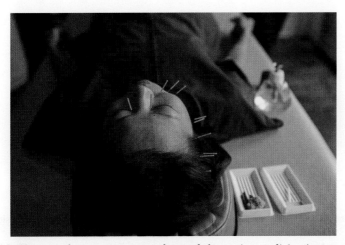

Figure 14.3 The use of acupuncture as a form of alternative medicine is commonplace.

Hard-to-Reach Populations

Health care often uses the term **hard-to-reach population** to describe the unique attributes of groups of patients who have obstacles to patient engagement and treatment adherence. Patients who are considered a part of the hard-to-reach population may include illicit drug users, people living with HIV, people from sexual minority communities, and homeless people. They may also include patients with limited financial resources, transportation challenges, low literacy levels, low socioeconomic status, and an inability to understand and/or speak English. Due to the added challenges, these groups of patients may have limited access to health care and thus are less likely to have had preventive services and regular sources of medical care and are less likely to understand medical jargon or processes. They may also have different approaches to coping with health issues. Health care professionals need to be aware of these differences and their challenges and be ready to accommodate.

Hard-to-reach patients deserve the same respect, time, and information as other patients. It is also important to consider that these patients may have greater health care needs than other patients due to lack of resources and/or preventive care and thus need more time with the provider. Be sensitive to these needs when working with this population. For example, when medication is being prescribed, health care professionals need to think about the cost of the prescription for the patient. Does the office have samples of the medication? It is also helpful to have a list of community resources to provide to patients, such as prescription drug programs that offer discounts to people with lower incomes.

Patients who do not speak English or for whom English is a second language have a unique set of circumstances, which presents significant communication barriers. For these patients, you can find out if there is an English-speaking family member or friend who can help serve as an interpreter (Fig. 14.4). If you use this approach, however, make sure that the patient agrees to have the person involved prevent any violation of confidentiality.

If someone is not available to interpret, speak slowly and clearly, although be cautious that you do not speak so slowly as to insult the patient. Focus on using simple phrases, and avoid slang or expressions that may be misinterpreted. Another approach is to use gestures and "act out" what you are trying to explain or use pictures. Sometimes writing the message is easier for some patients to understand.

If you find that you are frequently in this situation, it is helpful to learn a few words in the language that is most commonly used among your patients. Just a few words can go a long way, at least in communicating that you care and that you want to make

hard-to-reach population a group of individuals who may be transient, homeless, have mental illness, or have socioeconomic disadvantages and may be harder for health care professionals to reach for purposes of health care follow-up and treatment adherence.

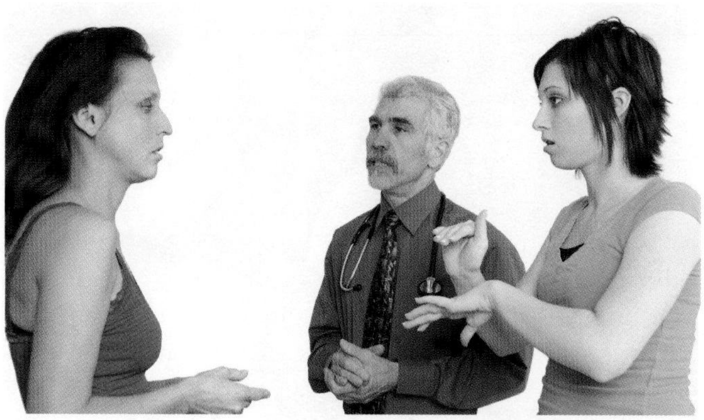

Figure 14.4 A younger family member acts as an interpreter for the physician.

your patients as comfortable as possible. If all else fails, you may request the services of a professional interpreter. Interpreter services are now available over the telephone or through video.

Patients in Pain

Pain is one of the most common reasons for a patient to see a health care provider. For patients in pain, the best first step is to try to help the patients get as comfortable as possible and provide them extra time during the patient visit. As with the other patients described earlier, it is recommended that you speak slowly, using simple phrases, and focus on one key point. Avoid asking more than one question at a time, and then give the patient time to respond. You may need to repeat the question to ensure that the patient understood. It may be helpful to give them written instructions that they can refer to later at home. If you have a patient in pain who frequently visits your office, try to schedule appointments when the patient experiences the least pain or discomfort.

Verbal Communication

Now that we have identified the various barriers to communication, next we will review the different approaches that can be used to communicate health care information to patients. First, we will discuss verbal communication and nonverbal communication. **Verbal communication** is simply sharing information, thoughts, and feelings through speech. The most common examples of this are through conversations over the phone and during patient visits.

verbal communication sharing information, thoughts, and feelings through speech.

Phone Etiquette

One of the most frequently used forms of verbal communication in health care is done over the phone. Oftentimes, communication by phone provides the patient with the first impression of a health care organization, and it all begins with how the phone is answered. Whether the phone call is to schedule an appointment, refill a prescription, or provide critical health information regarding treatment, the phone call can have a positive or negative impact on the overall business. Excellent phone etiquette is one of the most important tools to prevent a loss of patients, or patient attrition. Put yourself in the patient's shoes and consider what happens when the phone rings and rings. One begins to question whether the medical office will ever answer the call, whether the practice is understaffed, and what the quality of patient care and attention provided will be like. For example, if patients have to leave a message, they expect this message to be returned. As the health services manager, always be aware of patients' expectations.

Answering the Call

A best practice is that all phone calls should be answered by the third ring. All employees in the health care organization should work toward this goal, not just the front desk receptionist. Otherwise, if the call is not answered, the patient may hang up and call again, which just creates another call for you to handle later. Or, worse, the patient may not call back and will find another provider. Once you answer and have to put the caller on hold, always ask first and wait for a response before doing so. Just pausing that extra moment indicates that you care about the caller and his or her time.

The telephone greeting should be friendly and professional. It helps to smile when answering calls, as this improves the likelihood that your voice is conveying the same friendliness and energy. It has been shown that people can sense whether a speaker is smiling or frowning. Make sure to speak clearly using a moderate volume and speed. Although people like to hear the sound of their own name, health care professionals need to exercise discretion when mentioning the name of the caller and/or patient to protect confidentiality. At a minimum, avoid using both the patient's first and last name over the phone in case your conversation is overheard.

Offer to take a message if you cannot handle the call immediately. For example, if you are going to need to have another staff member answer the patient's questions, take a message. Otherwise, the caller may be placed on hold and left waiting for a long period. This may create extreme frustration for the patient. Taking messages also helps health care providers work more efficiently, as calls can be addressed in batches, thus avoiding interrupting work flow, which can often be a cause of medical errors. If you have taken a message, ensure that the call has been returned. Remember the importance of following through on promises and the role of dependability in building patient trust. The worst situation is not returning calls, which suggests the business does not care about its patients, leading again to patient attrition. The more efficient the work processes are, the more quickly you can help patients get the care they need.

Confirming Appointments

Using reminder calls or emails can reduce the number of no-shows and cancellations. However, do not include too much information in these communications. For example, if you must leave a voicemail message, keep it brief and succinct. If the message is too long, key pieces of important information may be lost or perhaps not even heard.

Test Results

Often patients will call the medical office for their test results. Make sure that the health care provider has seen the test results first and given permission to share them with the patient. Office policies should indicate which health care personnel can deliver test results and other medical information to patients. If the test results are unfavorable, the health care provider should share the results directly with the patient and give further instructions to the medical staff. Any questions regarding test results should be addressed by the health care provider, and the staff should show caution on not going beyond their scope of practice. As a general rule of thumb, the best approach for handling positive or abnormal test results is to schedule an appointment for the patient with the health care provider, as serious news is best delivered in person rather than over the phone. Sensitivity and tactfulness must be used in answering and managing these types of calls.

Health care professionals should also be careful that they properly identify patients before giving out any test results over the phone. The health services manager and all other health care personnel need to be aware of federal and state laws and regulations regarding the release of any medical information to someone other than the patient, including patients who are minors. Sharing information with individuals other than

TAKE AWAY ● · · · · · · ·

Excellent phone skills are among the most important communication skills in the practice.

the patient without authorization may be considered a breach of confidentiality and violate the privacy rules of HIPAA.

Some health care organizations may use the patient's date of birth or other types of personal information known only to the patient to be used as a form of identification. Other organizations may even use a special password or code that patients must provide before confidential information is released. It is recommended that health care professionals obtain at least two pieces of identification before sharing confidential medical information.

Billing

Patients may be calling to discuss their billing concerns. If billing matters are handled by another staff member or external company, tell the patient that the call will be transferred. (Some ambulatory care facilities use external agencies, in which case you may need to provide the caller with that entity's phone number.) If your organization is responsible for billing, politely ask patients to hold while you obtain their billing record. Once you have their information in front of you, thank them for waiting and tell them that you are able to answer their question(s) now. If there was an error, apologize and let them know that a corrected statement will be sent in the mail as soon as possible.

Ideally, patients should be given information on charges and fees before or when services are rendered. This practice will reduce the number of billing calls. However, fees vary widely among different facilities, and it is often impossible to quote an exact fee before services are incurred. So, in these situations, patients should be given an estimate of what they may expect to pay overall and at the time of the initial visit. After giving patients an estimate, remind them that the rate may vary based on any tests ordered and their results and the diagnosis made by the health care provider. If the facility requires the copayment to be paid at the first visit, make sure this is communicated to the patient. If it is office policy to regularly discuss fees over the phone, it is best practice to create a script that staff members can use when needed.

Closing the Call

When closing the call, use the same friendly tone you used to begin the phone conversation. Ensure that any instructions or medical information has been understood by the patient. Remember to avoid using any medical terms or abbreviations that the patient may not understand. Repeat key pieces of material discussed during the call to confirm the caller has understood the information. Make sure to ask if the patient has any other questions and thank the caller for the phone call before saying goodbye.

Triage and Call Flow Management

All health care organizations should be dedicated to improving patient satisfaction and quality of care by looking for ways to improve the patient experience. This begins by establishing performance targets to be monitored on a regular basis. To improve the quality and efficiency of the phone management system, a *needs assessment* should be performed. A **needs assessment** is a process used by organizations to determine priorities and "gaps" between current conditions and desired goals to make organizational improvements or allocate resources. A needs assessment can be used to evaluate how many calls the business receives each day, the peak times for calls, and how many calls may be lost due to long hold times. After establishing existing call volume, each business should evaluate the types of calls received. For example, if most of the calls are nonurgent matters, it may make the most practical sense to move these callers to each health care provider's voicemail box. Another performance measurement is to establish the monthly average and then gather the next month's data and see if you have improved upon that average.

needs assessment process used by organizations to determine priorities and "gaps" between current conditions and desired goals.

The phone system should allow patients to be triaged directly to billing and referral staff. Similarly, it is helpful to have patients directly connected to clinical staff for prescription refills. Regularly review the types of calls you receive and determine if a specific type of call could be reduced by creating another form of communication. For example, if the medical office requires injury reports from nursing homes each week, consider having those reports received as a fax or email rather than as a phone call. Or a special email box that goes directly to medical billing staff could be created solely for billing questions.

Patient Visit

When interacting with patients, all verbal communication should be clear, concise, sincere, polite, honest, and respectful. Health care professionals need to remember that patients enter the health care system under duress and emotion. Effective verbal communication with patients includes both active listening skills and sharing of information. Good patient relationships are created through the health care professional's ability to ask questions with kindness and to communicate information in a manner that does not frighten but shows interest and provides security and trust. Health care professionals should have empathy and compassion for the experiences of the patient, and they should be able to convey a response that is fully comprehensible and not bogged down in medical jargon.

By making sure that patient education is clearly understood, the health care professional increases the likelihood that patients are engaged in their own health care. More than ever, patients want to be active participants and decision makers in their own health care. Many are interested in preventive health behaviors, such as diet and exercise, and some will likely have done preliminary research on the Internet before seeing the health care provider. To be effective patient educators, health care professionals need to assess the patient's needs, concerns, preferences, limitations (e.g., low health literacy or mental capacity), and readiness to learn. The first step for health care professionals is to figure out what the patient already knows and then set health education goals. Patient education may be related to promoting wellness, preventing illness or disease, providing rehabilitation, and improving coping skills.

> **TAKE AWAY** •·········
>
> Health care professionals must remember that patients come to the practice under duress and emotion.

Nonverbal Communication

As described earlier, effective communication skills help health care professionals identify patients' health care needs more accurately, improve health outcomes, and improve patient satisfaction. In addition to verbal communication, effective communication includes nonverbal communication. **Nonverbal communication** is communication that occurs without language. It can be used to provide patients reassurance, exchange emotions, manage impressions, and share information. When verbal communication is unclear, nonverbal expressions can enhance the exchange of information in a health care setting.

Some examples of nonverbal communication include:
- Facial expression: smiling, frowning, eyebrow raising, or sustained eye contact
- Body posture: whether arms or legs are crossed or uncrossed
- Interpersonal distance: leaning forward
- Gestures: moving head or limbs, such as giving a "thumbs up" or clenching one's fist
- Tone of voice: pitch, volume, monotony, and rate of speech
- Touch

Sometimes nonverbal cues do not align with the message being expressed in words. When verbal and nonverbal cues are contradictory, most people are more likely to believe that the nonverbal cues are more telling because nonverbal communication is instinctive and likely to be sincere.

> **nonverbal communication**
> communication that occurs without language, such as body posture, gestures, facial expressions, gazes, eye contact, and tone of voice.

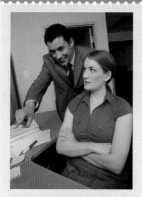

CURRENT TRENDS IN HEALTH CARE

Nonverbal communication is critical in the health care industry because it provides more accurate information between the patient and health care providers. A UCLA study found that 7% of information is relayed verbally, whereas 38% is communicated by voice tone and 55% by gestures and posture.

A 2002 study demonstrated that physicians who made significant eye contact, focused on the patient instead of the patient's chart, displayed concerned facial expressions, leaned in toward the patient, were seated approximately 2 feet from the patient, and smiled were more likely to establish patient trust than those who did not.[2] Studies have also shown that the length of the patient visit is correlated to patient trust—the longer the visit, the greater the trust. There are even studies that suggest understanding patients' nonverbal cues may be the best way for the provider to detect accurate patient pain levels. Patients who are able to trust their provider are more likely to actively participate in their care and be compliant with their treatment plan.

Written Communication

> **written communication** sharing information through written documents, such as emails, business letters, memorandums, and meeting agendas and minutes.

Another form of nonverbal communication is through **written communication**, which includes emails, business letters, memorandums, and meeting agendas and minutes. It is critical that written documents be accurate, clear in the message they are conveying to the reader, and professional in the tone and language to preserve the reputation of the health care organization. Written communication is also important because the words used are recorded and permanent and often considered legal documents. In the health care setting, some written communication shares confidential patient information. Thus all health care professionals must be cautious of what data and patient information are shared and with whom they are shared.

Email Etiquette

As with other business settings, the health care industry continues to transform and move toward more advanced technology. One of the more significant examples of this is the way health care professionals interact with patients by email and online. Currently, email is universally used for both professional and personal reasons to communicate and exchange information quickly and effectively. Thus poor email etiquette has the potential to sabotage both your personal and your professional reputation. If you are a new employee, it is always beneficial to talk to your supervisor about any specific email etiquette used by your health care organization. Just as any other forms of communication, emails are a reflection of you and your employer.

This section will further discuss common mistakes that are made in email communication and ways to avoid damaging your business' reputation.

[2]Aruguete MS, Roberts CA. In: Psychological Reports. Dec 2002, Vol. 91 Issue 3, p793, 14 p.; Ammons Scientific, Ltd.

Email or Phone Call

The first consideration when writing an email is to decide whether email is the best method of communication for the information you are sharing. When a message has multiple pieces of information that require explanation or negotiation, you should pick up the telephone instead. Otherwise, an email may generate several "back and forth" emails and create added confusion and wasted time. If timing of communication is critical, such as last-minute cancellations of meetings or appointments, a phone call may be warranted to ensure timely delivery. Another instance when an email may be inappropriate is when bad news needs to be communicated.

Replying to Incoming Email

In general, you should reply to any incoming email. Even if you do not know how to respond to the email immediately, it is better to send a note to the sender stating that the email has been received than to send no response at all. Without a reply or an email received receipt, the sender is left wondering whether you received it, whether you have forgotten it or ignored it, or why a response is taking so long. If more time is required to answer the sender's email, the best approach is to respond with an estimated timeline as to when you expect to reply, such as: "I should have an answer for you by early next week." Response times will vary based on the content of the incoming email, but often email responses should be sent within 24 to 48 hours.

If an incoming email triggers an emotional response from you, such as anger, it is recommended that you do not respond immediately. If time permits, "sleep on it" and wait until the next day to respond, or at a minimum, take a moment to catch a breath to prevent an emotional or inappropriate response. Remember emails last forever. When responding, make sure to address all issues from the incoming email and answer all questions.

Before hitting "send," consider whether the information being conveyed is related to the business or is personal. Emails coming from the health care staff should always be business related. You should ask yourself whether you would be comfortable sending the message using company email and whether the information should be shared outside of the office.

Subject Line

When sending an outgoing email, it is a good practice to ensure your subject line conveys a summary of the email message. The subject line should be descriptive, but short and concise. If the email contains a date or deadline, include this in the subject line. Table 14.1 shows examples of poor and effective email subject lines.

Message Content

The goal of your email is to convey accurate and timely information to the reader. When creating your email, the communication should be clear and with the most

TAKE AWAY
Generally, the practice should respond to all emails.

TABLE 14.1

EXAMPLES OF EMAIL SUBJECT LINES

Poor Email Subject Lines	Effective Email Subject Lines
Greenville Healthcare Conference	Invitation: Greenville Healthcare Conference: Aug. 12-14
Monthly Report Due	Monthly Budget Report: Due to John Smith Jan. 2
Interesting Article	FYI: Article with Tips on Health Care Communication with Elders
Action Needed!	Action: Decision on Billing Vendor Needed by Oct. 1

important points at the top of the message. The reader should not have to dig through the full email or, even worse, have to reread the email to get the main information. The purpose of the email should be stated in the first or second sentence. Later in the email, you can provide more detailed information or additional context. You may even indicate that "additional details are described below." When creating the email content, here are a few additional tips:

- Indicate at the beginning of the email whether or not the recipient needs to take some action.
- Avoid responding with "OK." For example, if your supervisor emails you about an office issue and you respond with "OK," you may come across as flippant or curt. If you are trying to respond quickly from your phone, it may be better to wait until you are at a computer before responding so you can provide a more thorough response.
- Avoid jargon, medical terminology, and abbreviations in emails to readers who may not be as familiar with the health care industry as you are. Be aware of your audience and write out abbreviations.
- Avoid emoticons, text abbreviations such as LOL or OMG, and multiple exclamation points. Using these will make the sender and the employer appear unprofessional.

Most readers appreciate the use of bullet points for more detailed information and easier reading. This allows readers to do a quick skim of the email and get to the main points if they are short on time. It is also easier to read if the writer includes space between main points of information. A good rule of thumb is to limit paragraphs to no more than five sentences.

One of the most common pitfalls in emailing is interpreting a writer's tone in an email. So be cautious when using sarcasm and/or humor in emails. If you have any question about how something might be received, it is better to leave it out or make different word choices. Always go out of your way to ensure an email is polite, professional, and courteous with the use of "please" and "thank you." Also, avoid using all caps or lowercase letters—all caps may be interpreted as the sender yelling, and the use of all lowercase may imply a lack of urgency or laziness from the sender.

Health care professionals must be aware that much of the information they are communicating is confidential in nature. Therefore you should always check with your supervisor on your organization's policy regarding emails to ensure compliance with the HIPAA guidelines. Some health care facilities may have standard privacy language that is included in all email correspondence that provides contact information in the event that the email is sent to the wrong address.

Closing and Signature

Professional emails should always include a closing and signature that provides your full name, title, company, and other contact information, such as a phone number. A more formal business closing may use "Sincerely" or "Best regards" before your signature. Alternatively, "Thanks" is often an acceptable way to close a business email.

Proofreading

Before sending the email, it is a best practice to always proofread it. A well-written email is one that uses appropriate capitalization, punctuation, grammar, and spelling. One tip is to read your email out loud before sending it. Health care personnel should also double-check the spelling of names and addresses to ensure accuracy and to avoid sending the email to the wrong person or having it "bounce" back or returned.

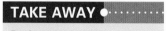

TAKE AWAY

Professional emails should close with the sender's contact information.

Carbon Copy and Blind Carbon Copy

In addition to the main recipient, some professionals will often use **carbon copy (cc)** when they want to include someone on the email for informational purposes only and are not expecting the cc'd recipient to respond. Similarly, **blind carbon copy (bcc)** may be used to include someone for informational purposes, but his or her identity is not shared with the other recipients. Oftentimes, "bcc" is used to send an email to the entire list of recipients but to keep the identity and email addresses of all recipients hidden.

Reply to All

The "reply all" should only be used when, in fact, everyone on the email truly needs the information in the response. It may be appropriate to only reply to the sender and then manually add the addresses of only some of the other recipients. Also, never reply all on an email where you were blind copied (bcc'd), since the original sender used bcc to keep your identity confidential. If you reply all, then you reveal your identity. The bottom line is that it is important to take the extra time to be cautious about sending your emails to the right people.

Forwarding Emails

When forwarding an email, your message, with your signature, should be above the forwarded email. Do not mix your text with the forward message, which can be confusing. Avoid making any changes to the forwarded email, unless you want to reduce the length of the text in which case you can use "…" to let the reader know you have removed a portion of the text. It is also important to "clean up" the forwarded email by removing any unnecessary carets, such as ">," or poorly formatted line breaks. Also, consider removing any email addresses from the forwarded email to protect the initial sender's privacy.

Attachments

When it comes to adding attachments, such as a document or a photo, to an email, consider the size of the attachment. It may be appropriate to provide a warning if you are sharing a significantly large file, such as something over 5 MB. You may want to ask the recipient if it is okay to send a file that large or whether there is a better time of day when there is less email traffic. It can also be helpful to use email tools that ensure your emails always include subject lines and attachments if you include the text "attachment enclosed."

Professional and Formal Business Letters

Health care professionals frequently use **business letters** as a form of written communication with patients, colleagues, and other professionals. It is important that these letters are courteous, written clearly, and articulate the main points of the communication at the beginning. Most business correspondence, such as drafting business letters, will be the responsibility of the health services manager. Thus the health services manager should be prepared to draft the following types of business letters:

- Appointment reminder letters
- Patient billing letters
- Referral letters (referring patients to another provider)
- Excused absence letters (for students or employees to document the reason for absence from school or work)
- Office announcement letters (such as changes in staff, insurance, hours, or other office protocols).

All formal business letters should be written on letterhead and typically have 1-inch margins on each side. Spacing throughout the letter should be consistent, either using

carbon copy (cc) a sending option used in email in which the sender wants to include someone on the email for information only and is not expecting that individual to respond.

blind carbon copy (bcc) a sending option used in email in which the sender wants to include someone on the email for information only, but the individual's identity is not shared with other recipients.

business letter written forms of communication for external parties. Business letters are often more formal and structured and include more background information than memorandums.

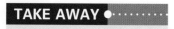

TAKE AWAY ●·········

Letters have a standard format.

single-space or double-space. To ensure readability, the letter should use a simple font, such as Times New Roman or Arial. Avoid overusing bold and italics for emphasis. Each letter should include seven key pieces, in order from top to bottom:

- Business's address
- Current date
- Recipient's address
- Greeting
- Main body
- Closing
- Signature

Fig. 14.5 shows an example business letter.

Business Address

It is common practice for businesses to have their address on the letterhead. However, if this is not the case, the letter should include the sender's address at the left margin, 1 inch from the top of the letter. Use single spacing and include the clinic or business's name, street or P.O. Box address, city, state, and ZIP code. It is not necessary to include the individual health care provider or employee's name because the author will be signing the letter at the end.

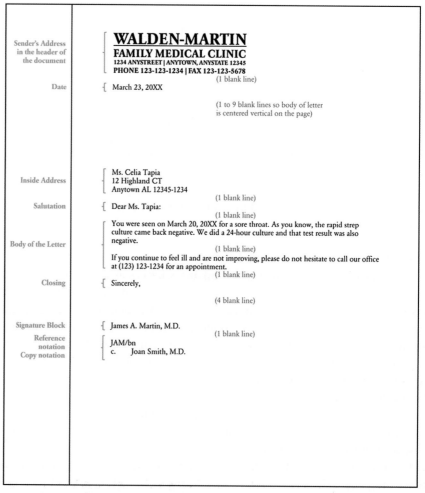

Figure 14.5 Example business letter. (From Proctor D, et al: *Kinn's the Administrative Medical Assistant*, ed 13, St. Louis, 2017, Elsevier. p. 116.)

Date of Letter

The date of a letter should reflect the date the letter was written, and it should be spelled out, such as December 15, 2016. If using letterhead, it should be inserted on the second line after the letterhead. Or, if not using letterhead, it should be on the second line below the business address.

Recipient Address

The address of the recipient should be left-justified. Allow for one blank line between the date line and the recipient address. This address should include the recipient's name and title on separate lines, followed by the department or agency where they work, then the street address, city and state, and ZIP code. Two-letter state abbreviations should be used. Always include the recipient's name or the guardian's name in the case the letter is going to the household of a minor.

Greeting

The greeting is also left-justified and placed on the second line below the recipient's address. The greeting should always be formal in business letters beginning with "Dear" and followed by the person's title (i.e., Mr., Ms., Dr.), his or her name, and a colon. For example, "Dear Dr. Jones:" may be the greeting. When addressing letters to women, try to use the recipient's preferred title. If you do not know her preference, use "Ms." If the gender is unknown, you may use the first and last name without a title or use the generic phrase "To Whom It May Concern."

Main Body

Two lines below the greeting is where the main body of the letter begins. In general, business letters tend to be short. The first part of the letter is a gracious opening clearly defining the purpose of the letter. Any remaining paragraphs should support the main point of the letter, with any action to be taken described at the end of the letter.

Closing

The closing of the letter should be left-justified and formal. It should be two lines below the body of the letter. Generally, letters close with "Sincerely." The closing should always be capitalized and followed by a comma. If the closing has multiple words, capitalize only the first word, such as "Best regards."

Signature

Formatting should include four line spaces where the sender will sign. Under the signature should be the typed name, title, and credentials of the sender. The title should be capitalized and placed directly below the name.

Form Letters

In this digital age, health care offices may use form letters to save time. Form letters created by different word-processing software can be personalized with patients' names and addresses and even personal case notes. However, if you are using a form letter, it should be personally signed if possible.

Memorandums

Business letters and **memorandums (memos)** are both forms of business communications with the intent to inform and make requests (Fig. 14.6). However, there are several differences between business letters and memos, with the most significant difference being the audience. Business letters are written forms of communication for external parties (outside the organization), whereas memos are written for internal colleagues and staff. Memos are

memorandums (memo) written form of communication for internal parties, often less formal and structured and include less background information than business letters.

Friendly Town Clinic

Memorandum

To: Patient Access Staff
From: Clinton Thomas, Health Care Administrator
CC: Dr. Hill; Dr. Burger; Dr. Lowdermilk; Amy Anslet, APRN
Date: May 15, 20XX
Subject: Painting scheduled June 29-30

We have scheduled Roberts Interiors to paint the interior walls of the facility beginning Friday night and ending Sunday evening. The crew of four will begin after close of business 6:00 pm Friday June 29 and work all night. The office will be open for our regular Saturday hours (9:00 am to 3 pm) during which no painting will be done to ensure regular patient flow. The crew is to continue work Saturday after closing and finish before the office reopens on Monday, July 2. Roberts Interiors will paint all rooms in the facility, except the exam rooms. You will not be responsible for moving any furniture, however, please ensure work spaces are neat and tidy.

This painting is scheduled from the evening of Friday June 29 until Sunday night, July 1. while the office is closed.

123 FIRST ST, FRIENDLY, PA 18611
T (123) 456-7890 F (123) 456-7899

Figure 14.6 Memorandum.

less formal and less structured than business letters, and the tone is more conversational. Memos also include less background information than business letters.

Formatting for memos is simpler than business letters, with only four required pieces: "To:"; "From"; "Date"; and "Subject." Most word-processing software have memo templates that make creating one very easy, although many businesses have created preformatted standard templates to be used within their organization. Memos also omit the mailing address and return address, as well as the opening and closing.

Memos are used to share information to solve problems and/or assist in decision making by analyzing issues and making recommendations. By using memos, organizations can avoid time-consuming meetings. For example, memos can be used to convey routine office information, such as protocol changes; discuss personnel changes; give instructions to staff; seek clarification; or share feedback.

Effective memos are efficient, persuasive, concise, and focused. Memos should only provide necessary information and should avoid being too "wordy." Memos should be short and focus on a single subject. Although memos are professional business documents, the tone of a memo is generally more informal and conversational. Box 14.2 lists some common mistakes made when crafting memos.

Heading

The heading should include the word "Memorandum" or "Interoffice Memorandum" followed by the four elements described earlier:

1. The "To:" line should include the recipient's name and business title, omitting titles of Mr., Ms., Mrs., and Miss. For several recipients, separate each name with a comma, or each name can be on its own line.

TAKE AWAY

Memos help the practice avoid time-consuming meetings.

| BOX 14.2 | COMMON MISTAKES IN WRITING MEMOS |

- Avoid "burying" the main point in the middle or end of the memo. There should be a summary at the beginning that highlights the main point of the memo.
- The memo should be organized and succinct. A reader should be able to skim it and be able to get a good idea of what the memo is about. Sometimes using headings can help the reader skim the key points of the memo without reading it completely.
- Memos often make recommendations. Oftentimes, the author does not provide sufficient evidence of support for the memo's recommendation. Never make a recommendation without evidence to support it.
- Some memos are written like academic papers with long sentences and difficult-to-understand vocabulary, when they should be short, concise, and easy for everyone to understand.

2. The "From:" line should include the sender's name and business title. The sender may choose to initial the memo next to his or her name before the memo is sent to signify the authorization of the memo.

3. The "Date:" is the date the memo was written, which should be spelled out.

4. The "Subject" is the main topic to be covered in the memo. The subject line in memos follows many of the same rules of thumb as the subject line in an email, as discussed earlier. It should be clear and concise. Keep in mind that the subject line usually determines whether the recipient will actually read the memo or not.

Body or Content

When preparing to write the memo, you should identify the problem, the reasons the memo is needed, and any action you wish the reader to take after reading the memo. Then the writer can begin providing appropriate background information and supporting data in the body of the memo.

The first paragraph of a memo sets the tone and can provide the reader with an outline of what will be covered in the memo. Use clear and concise sentences with smooth transitions to summarize the memo in the introduction, focusing on the major points that need to be communicated. Then discuss the background of the issue and provide any supporting evidence. This is where the writer needs to prove a point, analyze options, address counterarguments, and support recommendations, if appropriate.

Informational memos should focus on summarizing information and outlining options and considerations in the body of the memo. Action memos summarize information and provide recommendations for the reader. After sharing this information with the reader, memos should provide a clear and concise closing summary that reminds the reader of the key points of the memo.

Formatting

Just like business letters, there are standard formatting guidelines for memos. The headings should be left-justified, using boldface, and capital letters followed by a colon. The information added afterward should be in regular font. Then you want to allow for two to three blank lines between the heading and the body of the memo. The memo body should be single-spaced and also left-justified. Lastly, just like business letters, memos should use margins of 1 inch on each side.

> **TAKE AWAY**
> Memos have a standard format.

Distribution

Memos can be distributed in hard copy or electronically. In today's current work environment, it is more common for memos to be sent as attachments to emails or posted on office intranet sites. However, hard copies of memos may be sent through interoffice mail and/or be posted to centrally located office bulletin boards.

TABLE 14.2

TERMS USED IN MEETINGS

Term	Meaning
Ad hoc	Arranged for a single purpose or work product
Adjournment	Closing or ending of a meeting
Amendment	A proposal to make a change
Quorum	The minimum number of attendees needed to proceed with the meeting
Subcommittee	Small subgroup of meeting attendees to deal with a specific project appointed by the larger committee
Unanimous	When all meeting attendees (or members) vote in favor of something

Meetings

One of the most important opportunities for business communication is during meetings. Meetings are successful if they are well organized, well led by a chairperson, and serve a necessary and focused purpose. Attendees need to be considerate of others and make sure everyone is heard. It is highly recommended that all businesses establish a policy for the use of cell phones during meetings. Cell phones often provide distraction from what is being discussed and should always be on silent during a meeting. All attendees should agree not to send or read text messages during the meeting, as it is disrespectful to others who may be speaking. If a call needs to be taken, it should always be taken outside the meeting room. Table 14.2 list several common terms used in formal meetings.

Agenda

agenda a list of what will take place during a meeting, often sent to meeting participants to prepare before a meeting.

Every meeting should have an agenda. An **agenda** lists what will take place and be discussed during the meeting. Ideally, the agenda should be sent with the meeting invitation. Agendas promote meeting efficiency because participants can prepare ahead of time for the topics to be discussed. Productive meetings are those that are focused on what needs to be achieved, and an agenda can help do this. Fig. 14.7 provides an example of an agenda.

Agendas generally include the following items:
- Date and time of the meeting.
- Location of the meeting.
- List of meeting invitees and any materials they should bring.
- Topics to be discussed. Topics that were previously discussed should be referred to as "old business"; topics that need to be discussed at the meeting should be referred to as "new business."
- List of any guest speakers.
- Attachments may also be added if there are background materials participants should read ahead of time. If attachments are used, it is helpful to identify on the agenda which attachment goes with which topic to be discussed.

Minutes

minutes a summary record of what took place at a meeting.

During a business meeting, a staff member should be assigned to "take minutes." Meeting **minutes** are a summary record of what took place and what was discussed at a meeting (Fig. 14.8). Meeting minutes typically show:
- Who attended and participated in the meeting, as well as those who were absent
- The date and time the meeting was called to order

```
AGENDA
Internal Medicine Specialists
Thursday, January 5th, 2017 at 8:00 AM
Conference Room A


CALL TO ORDER

I. Opening Remarks – Dr. Smith

II. Approval of December 21, 2016 minutes – Judy Milton

III. Further discussion of draft inventory survey - Louise Parker

IV. Presentation of most recent Administrative Report - Louise Parker

V. Presentation of most recent Budget Report - Tim Wilton

VI. Announcements - Dr. Smith

VII. Discussion of next steps and confirmation of next meeting date/time
- Dr. Smith

VIII. Other Business

ADJOURN
```

Figure 14.7 Agenda.

- Documentation that minutes from the previous meeting were approved and accepted, identifying any amendments made to those minutes
- A summary record of issues that were discussed
- A description of announcements and decisions that were made
- The time the meeting adjourned
Meeting minutes serve multiple purposes, including:
- Creating documentation for any potential auditing, accrediting, or regulatory purposes with a signature of the person who created the minutes.
- Allowing those invitees who missed the meeting to see what happened.
- Providing a resource for the next meeting's agenda, including the date, time, and location of the next meeting, if a follow-up meeting is needed. Specifically, the minutes will highlight any outstanding action items to be covered at the next meeting.
The staff member who takes the minutes may be asked to perform additional duties, such as:
- Arrange the meeting date, time, and place
- Send the invitation to potential attendees
- Draft the agenda
- Circulate the agenda to attendees (ideally with the meeting appointment)
- Take notes at the meeting
- Draft, proofread, and get approval of the minutes
- Circulate minutes to all invitees (including those who did not attend the meeting)
In some cases, the assigned staff member may be the health services manager, the front desk receptionist, or an administrative assistant.

January 2017 Staff Meeting Minutes
Internal Medicine Specialists

CALL TO ORDER
An Internal Medicine Specialists' staff meeting was held in Conference Room A on Thursday, January 5, 2017. The meeting was called to order by Dr. James Smith at 8:05 a.m.

ATTENDANCE
Dr. James Smith, Dr. Anna Cambell, Dr. Madison Anders, Louise Parker, Tim Wilton, Judy Milton, Pamela Sota, and Mike Layton were in attendance. Dr. Anthony Kasik and Amber Ryder were absent.

I. Opening Remarks - Dr. Smith thanked all staff members for their assistance in transitioning the last portion of patient records into the new database.

II. Approval of December 21, 2016 minutes - The minutes from the month of December were read by Judy Milton and approved.

III. Further discussion of draft inventory survey - Louise Parker presented the latest changes made to the draft inventory survey. Tim Wilton suggested that the cost of inventory items be totaled and reported at each staff meeting in the future. It was agreed that this information will be added to inventory reports for staff meetings beginning in February 2017.

IV. Presentation of most recent Administrative Report - Louise Parker presented the Administrative Report for December 2016. The only notable item in the report was longer call hold times. Louise recommended that the staff consider why the call hold times were longer for this month and come back to the next staff meeting with ideas for improvement.

V. Presentation of most recent Budget Report - Tim Wilton presented the Budget Report for December 2016. During the presentation, Tim reminded all staff that budget requests for 2017 are due to him no later than January 6, 2017.

VI. Announcements - Louise Parker announced that Amber Ryder will continue to be out on medical leave until January 12, 2017.

VII. Discussion of next steps and confirmation of next meeting date/time - Dr. Smith stated that the next meeting will be held on Thursday, February 2, 2017.

VIII. Other Business - Louise Parker reminded staff members that the office will be closed on January 16, 2017, in observance of Martin Luther King Day and on February 20 in observance of Presidents Day.

ADJOURN
Dr. Smith convened the meeting at 8:49 a.m.

Figure 14.8 Meeting minutes.

LEARNING CHECKPOINT 14.2
Effective Communication

1. A woman sees the physician in the parking lot and asks about how to care for her husband's cast. Why does the physician suggest they speak in the exam room?

   a. They may not be able to hear each other well.
   b. The location is not private.
   c. The woman may not understand the physician's body language.
   d. a and b

2. Because the practice is in a community with a large Hispanic population, the health services administrator, Sarah, makes sure she has a Spanish-speaking team member on staff during operating hours. This is an example of:

   a. nonverbal communication
   b. cultural competency
   c. communicating with a hard-to-reach population
   d. acting on a needs assessment

3. How can an organization reduce the number of billing calls?

   a. Insist that patients discuss the matter in person.
   b. Provide an estimate before or when services are rendered.
   c. Use a friendly tone.
   d. Refer the patient to their third-party payer.

4. Which is an example of nonverbal communication?

   a. Greeting the patient
   b. Asking the patient to "please hold"
   c. Discussing the weather
   d. Smiling

5. What is the last step before sending an email?

   a. Cc-ing or bcc-ing
   b. Proofreading
   c. Closing
   d. Signature

6. Which type of communication is only used internally?

   a. Memorandums (memos)
   b. Business letters
   c. Emails
   d. Nonverbal communication

CASE STUDY

To help address her staff's challenges, Zeina provides a training for her staff on cultural competency and how to effectively communicate with Stella and other patients with similar challenges. The training includes strategies to communicate with the elderly and patients with language barriers, such as scheduling appointments to allot for extra time, speaking slowly and clearly, and using actions and gestures to act out instructions to patients. An additional strategy includes having a family member of Stella's accompany her to appointments to assist as an interpreter.

REVIEW QUESTIONS

1. What is professionalism?

2. Why is effective communication especially critical in the health care industry?

3. Name two barriers to effective communication.

4. What are the communication challenges for special populations?

5. What is verbal and nonverbal communication, and how are they different?

6. How are business letters and memorandums (memos) different?

7. Name the seven parts of a business letter.

8. What is typically included in a meeting agenda?

9. What is typically included in meeting minutes?

CHAPTER 15

MARKETING*

CHAPTER OUTLINE

INTRODUCTION
MARKETING NEEDS OF
  THE HEALTH CARE
  PRACTICE
  Identifying Customers
  SWOT Analysis
    Strengths and Weaknesses
    Opportunities and
      Threats
MARKETING TOOLS
  Community Involvement
  Automated Phone Calls
  Newsletters and Blogs
  Print Ads in Magazines and
    Newspapers
  Internet Reviews
  Social Media

Websites
  Choosing a Website Name
  Creating a Site Map
    Home Page
    About Us Page
    Testimonials or Information
      Page
    Specials Page
    Contact Us Page
  Designing Pages
  Increasing Website Traffic
PUBLIC RELATIONS
  Addressing Bad Press
HIGH-QUALITY CUSTOMER
  SERVICE
  Patient Loyalty
  A Helpful Attitude

Identifying With Patients
What Do Patients Expect?
Patient Surveys
Problem Patients
"WELCOME TO OUR OFFICE"
  PACKET
  Introduction to the Medical Office
  Missed Appointments and
    Cancellation Policy
  Medical Office's Financial Policy
  Patient Portal
  Patient Instruction Sheets
  List of Community Resources
LEGAL AND ETHICAL ISSUES

VOCABULARY

advocate
blog
cost–benefit analysis

liaison
marketing plan
site map

social media
SWOT analysis
target market

CHAPTER OBJECTIVES

After completing this chapter, the student should be able to do the following:

1. Define a marketing plan and discuss its purpose.
2. Explain the use of a SWOT analysis.
3. Review the marketing tools used to market a health care practice.
4. Distinguish between advertising and public relations.
5. Explain how to successfully deliver high-quality customer service.
6. Review the importance of the new patient information packet, and develop a current list of community resources related to patients' health care needs.

---

*The editors wish to acknowledge writing in Niedzwiecki B, et al: *Kinn's The Administrative Medical Assistant: An Applied Learning Approach*, ed 13, which forms the basis of this chapter.

INTRODUCTION

As we have discussed in previous chapters, a health care practice is a business. Therefore success lies in bringing in new patients and retaining current patients to maintain cash flow. Marketing and customer service are both essential for a health care practice to grow. *Marketing* is the process of informing the local community of a product or service, or, in this case, the medical procedures and services the health care practice provides. Once customers visit the practice and become patients, providing excellent customer service can enhance their experience so they want to return.

Marketing can be expensive yet ineffective at increasing patient traffic if it is not planned well. Some health care practices work hard to attract patients in the community, but then lose the patients' business through poor customer service. Customer loyalty ensures the longevity of a health care business. Therefore it is essential for the health care practice's survival to develop and execute a well-thought-out marketing plan and build loyalty through customer service.

CASE STUDY

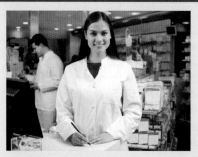

Monica had been working at Plus Care Clinic for several years as a medical assistant before being promoted to a health services administrator at the clinic. Recently, Plus Care added a walk-in urgent care clinic to serve patients with minor illnesses and injuries and chronic conditions, like diabetes and asthma management, and provide physicals and vaccinations. Shivaughn, the clinic's nurse practitioner, is aware that effective marketing is essential to growing the clinic. She regularly praises Monica for her customer service skills, so she has asked Monica if she would be willing to assume some marketing responsibilities for the practice. Shivaughn knows that Monica is comfortable using the Internet and is social media savvy. Monica is excited about this opportunity.

Shivaughn has suggested a small budget and a few marketing tools that Monica may want to implement. In turn, Monica has suggested some updates to staff members' training to improve their customer service skills and, hopefully, increase patient traffic.

MARKETING NEEDS OF THE HEALTH CARE PRACTICE

There are many ways to market a health care practice, but which strategies are best to attract new patients? A TV commercial or billboard near a freeway is a common way to promote a business because of the large number of people it can reach. However, this type of marketing may not be effective, especially for small businesses, and it can be very expensive, costing several thousand dollars for a short period of exposure.

A health care practice can also print business cards for about $20 and then have someone leave a card at all the stores in a retail center. Although relatively inexpensive, this method does not ensure that the right people are being reached. Table 15.1 lists some of the ways a health care practice can market its services and their relative costs.

Before investing too much time and money into any form of advertising, the health care practice should develop a **marketing plan**. A marketing plan is a formal analysis, strategy, and list of actions the health care practice will undertake to best promote

○ **marketing plan** a formal analysis, strategy, and list of actions the health care practice will undertake to market itself.

TABLE 15.1
MARKETING STRATEGIES FOR OUTPATIENT SETTINGS

Strategy	Cost
Maintain a professional website	$$$
Manage an active Facebook, Twitter, Instagram, and/or other social media handle	No cost
Actively participate in community health fairs and events	$
Mail yearly checkup reminders	$$
Purchase billboard or magazine advertisements promoting the medical office	$$$$
Invite the public to an open house	$

itself. This chapter will discuss important key factors and strategies to consider when marketing a health care practice and creating a marketing plan.

Identifying Customers

Customers who purchase products or services are central to any marketing effort, and in the case of a health care practice, the customers are the patients. The most important element of the marketing plan is to identify the **target market**; this is the group of people most likely to need the services or products offered by the health care practice. Reaching the target market means that the targeted groups are made aware of the health care practice and what it offers.

The first step in identifying the target market is to determine who will need the medical procedures, services, and products the health care practice offers. For example, a practice that has a high number of older adults as patients would benefit from an audiology clinic, or a weight loss clinic would benefit from having a nutritionist and dietician on staff.

To understand the target market, the health care practice can review the demographics of its current patient population. It may find, for example, that most of the patients for the urgent care clinic come from the 78253 ZIP code. A public health clinic may find that most of its patients are between the ages of 20 and 25. It is a good idea for the health services administrator to keep a spreadsheet file for all patients with the following fields:
- Reason for visit
- Patient's age
- Employment
- ZIP code
- Gender
- Marital status
- Ages of children
- How the patient found out about the health care practice

These demographics provide the details of the health care practice's specific target market and will help in developing an effective marketing plan.

SWOT Analysis

One effective tool for businesses is the **SWOT analysis** (Fig. 15.1). A SWOT analysis provides an evaluation of the business environment in which the health care practice operates. The acronym SWOT stands for:

S – Strengths
W – Weaknesses

target market the groups of people most likely to need the medical services the health care practice offers.

TAKE AWAY

Reaching the target market means that the targeted groups are made aware of the practice and what it has to offer.

SWOT analysis an evaluation of the business environment that identifies an organization's internal strengths (S) and weaknesses (W), as well as external opportunities (O) and threats (T).

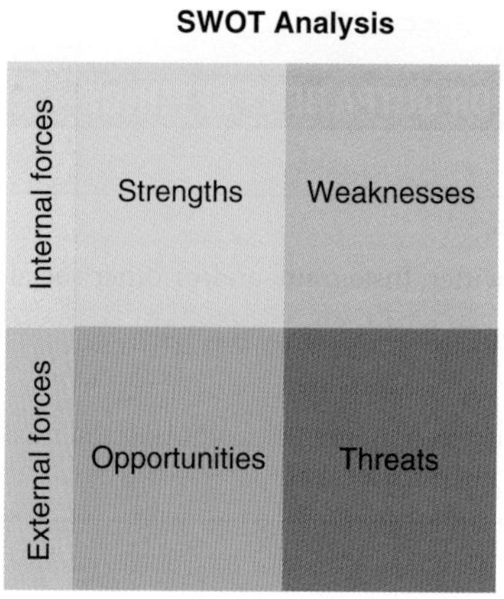

SWOT Analysis

Figure 15.1 A SWOT analysis can be done to define the target market.

O – Opportunities

T – Threats

This tool evaluates how economic forces affect the health care practice internally and externally. The strengths (S) and weaknesses (W) categories evaluate internal organizational resources, and the opportunities (O) and threats (T) categories evaluate external economic forces.

Strengths and Weaknesses

The strengths of a health care practice are the advantages it has over its competitors, such as in the following categories:

- Reduced patient wait times
- Advanced medical techniques and health information technology
- Flexible appointment hours
- Patient information web portals

Conversely, the weaknesses category evaluates whether the health care practice's competitors are better in any of these categories. For example, a competing urgent care clinic may have extended hours, accept more insurance plans, or is more accessible by public transportation.

No health care practice can build only strengths. The expense of offering every benefit or service to patients would cost more than the revenue generated, even if it captured all the patients in the target market. Therefore the health care practice needs to perform a **cost–benefit analysis**, which is an assessment that weighs the benefits of attracting patients against the costs required. For example, a health care practice could invest in an in-house magnetic resonance imaging (MRI) machine, which would cost about $7500 a month in lease payments over the next 5 years. But how many patients will use the machine in a month or even a year? How much revenue will the equipment generate for the practice? What are the other advantages to patients receiving an MRI in-house compared with referring them? In general, after fixed and direct costs are accounted for, 85% to 90% of the reimbursement must be profit for the practice to benefit from having an MRI machine.

Opportunities and Threats

Opportunities review the prospect of increased business due to external forces. Health care facilities generally have little or no control over the external market environment; however, a practice that recognizes the few opportunities that exist can improve its

cost–benefit analysis an assessment that weighs the benefit of attracting patients against the cost required.

internal strengths. Likewise, disregarding changes in the market and any health care trends and regulations can worsen a practice's weaknesses.

Some examples of opportunities include:

- Medical technology that reduces the cost of health care and hospital stays
- The increased number of Americans with health insurance due to the Affordable Care Act
- Electronic management of patient information, which reduces the time needed to care for each patient
- Public health campaigns, which highlight the importance of seeing a health care provider for specialized care

Threats are external factors that can damage the long-term viability of a health care practice. For example, a threat is ignoring the integration of electronic health record (EHR) systems into the practice. EHR systems facilitate the delivery of quality health care to patients and can support the continuity of patient care through collaboration among different health care providers. Although the implementation of electronic systems in health care facilities can be initially expensive, the long-term market outlook for them is good and is an important part of staying compliant with the Health Insurance Portability and Accountability Act (HIPAA) security standards.

TAKE AWAY ●·········

A SWOT analysis provides an evaluation of the business environment.

■ LEARNING CHECKPOINT 15.1
■ Marketing Needs of the Health Care Facility

1. The _____ analysis weighs the benefits of attracting patients against the costs required.

2. What does the acronym SWOT stand for? _____

MARKETING TOOLS

As mentioned earlier, some marketing strategies can be quite expensive and yet ineffective. Thus it is important to clearly identify the target market to then develop effective marketing tools. Marketing tools are techniques, materials, or strategies used to promote a product or service. Some marketing tools may use a more concentrated marketing strategy, where marketing efforts focus on only one very defined and specific market segment. There are a number of marketing tools that can effectively increase patient volume.

Community Involvement

It is important for health care practices to be involved in their local community and participate in community outreach. Not only does this help with increasing visibility of the practice and is considered "free" marketing for the practice, it also helps build patients' trust and loyalty.

Some health care practices participate in local health fairs offering free health screenings, partner with farmers' markets to promote healthier eating, or sponsor a local 5K run/walk to encourage exercising. The health care practice may also sponsor specific charities annually or donate time and money to local nonprofit organizations. Additionally, staff members can get involved by attending public community events and chamber of commerce meetings. The more the public views the health care practice actively participating in the community, the more likely they will become patients at the practice.

Automated Phone Calls

Automated phone systems are a popular means of communicating with a large number of patients. These communication systems are efficient in that a computer dials multiple phone numbers at the same time and plays a recorded message. Similar systems can send out text messages since many patients use their cell phones as their primary phone line. The automated phone call can be used for appointment reminders, which would be effective in reducing patient no-shows and loss of revenue.

A health care practice can also use the automated phone system to contact existing patients if the practice is planning to relocate. An automated call could be initiated to notify all patients that the practice will be moving after a certain date, what the address of the new location is, and even prompt patients to "Press 1" if they need to schedule an appointment. The same principle could be applied to news about an upcoming health fair or a special seminar about a certain illness.

> **TAKE AWAY** ●·········
>
> Automated call distribution is a popular means of communicating with large numbers of people.

Newsletters and Blogs

Another effective marketing tool is publishing a newsletter or having a blog. Health care newsletters are a cost-effective way to keep in contact with both patients and referring providers on a regular basis. Newsletters can be sent by mail or, more commonly, electronically as an e-newsletter. E-newsletters are more cost effective because they offer a quicker form of communication and are less costly because they do not require postage. Regardless of the format, newsletters should be sent regularly, typically every month.

The newsletter's content should focus on educating patients about health issues important to them and inform patients about health conditions that the provider commonly sees in the practice. For example, as an introduction to outdoor summer activities, the newsletter may promote healthy sun habits, such as wearing hats, sunglasses, and sunscreen. Or, in the fall, the provider can publish a newsletter to discuss ways to avoid catching the flu and may include a short video on how to properly wash hands to prevent the spread of disease. However, providers should be cautious of providing medical advice in the newsletter.

A **blog** is an online journal that providers can use to share their experiences in caring for patients. Usually, providers do not follow a schedule for blog posts; they post when they have an experience to share in regard to prevention, any new health trends, or an experience that patients would benefit from reading. For example, a provider may write about a patient who came in with a second-degree sunburn and how the patient suffered through an unfortunate incident that could have been prevented. Or ambulatory surgeons can post surgical videos to their blogs to inform patients of the services they provide. If a patient's case is discussed in the newsletter or blog, it is imperative that any identifying information about the patient is removed to protect the patient's identity and to uphold all privacy and confidentiality rules established by HIPAA.

○ **blog** an online journal that providers can use to share their experiences in caring for patients.

Print Ads in Magazines and Newspapers

Marketing through print ads, such as magazines, newspapers, or mailers, have been the traditional method of advertising and can still be very effective in reaching a target market. Print ads are usually expensive, but they are able to reach a wider audience.

> **TAKE AWAY** ●·········
>
> It is important to ensure that the target market can be reached by advertising in newspapers and magazines because it is significantly more expensive and reaches a wider audience.

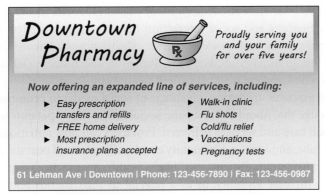

Figure 15.2 A mailer promoting the health care practice.

Thus a cost–benefit analysis needs to be done to ensure that whatever print ad is invested in is an effective marketing strategy.

Mailers are postcards or flyers that are mailed directly to hundreds or thousands of households in a geographic area (Fig. 15.2). This practice can be costly, and the mailer may be wider than the target market, possibly making the strategy not cost effective. Further, the more specialized the services the health care practice offers, the less likely it is that a mailer campaign would reach the target market.

The effectiveness of a print ad marketing strategy should be routinely evaluated by asking new patients how they learned about the health care practice. If a significant percentage mention the magazine or newspaper ad, the target market was reached, and the benefits would outweigh the costs of the print ads.

Internet Reviews

Nowadays, it is common for consumers to read customer reviews on various websites before patronizing a business. Businesses with more and better reviews tend to attract new customers. A health care practice has many opportunities to build a strong reputation through Internet marketing because patients can post reviews of their experiences on many different and popular websites. The key is to ask every patient before he or she leaves to post a review of the services that the patient received. Some health care practices will even send out a follow-up email requesting that the patient provide a review. As the number of reviewers and positive reviews grows, the potential for new patients will also grow.

A health services administrator can take responsibility for monitoring customer reviews on websites to confirm that the reviews are mostly positive. Some websites allow businesses to address negative comments, so the health services administrator should be ready to post a reply, such as, "We're sorry that you feel you did not receive the care that you deserve. Please feel free to contact me to discuss how we could have improved your experience. Thank you for your feedback."

Social Media

Social media, such as Facebook, Twitter, and YouTube, allow for two-way communication between a business and the consumer. Social media outlets promote the business, and customers can respond positively or negatively about the service they received. In contrast, traditional media outlets, such as newspapers and magazines, allow only limited ability to respond. A person can write a letter to the editor of a newspaper, but the

social media Internet-sponsored, two-way communication between individuals, between individuals and businesses, or between businesses.

letter does not provide an immediate two-way exchange. Social media is considered a blending of technology and social interaction that can create an effective marketing tool. For example, many health care practices' websites now have icons that have links to Facebook, Instagram, Twitter, YouTube, Pinterest, and other social media sites to promote interaction and create loyal patient relationships.

Health care practices are taking advantage of social media to promote the services they offer. Just like the "About Us" webpage, social media allows patients to gain insight into the medical care and services delivered. Providers can post nutritional counseling videos on YouTube, announce a community event on Twitter, and post the event pictures immediately on Instagram. Patients can "like" a health care practice's page on Facebook as a review, to increase visibility, or as a referral to their friends and family to the practice. Social media can bring the provider–patient relationship closer even without the provider directly interacting with the patient.

It is easy to understand how a well-planned social media marketing approach can positively affect the financial health of a practice. A health services administrator who can promote the health care practice on social media in a professional way is a valuable asset to the practice.

Websites

One of the most popular and beneficial marketing tools for the health care practice is a professional website. A part of the marketing budget needs to be dedicated to the cost of having a web developer create a website and maintain it on a monthly basis.

Five basic steps are involved in building a website for a medical practice:
1. Choosing a website name
2. Creating a site map
3. Designing the pages, including graphics and written content
4. Increasing traffic to the website
5. Using social media to increase public awareness of the website.

Choosing a Website Name

Choosing a website name should be part of the health care practice's marketing strategy. Patients should commonly associate the website name with the health care practice. The ideal website name is typically 7 to 15 letters and is related to or should include the practice's name. The Internet has been around for some time, so many website names may have already been taken. Therefore an Internet search should be done to check the availability of the preferred name before it is given to the webpage developer. Most website addresses begin with *www.*, followed by the name with no spaces, and then end with *.org, .com,* or *.net.* The following website endings should not be used for a health care practice or any other kind of business: *.gov,* which is for government sites, and *.edu,* which is for educational institutions.

There is no requirement that the website name reflect the provider's name or the name of the health care practice. But it is a best practice to do so in order for patients to easily locate the practice on the Internet. For example, Plus Care Clinic may have the website: www.pluscareclinic.com. Some practices may even identify themselves as the local specialist, as in: www.pluscareclinicnyc.com.

Creating a Site Map

An organized **site map** makes the website more user friendly. When the website is designed, it is important to identify which informational pages should be included. A standard website has a Home page, an About Us page, a Testimonials or Information page, a Specials page, and a Contact Us page.

Home Page

The Home page is the introduction to the entire website. It is the first page viewed when the patient types the website into the address bar. The purpose of the Home page is to introduce the patient to the health care practice. Design is a key element of this page. Colors should be appealing to the eye, and there should be a balance of images and content.

The Home page should contain the practice's name, the address, phone number, and any social media handles. The links to other pages, or the navigational menu, on the website should be presented vertically or horizontally along the webpage. Most health care practices have a link to a patient portal, which provides access to the patient's personal health records and offers a way to directly communicate with the practice; the user name and password to access the patient portal are assigned by the practice. Often, there is a link to new patient forms on the Home page.

About Us Page

The About Us page offers a unique opportunity to introduce all the providers in the health care practice. Many websites include photos of the health care providers, medical team, and support staff. Profiles are often included, with the health care providers' education, certification, specialties, years in practice, and a personal note. These profiles are an effective marketing tool in that they inform potential new patients about who the providers are, the types of services the health care practice offers, and the type of care the patient can expect to receive.

Testimonials or Information Page

The Testimonials or Information page is an opportunity for the practice to customize its website. Some health care practices prefer to include positive patient reviews about the practice; the page could also have a link to a public reviewer website with additional reviews. Other health care practices use the page for more informational purposes, such as for a monthly e-newsletter or any research papers a provider in the practice has published. The content of this page is often left to the discretion of the medical staff.

Specials Page

Often, the Specials page is used to attract more patients by offering specials for various services, such as discounts or special offers. These specials may be good options for people who are uninsured or underinsured and need more affordable medical services. For example, the practice can offer a special for flu vaccination at a discounted price, advertise a new cosmetic surgery procedure, or offer free nutritional supplements for new patients. Offering specials not only attracts new patients, but it also shows that the health care practice is invested in the well-being of the community.

Contact Us Page

The Contact Us page contains a form that patients can fill out and submit to request a staff member contact them. This page is distinct and separate from the patient portal because it is not designed for answering questions about the patient's medical condition or treatments. Instead, patients might use this contact form to submit a compliment or complaint, ask billing questions, or ask if their insurance is accepted. The contact form may also be used to inquire about employment at the practice.

Once the form has been filled out, the data collected are sent to the health care practice's e-mail address associated with the webpage. The health services administrator or another staff member should be assigned to check this email account regularly to ensure a timely response.

Designing Pages

Once the site map has been created, the web developer can begin brainstorming ideas about what the site will look like on the computer screen. Attention should be paid to graphics, color choices, animation, and fonts. These elements enhance a website's look and should be kept in balance. For example, smaller fonts make the text difficult to read for patients with poor vision. Too many graphics crowd out the content of the website. The navigational menus should be designed so that viewers can move easily through the site. Most users appreciate a means to go back to the page previously viewed, and they may become frustrated with sites that have an excessive number of pop-up boxes. Consistency is important, so it is a good idea to keep the same design theme on each page of the website.

Photographs, graphics, and video can personalize the website, but be careful not to overdo them. Larger graphic files can take time to download. Most users will not wait longer than 10 seconds for a webpage to load before clicking elsewhere. Graphics can be found from websites that license stock photos. Always respect any copyrights that are designated on any graphic file used. Some websites offer these files for free or charge a small fee.

The most important part of the website is the text, which should be developed by the health services administrator and the provider. It has been said that every word in a book must add to the story, and this is a good way to look at the text in a website. Avoid too much repetition, and remain clear about what is being communicated on the site. Headings and titles help clarify the theme of each page. Use a spell-checker before uploading any text and making it available for public viewing.

Hyperlinks are words or graphics on a webpage that, when clicked, take the viewer to another page or another website. To add a hyperlink, simply highlight the text field or graphic, select the hyperlink icon, and specify the destination address, or the *uniform resource locator* (URL). Always include the full URL to ensure that the link directs the user to the desired page.

Increasing Website Traffic

A well-organized website has no value if patients are not aware that it exists. When patients search for health care practices in their geographic area on a search engine website, the practice's website should pop up. In order for the search engine to pick up the website, the web developer will include appropriate keywords into the website developer code. All health care practice websites should include keywords such as the practice's city, state, medical specialty, types of insurances accepted, and so on. These keywords are not viewable on the website but are included in the design code.

Website traffic should be monitored on a regular basis by the health services administrator or an appointed staff member responsible for patient relations or marketing. Counters often can be added to the website that indicate how many people have viewed it. This helpful tool allows the practice to track how many people are viewing which pages. A sharp decline in traffic may indicate a technical problem with the website, so it is important to monitor website traffic regularly and ensure that all webpages are working properly.

TAKE AWAY ● · · · · · · · · ·

Make sure the health care practice's webpage shows up in a list of search engine results, such as Google.

▪ LEARNING CHECKPOINT 15.2

▪ Marketing Tools

1. Which marketing tool is interactive?

   a. Internet review
   b. Social media
   c. Automated phone calls
   d. a and b

LEARNING CHECKPOINT 15.2—cont'd

Marketing Tools

2. Which term is a list of all the links on a website?

    a. Site map
    b. Blog
    c. Marketing plan
    d. Home page

PUBLIC RELATIONS

There are similarities and differences between advertising and public relations. There's an old saying: "Advertising is what you pay for, publicity is what you pray for." As discussed earlier, advertising involves marketing or promoting a brand, a product, a service, or a business to increase revenue through the use of many different tools and strategies, such as the Internet, print ads, newsletters and blogs, and telecommunications. Public relations is related to advertising in that it often employs the same tools and strategies; however, it is more focused on maintaining the image of a business or individual. Thus public relations is more directly related to creating or changing attitudes, beliefs, and perceptions by influencing people. The person who is controlling public relations will dictate if it is a positive or negative image.

For example, the health care practice may release a press release about receiving an award from the local chamber of commerce or that one of its physicians was honored by the medical board. This creates positive publicity about the practice, which is important for maintaining current patients and generating new ones. Patients are more likely to choose a practice or provider they heard or read good things about over those they have never heard of or have read something negative about.

However, public relations can produce a negative image if it is generated, for example, by a third party. For example, a prominent physician gets arrested for driving under the influence after causing a multiple-car accident. The local newspaper reports it, which gets picked up by the national media, and that gets circulated on social media, such as Facebook and Twitter. This generates a negative public relations image for the health care practice, which may result in current patients leaving the practice and a loss of revenue.

Addressing Bad Press

A health care practice may face a case of medical error, poor health care delivery, the leaking of personal health information, or some other negative publicity that has found its way into the national headlines. Because health care is a personal issue, negative health news stories can destroy the trust the community has in the provider and the health care practice.

As a first line of defense, the health care practice needs to establish a high standard of customer service in the practice. Many patients will overlook small mistakes if the medical staff is apologetic and takes responsibility for the error. If a medical error has been published in any type of media, it is wise for the practice to post an official apology statement on its website. This statement should not defend the actions of the provider and/or the practice, but rather express concern for anyone who was negatively affected

TAKE AWAY •·········

Public relations is focused on maintaining the image of a business or individual.

by the error. The statement should also inform the public of the practice's remediation and rededication to delivering quality health care to all its current patients. A copy of the statement can also be displayed in the reception area of the health care practice.

The health care practice and the provider must work to overcome the stigma and negative publicity. Greater participation in the local community can help win back patients' trust, but patience and diligence may be needed to rebuild a thriving practice. Depending on the severity of the situation and the amount of negative publicity, it may be wise for a health care practice to hire a public relations consultant to help improve its image in the community.

HIGH-QUALITY CUSTOMER SERVICE

Once a patient comes to a health care practice, the key is to retain the patient for his or her long-term health care needs. High-quality customer service is not only critical to retaining loyal patients; it also encourages them to refer their friends and family to the health care practice. Thus the delivery of high-quality customer service is also considered an effective marketing tool.

Patient Loyalty

The most effective way to increase the number of patients is word of mouth, or by referrals. When patients are satisfied with the treatment they receive, they often refer other patients to the provider. However, if they are dissatisfied, they may tell everyone they know about their negative experience, which may affect the practice's future business.

Because patients often have a choice about who provides their health care services, it is important that the health care practice become the patient's first choice. Some patients are so loyal to a certain provider that even if their health care coverage no longer pays for visits, they will continue to see that provider.

A Helpful Attitude

The provider and staff members should project a helpful attitude in every interaction with the patient. They should sincerely ask, "How may I help you?" and then take steps to assist the patient in whatever way possible (Fig. 15.3). Instead of pointing in the

TAKE AWAY

High-quality customer service retains patients and prompts patients to refer their friends and family so that they can receive the same quality of care.

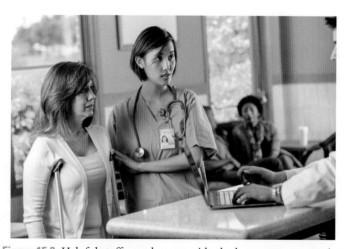

Figure 15.3 Helpful staff members provide the best customer service.

general direction of the radiology department, a staff member should take the patient there and introduce him or her to the front desk receptionist.

As stated in Chapter 14, telephone skills are also very important, as the telephone is usually the first impression of the ambulatory care office. Instead of telling a patient on the telephone, "Ann handles the insurance billing. I'll transfer you to her," say, "One moment, Mrs. Brown, let me see if Ann is at her desk." Place Mrs. Brown on hold, call Ann, and let her know that she has a call. Then return to Mrs. Brown, tell her that Ann is at her desk, and transfer the call at that time.

Be courteous and kind to every patient and visitor to the office. Good customer service must be one of the primary goals of the practice's medical staff. Patients count on staff members to be reliable and available to help them to the best of their abilities.

The health services administrator should emphasize to all staff members the importance of delivering quality customer service. Staff meetings should be scheduled regularly to discuss customer service failures, review how those situations should have been handled, and recognize staff members who display high-quality customer service.

Identifying With Patients

Patients appreciate staff members who can be empathetic with the problems they are facing. This is especially important when a patient is upset or angry. For example, if a patient comes to the office complaining that charges were placed on his account for procedures that were not performed, the health services administrator may respond with, "Mr. Roberts, I understand that you are upset about these additional charges. Let me do some research on your account and I'll let you know what I find out as soon as I can."

No matter how upset the patient may be, it is important to identify with the patient. Always acknowledge and restate the patient's concern. It shows that the staff member is listening and is interested in resolving the problem.

Remember, it costs much more to recruit new customers than to keep existing customers. Providing helpful, personal service impresses even the most difficult patient. To patients and visitors to the clinic, each member of the medical staff represents the entire practice.

What Do Patients Expect?

The medical staff should always remember and follow the Golden Rule: "Do unto others as you would have them do unto you." Patients expect their concerns to be met with responsiveness, which means that medical staff should have a caring attitude (Fig. 15.4). They also expect the medical staff to be knowledgeable about their field or specialty. For example, a medical insurance biller should know more than just the basics of insurance filing. The health services administrator should have a certain degree of authority to handle problems and complaints. Patients also expect confidentiality and trust from the medical staff. They expect an organized office that runs on schedule. They also expect that if a staff member states that he or she will do something, it will be done.

Friendly staff members are the best marketing tool. A smile is an excellent way to make patients feel welcome in the medical practice.

Patient Surveys

There is no better way to understand the quality of the care delivered than by asking the patients themselves. A patient survey is a very effective tool for a health care practice

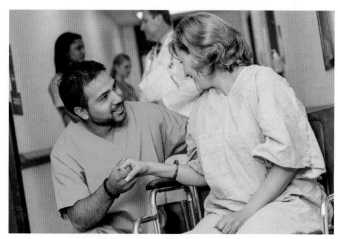

Figure 15.4 Friendly staff members are the best marketing tool. A smile is an excellent way to make patients feel welcome in the medical practice.

to evaluate the level of quality provided to their patients (Fig. 15.5). Patient surveys can be mailed, emailed, done by telephone, or posted in the patient portal. In general, patients unhappy with the care they received or who had a negative experience are more likely to submit a patient survey than patients with positive experiences. Regardless, all patients should be encouraged to complete the survey to get an accurate picture. The health services administrator can send friendly reminders to patients to complete the survey. Some health care practices have even offered a small honorarium or token for completing the survey, such as a $10 gift card to a local coffee shop.

Successful health care practices take these surveys seriously by addressing patients' recommendations and concerns. The health services administrator should review some of the responses during monthly staff meetings to discuss any changes that can be implemented to improve customer service. For the most part, surveys are anonymous. However, if a patient identifies himself or herself and presents a specific concern, the health services administrator should contact the patient immediately to offer a resolution.

Problem Patients

Most patients are genuinely concerned about their health and are quite cooperative. However, some patients can be quite challenging for the provider and the medical staff and require extra patience and understanding. Types of "problem" patients may include those who are:

- Complainers
- Angry
- Needy
- Demanding
- Violent
- Nonpaying
- Noncompliant
- Drug seeking
- Reschedulers

The health services administrator may act as a **liaison** between the patient and the providers or medical staff when issues arise that are somewhat complicated or need more time to resolve. Some patients may feel ignored or mistreated by the medical

liaison an individual assigned to communicate between multiple parties.

Thank you so much for visiting Clear Skin Dermatology! We want to ensure your experience with us was excellent! Your experience is important to us, so please share your thoughts by completing this survey. All surveys are confidential and are used to improve our service only. Thank you so much for your time and we look forward to caring for you soon!

	YES	NO
1. Is the location of our office convenient?	☐	☐
2. Do you find our reception area comfortable?	☐	☐
3. Do you feel relaxed in the reception area?	☐	☐
4. Do you find our front office personnel (Receptionist, etc.)		
Friendly?	☐	☐
Courteous?	☐	☐
Rude or indifferent?	☐	☐
5. Do you find our business personnel (practice manager, billing specialist, etc.)		
Friendly?	☐	☐
Courteous?	☐	☐
Rude or indifferent?	☐	☐
6. Are phone calls handled in a prompt, courteous, competent manner?	☐	☐
7. Do we provide adequate help with your insurance?	☐	☐
8. Have you received a copy of our financial policies?	☐	☐
9. Have our payment and billing policies been explained to your satisfaction?	☐	☐
10. Do you find our nurses and other clinical allied health workers:		
Friendly?	☐	☐
Courteous?	☐	☐
Rude or indifferent?	☐	☐

Comments/complaints: _____
_____
_____
_____

Figure 15.5 Sample patient survey.

staff. Others may have a general lack of trust that makes complying with the provider's orders difficult for them. Cultural differences, social issues, and financial problems can all affect a patient's compliance and attitude.

The health services administrator and the medical staff should serve as patient **advocates**; however, they can never withhold information from the provider, even if the patient requests it. For instance, if a patient tells the health services administrator that he has been smoking, although he told the provider he quit, this information must be presented to the provider and documented in the patient's medical record. The medical staff should respectfully inform the patient that they are ethically and professionally obligated to share all information collected with the provider.

"WELCOME TO OUR OFFICE" PACKET

Another effective tool is creating a "Welcome to Our Office" packet to new patients that explains the operational and service aspects of the practice. The provider and staff can compile a patient information booklet, which can reduce the number of patient calls to the health care practice by an average of 20% to 30%. It also can reduce misunderstandings and forgotten instructions. The packet should be custom tailored to the specific practice.

TAKE AWAY

Cultural differences, social issues, financial problems, or psychological problems affect patients' attitudes and compliance.

advocate an individual who represents and supports the patient when health care decisions are made.

TAKE AWAY

The "Welcome to Our Office" packet can reduce misunderstandings and instances of forgotten instructions.

Introduction to the Medical Office

The welcome packet should begin with an introductory letter. The information on the introductory letter should be the same or similar to what would be found in the "About Us" webpage on the practice's website. The health care practice's letterhead should be used, which includes the address, contact numbers, website, and/or any social media links.

A statement of philosophy frequently is included in the introduction, followed by a description of the practice. Consider this example:

> The physicians and staff would like to welcome you to our office. We work as a team with the goal of providing prompt and quality care to improve your health. We are always working to improve our care and service in any way possible. Our practice is limited exclusively to dermatology and related disorders. Therefore it is important for each patient to have a primary care provider, such as a pediatrician, a family provider, or an internist, to oversee your primary medical care. Our role is most effective as a consultant to your primary care provider.

The introductory letter should list all the providers in the practice; their educational backgrounds, training, and board certifications; and what their specialties are. List the names of key clinical and administrative staff members, such as registered nurses and nurse practitioners, medical assistants and the health services administrator. Provide the practice address, a map of how to get there, and information about the parking facilities.

Missed Appointments and Cancellation Policy

The office policy regarding missed appointments and cancellations, telephone calls, and the function of the answering service should also be mentioned in the welcome packet. For example:

> We always strive to answer your telephone calls as quickly as possible. But at times you may be asked to wait as we finish handling prior patient calls. Your call is important to us, and we appreciate your patience. If you wish to speak to a physician, the receptionist will take your information, and the physician will contact you during the next available break or at the end of the office day. If this is an urgent situation, please inform the receptionist, and he or she will inform the physician. Our triage nurse and the medical assistant are also available to help you. Patients can also use the "Ask the Provider" email service located on the "Contact Us" page on the website.
>
> *If this is an emergency, please hang up the phone and call 911.*

Medical Office's Financial Policy

It is important to detail the health care practice's policies on billing and collection procedures, making it clear that patients are responsible for their financial portion of the fees. If payment is expected at the time of service, add this information to the welcome packet. Keep the language simple and straightforward so that the message is clear:

> We ask that our services be paid for at the time they are rendered. If you are referred to an outside office for laboratory testing or special x-ray procedures, you will be billed separately by that office. We will bill your insurance on your behalf. Thank you for accepting financial responsibility for the amount assigned by your health insurance, such as your coinsurance and/or deductible.

Patient Portal

Patients should be granted access to their patient portal through the health care practice's website. The username and password are assigned at the patient's first office visit. Using the patient portal, patients can gain access to their laboratory reports, test results, consultation reports, and any other medical encounter records.

Patients can also request pharmaceutical refills, update health insurance information, and request an appointment through the patient portal. However, patients should be aware that the patient portal manages medical records for the health care practice and not for any other specialists, laboratories, or hospitals associated with or referred by the provider.

Patient Instruction Sheets

In most health care practices and specialties, many medical procedures are performed over and over again. In addition to providing verbal instructions to the patient, the practice can create written instructions (Fig. 15.6) that can be reviewed with the patient and then uploaded to the patient portal. The following are some suggested topics for patient written instructions:
- Preparation for an x-ray procedure or laboratory tests
- Preoperative and postoperative instructions
- Dietary guidelines

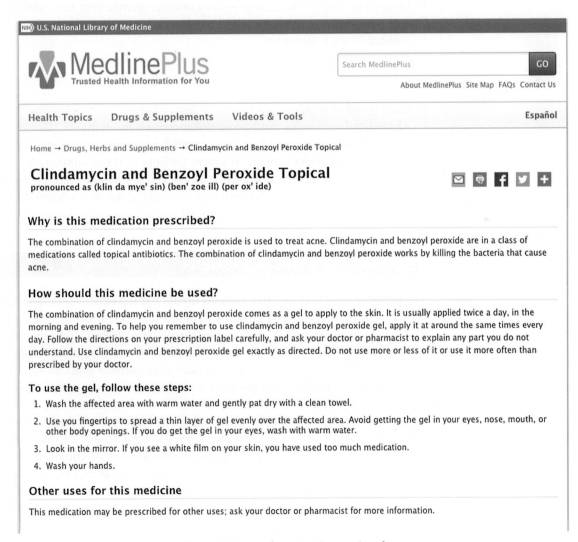

Figure 15.6 Sample patient instruction sheet.

- Performing an enema
- Preparing for a sigmoidoscopy or colonoscopy
- Taking medications
- Using a cane, crutches, walker, or wheelchair
- Care of casts
- Exercise therapy

List of Community Resources

Community organizations can collaborate with health care providers to meet the patient's health needs. As an active participant in the health of the local community, the practice should generate a list of community resources to assist patients in their efforts to improve their health. These resources can represent a wide variety of services, such as:
- Meals assistance and food banks
- Adult day care services and centers
- Grief support groups
- Chronic disease support groups
- Domestic violence and abuse resources and emergency shelters
- Medical equipment suppliers
- Home health care centers
- Long-term health care facilities—for example, convalescent care, skilled nursing facilities, rehabilitation centers, and psychiatric hospitals
- Assisted-living information
- Hospice services
- Immunization clinics
- Smoking cessation programs
- Local board of health
- Alcoholics Anonymous and Narcotics Anonymous meetings.

In addition, local communities have many outreach programs. For example, the American Cancer Society provides support to cancer patients in the community by providing rides to treatment, lodging near treatment centers, and hair loss and mastectomy products. The health care practice should maintain an updated list of resources on a regular basis, but it should not be held responsible if the services are no longer available.

LEGAL AND ETHICAL ISSUES

The provider must take care that patients do not use the information in brochures or on the health care practice's website as a substitute for the provider's medical advice. The patient may interpret information on the practice's website to be an extension of the provider's advice, so make sure everything on the website is accurate. Before attaching a link to another website, the health services administrator must be sure the site is reputable. For example, using government websites is recommended since they are generally taken as credible.

The provider should carefully review all printed information used to promote the health care practice. Make sure there are no misleading statements. A disclaimer should be included to remind patients that the information given in brochures and on websites is for general use only. Patients should be advised to discuss specific issues with their health care provider or to use the "Ask the Doctor" feature.

◉ CASE STUDY

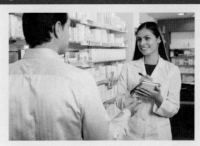

Monica is confident that a simple marketing plan will enable the practice to recruit a steady stream of patients to the newly opened walk-in urgent care clinic. She realizes that she first must determine the type of patients the practice currently serves. She has performed a SWOT analysis and reviewed the spreadsheet of patient demographics to identify a specific target market.

A monthly newsletter and the clinic's website are some of the marketing tools Monica plans to use to reach the target market. One of her first steps is to develop a newsletter with a calendar of special events and community outreach. The newsletter, which will provide health information and details about upcoming events, will be available both in print and online. Current patients whose email addresses are already in the clinic's database will automatically receive a computer-generated email message with a link that takes them directly to the online newsletter. Monica also has planned one special community event for each month of the upcoming year. The first will be an informational seminar on healthy diets to reduce cholesterol levels.

Monica plans to track the responses to each event promoted on the clinic's website to determine which marketing tools were most effective in promoting the clinic. The website's counter allows her to count the number of visits and to determine which pages are the most popular. Monica also has found that using social media for marketing has increased traffic to the clinic's website, which offers patients several options to educate themselves on health-related subjects and to find opportunities to participate in events that promote good health. Monica will keep Shivaughn updated on her progress and her marketing plan.

REVIEW QUESTIONS

1. How does identifying a target market help patients?

2. Conducting a SWOT analysis, the health services administrator at a vein center recognized that by the end of the year, many people have met the deductible of their health care plan and can pursue some health services at no out-of-pocket cost. Which part of the SWOT analysis is this?

3. Choose one of the marketing tools discussed in this chapter and discuss its advantages and disadvantages.

4. What are some ways a practice can overcome bad publicity?

5. How does the health services administrator help resolve issues with "problem" patients?

6. What information should be included in the "Welcome to Our Office" packet?

PEOPLE AND ORGANIZATIONAL MANAGEMENT

16 HIRING, TRAINING, AND EVALUATING EMPLOYEES
17 LEADERSHIP, MOTIVATION AND CONFLICT MANAGEMENT
18 PROJECT MANAGEMENT

HIRING, TRAINING, AND EVALUATING EMPLOYEES

Meredith Robertson

CHAPTER OUTLINE

INTRODUCTION
STRATEGIC HUMAN RESOURCE
   MANAGEMENT (SHRM)
RECRUITMENT STRATEGY
   Whom to Hire
   Advertising Channels
   Internal Recruitment Methods
   External Recruitment Methods
HIRING
   Prescreening
   Interviewing
   Selection
TRAINING AND DEVELOPMENT
   Onboarding
     Orientation
   Training and Development
     Diversity Training
PERFORMANCE REVIEWS
     Assessment
     Discussion

TERMINATIONS AND
   DISMISSALS
   Legal Framework
     Breach of Implied Contract
     Breach of Covenant of Good
       Faith and Fair Dealings
     Public-Policy Exception
     Discrimination
   Disciplinary Process
   Ending Employment
     Exit Interview
   Employee Turnover and
     Retention
   Improving Employee Retention
     Improving Employee
       Engagement
     Reducing Absenteeism
     Compensation and Benefits
     Career Growth and
       Opportunities

     Supportive Managers
     Organizational Culture
EMPLOYMENT LAWS
   Discrimination
     Civil Rights
     Disabilities
     Substance Addiction
     Discrimination Based on
       Genetic Information
     Discrimination Based on
       Pregnancy
   Family Leave
   Military Leave
   Wages
   Gender-Pay Differences
   Workplace Safety
   Sexual Harassment

VOCABULARY

360° review
Age Discrimination in Employment
   Act (ADEA)
comparative assessment
covenant of good faith and fair
   dealings
development
disparate impact
diversity
employee referral program
employment-at-will
Equal Employment Opportunity
   Commission (EEOC)
Equal Pay Act (EPA)
Fair Labor Standards Act (FLSA)
Family and Medical Leave Act
   (FMLA)

federal minimum wage
Genetic Information
   Nondiscrimination Act (GINA)
implied contract
job analysis
job announcement
narrative assessment
National Defense Authorization Act
   of 2008 (NDAA)
Occupational Safety and Health Act
   (OSH Act)
Older Workers Benefit Protection
   Act (OWBPA)
onboarding
orientation
passive candidate
performance review

Pregnancy Discrimination Act
   (PDA)
public-policy exception
reasonable accommodations
recruitment strategy
Strategic Human Resource
   Management (SHRM)
structured interview
Title VII of the Civil Rights Act
training
turnover
Uniform Guidelines on Employee
   Selection Procedures (UGESP)
Uniformed Services Employment
   and Reemployment Rights Act
   (USERRA)
whistle blower

CHAPTER OBJECTIVES

After completing this chapter, the student should be able to do the following:

1. Recognize the importance of human resources in the success of health care organizations.
2. Identify the key elements of a successful recruitment strategy.
3. Outline the steps included in the hiring process.
4. Describe the importance of onboarding, training, and development, especially as it relates to employee retention.
5. Describe the performance review process.
6. Understand the termination process and rights related to job terminations and dismissals.
7. Identify reasons employees leave organizations and how to improve and manage employee retention.
8. Understand key employment laws related to preventing discrimination and sexual harassment, family and military leave, fair compensation, and workplace safety.

INTRODUCTION

The health care industry is rapidly growing in the United States. However, as demand for health care professionals continues to grow, the supply of labor or human capital remains stagnant. The health care labor shortage is further exacerbated by the fact that many members of the current workforce will reach retirement age in the next 10 to 15 years. As discussed in Chapter 3, the federal government efforts to expand insurance coverage, the retiring of baby boomers (those born from 1946 to 1964), high employee *turnover* rates, and the increased life expectancy in the United States are all compounding the pressures on the health care system, thus creating the "perfect storm" for talent acquisition for health care organizations. Health care employers have to compete with potential employees who have more choices of places to work and who have the added convenience of Internet job boards in finding and comparing job opportunities. Therefore the importance of human resources in health care organizations may never have been more critical than now. Health care organizations must have a *strategic human resources management (SHRM)* plan to be competitive in recruiting and retaining the most talented employees.

● CASE STUDY

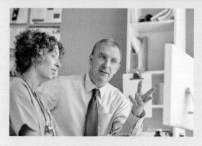

Molly has worked as Dr. Smith's clinic manager for 5 years. However, over the past 12 months, Dr. Smith has noticed that Molly has been struggling with some new software they've implemented to improve the clinic's electronic health records (EHR) system. Molly has consistently been a competent employee, but her lack of skills with the system is causing issues for the billing manager, Bob. As you read through this chapter, think about Molly's situation. If you were Dr. Smith, how would you handle her performance?

STRATEGIC HUMAN RESOURCE MANAGEMENT (SHRM)

In general, human resource management is the recruiting, hiring, and training of employees and providing them with the compensation, benefits, and development they need to be successful in their role within an organization. In comparison, **Strategic Human Resource Management (SHRM)** is the alignment of organizational strategic goals and objectives with the management of the organization's greatest investment—its employees. SHRM is designed to attract, develop, and retain employees for the benefit of both the employees and the organization.

Organizational leadership must first recognize employees as assets in which to be invested. The fact that the health care industry is a service industry requires organizations to realize that competitive positioning relies heavily on the skills and dedication of its employees. It is the customer service aspect of the health care industry that affects patient satisfaction and patient outcomes.

Additionally, successful health care organizations understand how critical a talented workforce is to the industry. They understand that investment makes an organization not only attractive to potential new employees, but helps maintain its current employees, thus reducing **turnover**—the rate at which employees leave an organization and are replaced. Organizations will lose any competitive advantage if they consistently lose current and/or potential talent.

Just as in any business, good strategic planning for health care organizations begins with an assessment of the environment. As discussed earlier, the changing dynamics of our population (the baby boomers retiring, longer life expectancy, etc.) are putting increasing pressure on the human resources function in organizations. As a result, organizations need to look at external forces: political and economic conditions; changes in federal and state laws, regulations, and policies; technological advances; changing needs of workers; declining reimbursement rates from public and private payers; increased competition within the industry; and labor shortages. Organizations may also face internal forces, such as budget constraints, which limit their ability to recruit top talent, pay competitive wages, and train staff. To respond to external and internal pressures in the health care environment, organizations need to assess their current positioning and consider what adjustments must be made to remain competitive. Many organizations will conduct regular internal audits to identify organizational strengths and weaknesses. For example, organizations may review company policies and procedures to ensure they not only remain compliant and competitive in the present environment, but that they also are equally prepared for the future and any changes to their business environment.

Finally, the leaders of the organization must come to consensus about the strategic direction of the organization as a whole. Leaders must determine the long-term and short-term goals for human resources that will be needed to help the organization meet its overall strategic direction. To meet the necessary human resources goals, it is important that all policies and procedures are aligned with and supportive of the organization's strategic goals. This applies to all functions of the human resources department, including the hiring process, training and development, performance appraisal systems, compensation and benefits, workforce retention efforts, and the recruitment strategy.

RECRUITMENT STRATEGY

The **recruitment strategy** is essentially the process of attracting talent or qualified applicants to the health care organization for current job openings. Recruitment includes the entire process of sourcing, selecting, and onboarding employees to an organization. It is often a function within the human resource department, or it may be the responsibility of an individual, such as a talent acquisition manager, director of personnel, a recruiting/sourcing manager, or even a health services administrator.

Strategic Human Resource Management (SHRM) the alignment of organizational strategic goals and objectives with the management of the organization's human resources.

turnover the rate at which employees leave an organization and are replaced.

TAKE AWAY

Successful health care organizations understand that a human resources investment makes an organization not only attractive to potential new employees, but also helps maintain its current employees.

recruitment strategy the process of attracting talent to the health care organization for current job openings.

Whom to Hire

The recruitment process begins with identifying the type of applicants an organization wants to attract. In most cases, especially in health care, organizations focus on the skills, education, certification or licensing, and the experience of applicants. The main objective is to draw in the most highly qualified individuals. Given the labor shortage described earlier, health care organizations may need to consider whether to focus on a particular subgroup of the workforce, such as older workers, former employees, former interns, temporary employees, or "passive candidates." **Passive candidates** are those who are not currently seeking a new position, but may be inclined to consider it if the conditions, such as compensation and benefits, are attractive enough.

> **Passive candidate**   An individual who is not currently seeking a new position but may be inclined to consider a position if the conditions were right.

Recruiting older applicants may be an appropriate recruitment strategy if a health care organization is seeking individuals with significant experience. To attract older applicants, organizations should design job opportunities with greater schedule flexibility, such as having job-share positions where two part-time employees are hired instead of one full-time employee. Also, hiring more experienced workers allows for greater mentoring opportunities and knowledge sharing with newer workforce entrants.

Another recruitment strategy focuses on hiring employees who have a better understanding of the organization's values and the position they are applying for. This may include former employees, interns, and referrals from current employees because they will have more awareness of the organization, the culture, and the specific needs of the position compared with other applicants. Hiring these individuals, assuming they possess all the necessary qualifications, may reduce employee turnover because they typically need less training and job transition time.

Advertising Channels

A major part of the recruitment strategy is determining where to find and tell the target population of candidates about a job opening. These "channels" of advertisement can be internal (promoting current employees) or external (seeking applicants from outside the organization). Internal approaches to recruitment include posting open positions on the organization's intranet site, promoting from within, or creating an employee referral program to take advantage of current employees' professional and personal contacts. External approaches to recruitment include using media advertising; using professional search firms, headhunters, or temporary staffing agencies; creating relationships with colleges and universities; targeting specific professional journals; posting openings on Internet job boards (industry specific or general); participating in electronic job fairs; and using social networking.

Internal Recruitment Methods

There are several advantages to internal recruitment. Typically, promoting from within allows managers to have better insight into an individual employee's skills, experience, and job performance. In internal recruitment, managers have an opportunity to observe a potential candidate over time, and employees are less likely to leave an organization than first-time hires recruited externally. The cost of internal recruitment and the time investment are also significantly less than external recruitment options. However, there are a few disadvantages with internal recruitment. If an organization is strategically trying to change its corporate culture or bring in new, innovative ideas, hiring from within is usually not ideal.

> **employee referral program**   a recruitment strategy that provides existing employees with financial incentives for referrals of potential job candidates.

To disseminate job openings, many organizations create **employee referral programs**, which give current employees a "finder's fee" or "bonus" for referring possible job candidates. For example, an organization may offer $500 to existing employees when their referral is hired. A common practice is to pay current employees half of the bonus up front and the other half after the new employee has remained with the organization for a set period, such as 6 months. Referral programs may also be a cost savings to the organization because employee referral programs are usually less expensive than the cost of print advertisements or hiring a search firm.

As mentioned earlier, referred applicants usually have a better understanding of the organization and the position. Referrals are also useful in finding passive candidates, as managers and other skilled workers may have contacts from association memberships or regional and national professional conferences and meetings. Plus, referred applicants tend to have better qualifications, better performance, and less turnover. However, organizations must not rely too heavily on word-of-mouth recruitment as it may result in a lack of diversity. As discussed later in this chapter, a company that excludes certain groups from its recruitment and hiring may be in violation of the laws of the **Equal Employment Opportunity Commission (EEOC)**.

External Recruitment Methods

External recruiting brings job openings to the attention of potential applicants outside of the organization. There are numerous approaches to external recruiting, so this section will focus on those that are most commonly used today. In the past, companies tended to rely on print media, such as the job classifieds or the "want ads" to garner applicant interest. Today's environment is far different. Most organizations have relied more on Internet sources and social media, which allow job seekers to connect online and post electronic resumes and applications.

Many employers advertise job opportunities through Internet job boards. There are different approaches to using this recruitment channel. Some health care organizations may choose to use an industry-specific job board to attract highly skilled applicants, whereas others may choose to use a general job board to attract a larger pool of applicants. Although job boards are cost effective and allow for rapid communication between job seekers and recruiters, they may become time consuming as there are so many resumes to be screened. Thus recruiters need to be cautious when selecting a job board. The job board needs to reach the targeted applicant pool the organization is seeking, and it should generate interest in the job opening.

Health care organizations are also starting to think about long-term solutions and creating a "talent pipeline." These organizations have strategically started thinking about working with universities and colleges to recruit graduates, for example, by offering internships. Internships have been particularly effective in finding candidates in particular health care specialties that are in high demand. Although developing long-term relationships with educational institutions is important, it is also important to gather data and assess whether each institution is providing employees that are best aligned with the strategic direction of the organization.

HIRING

Successful recruitment begins with an accurate and informative job announcement. The **job announcement** describes key elements of the position and expectations, which are identified through the process of job analysis. In a **job analysis**, the hiring manager identifies the skills, responsibilities, tasks, activities, training, experience, certifications, or licenses that are necessary for the success of the individual in a position. It is helpful for the hiring manager to gain insight from others, such as individuals who previously served in the role, other managers who oversee similar positions, or employees who are currently performing well in the position.

Equal Employment Opportunity Commission (EEOC) federal agency created by the Civil Rights Act of 1964 to enforce the provisions of the Civil Rights Act.

TAKE AWAY ● ·········

Most jobs are posted online.

job announcement describes the key elements of an open position within a health care organization and job expectations.

job analysis process by which the hiring manager identifies the skills, responsibilities, tasks, activities, training, experience, certifications, or licenses that are necessary for success in a particular job position.

After gathering data through the job analysis process, the hiring manager works with the human resources recruiter to develop a job description that will be used in advertising the position. One way to begin writing the description is to start with an existing job description and then edit it; or it may be determined that an entirely new description is needed. A new description does provide the manager an opportunity to rethink the key responsibilities and expectations for the new position. The recruiter and hiring manager should also consider, if applicable, the past successes or failures of previous searches for the same position. The final job description should include all of the requirements for the position, the expectations for success in the position, and information on who the new employee will report to.

Job descriptions should also include information that will be used in the selection process, such as experience, education, and any technical certifications and licenses. The hiring manager, recruiter, and others involved in the selection process will use the job description elements to screen and select candidates. It should also be noted that the job description is important because it is used as the basis for job orientation, training, and future performance reviews.

Prescreening

In most health care organizations, the human resources team takes the lead on prescreening applications and resumes to narrow down the applicant pool. This prescreening usually eliminates applicants who do not meet the minimum requirements for the position. Then the remaining candidates' resumes are reviewed with the hiring manager and search committee, if applicable, to sort candidates based on experience.

Oftentimes, candidates are sorted into three main categories: those who have limited experience and skills; those with reasonable experience and skills to adequately perform the job; and those candidates that the search committee finds are highly qualified with excellent skills who will "fit" into the new department and organization well. The hiring manager, recruiter, and search committee will then rank candidates to determine which should be interviewed; usually the top three to seven candidates are selected.

Interviewing

Interviews may be conducted over the phone, via video conferencing, or in person; or a combination may be used in different "rounds" of the selection process. For example, candidates may be initially screened with a phone interview and only the most qualified candidates are invited to interview in person (Fig. 16.1).

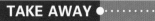

TAKE AWAY ●········

Prescreening usually eliminates applicants who do not meet the minimum requirements for the position.

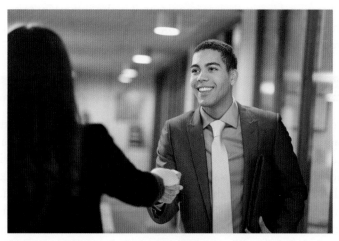

Figure 16.1 A candidate and a hiring manager meet for an in-person interview.

Video interviewing is becoming particularly popular and offers multiple benefits to both the organization and the candidate. It offers greater convenience because it just requires a computer or laptop, and an interview can be done from any location that provides Internet access. Video interviewing can be scheduled within a short period at the convenience of both the interviewer and the candidate, which saves both money and time.

Regardless of how the interview is conducted, the interview must have a planned and structured strategy for what information is needed from the interview conversations. Different organizations use different interviewing approaches. Most organizations tend to use **structured interviews**, which provide interviewers—whether just the hiring manager and human resources recruiter or a panel of interviewers—detailed and defined questions to ask. Series of questions are generally provided to interviewers based on the sequence of experiences provided in the applicant's resume, although others may use a questionnaire. One of the key advantages of a structured interview approach is that it ensures all applicants receive the same questions, thus promoting consistency and reducing future legal liabilities related to the hiring process.

As a final note, it is important for interviewers to consider the candidate's feelings and self-esteem. Remember, the interviewer is representing the organization. The candidate will be assessing their view of the organization, just as the organization is assessing the individual's fit for the position.

> **structured interviews** interviewing style in which interviewers have detailed and defined questions to ask during an interview.

Selection

After the interview is completed, the recruiter, hiring manager, and others involved (or search committee) will gather and discuss how well each candidate meets the selection criteria. The search committee reviews and discusses qualifications, such as each candidate's work experience, education, skills, interests, personality, and work references. The recruiter may also perform a social media background check on the individual by reviewing Facebook, Twitter, and other public information on the Internet. Finally, the hiring manager will select the candidate he or she wishes to hire, and human resources will extend the official job offer.

Job offers should be in writing or sent via email and include the position, start date, salary or compensation, signing bonus, moving allocation, benefits, and any other relevant information. Sometimes there is further negotiation between the candidate and the organization regarding start date, salary, benefits, and other concerns.

▪ LEARNING CHECKPOINT 16.1
▪ Recruitment and Hiring

1. _____ candidates are those who are not currently seeking a new position, but may be inclined to consider it if the conditions, such as compensation and benefits, are attractive enough.

2. In a job _____, the hiring manager identifies the skills, responsibilities, tasks, activities, training, experience, certifications, or licenses that are necessary for the success of the individual in a position.

3. A _____ interview is one in which an organization gives an interviewer detailed and defined questions to ask.

TRAINING AND DEVELOPMENT

With such significant transitioning of the workforce, the need for retaining talent, and the costs of hiring, more and more employers are going to great lengths to ensure that employees feel valued, respected, and comfortable in their new workplaces. It is critical that organizations focus on making the new hire transition as smooth as possible to optimize job performance and minimize employee turnover.

Onboarding

onboarding the process of helping new hires integrate into the organization, preparing them for job success, and becoming productive employees.

After successful recruitment and selection, most health care organizations will continue to support the new hire's assimilation into the organization through onboarding. **Onboarding** is the process of helping new hires integrate into the organization, preparing them for job success and becoming productive employees. Onboarding includes both the social and performance aspects of the new job, which may continue for several months after the start of the job.

Orientation

orientation overview of an organization for new employees, which may include organizational values, goals, objectives, policies and procedures, employee benefits, and mandatory compliance training.

The orientation is an important part of the onboarding process, and most employers require mandatory participation before starting the job. **Orientation** covers many different topics of importance for new hires, such as:
* Organizational values, mission, goals, and strategic objectives
* Policies and procedures (such as safety and security protocols)
* Dress code and codes of conduct
* Employee benefits
* Performance assessment process
* Disciplinary actions and grievances
* Opportunities for training and development
* Mandatory compliance training programs—for example, compliance with Health Insurance Portability and Accountability Act (HIPAA) confidentiality requirements, Medicare rules, sexual harassment, customer service, and communications

Orientation is also an opportunity for the human resources department to give new hires important documents such as the employee handbook and information on the Whistleblower Protection Act of 1989. Additionally, the orientation meeting may include an opportunity for new employees to meet coworkers and the senior management team for an overview of different departments within the organization.

Training and Development

Training and development should be considered an ongoing process for all organizations, as there are always new hires, new issues, changes in technology and information systems, ongoing licensure and certification requirements for clinical staff, and industry changes that may require different employee skill sets.

training teaching employees the necessary skills to perform their jobs successfully, focusing on the short-term needs of an organization.

Training focuses on short-term needs of the organization. Training may focus on a broad range of issues, such as training on:
* Patient safety
* Diversity awareness
* Sexual harassment
* Health care equipment
* Information technology software
* Customer service
* Interpersonal communication skills

- Leadership
- Managerial skills—for example, conducting performance reviews and hiring processes
- Other policies and procedures

Employee **development** is broader in scope and focuses on the long-term skills for individual employees. Every employee should have a well-thought-out employee development plan, which provides employees with opportunities and clear direction on how to increase their skills and advance their careers. It is important to ensure that the employee development plan is aligned with the organization's needs. Thus with a more expanded skill set, employees have more tools to help their organization forge ahead.

development long-term gains of skill for an individual employee.

Diversity Training

Diversity is an appreciation and recognition of individual differences, such as race, gender, age, religious beliefs, sexual orientation, and socioeconomic status. By raising awareness, diversity training helps employees at all levels within a health care organization to better understand and care for patients with different backgrounds. Diversity training also supports the inclusion of minorities and supports collaboration, which is critical in health care.

diversity an appreciation and recognition of individual differences such as race, gender, age, religious beliefs, sexual orientation, and socioeconomic status.

Diversity training may include:

- Appreciation and awareness of diversity
- The impact of cultural values and norms on communication
- Resolving conflict and building teams
- The business case for supporting diversity by the health care organization
- Managing individuals from different generations
- Strategies in attracting and retaining a diverse workforce and customer base
- Courses in cultural awareness for managers focusing on interviewing, hiring, selection, performance assessments, and coaching

TAKE AWAY

Diversity training helps employees understand and care for patients and each other.

■ LEARNING CHECKPOINT 16.2
■ Training and Development

1. Which type of training is for new hires?

   a. Orientation
   b. Onboarding
   c. Development
   d. a and b only

2. Which is a part of diversity training?

   a. Learning the names of supervisors
   b. Understanding cultural norms
   c. Discussing dress code and codes of conduct
   d. Learning organizational values, mission, goals, and strategic objectives

PERFORMANCE REVIEWS

One of the most important responsibilities of the human resources department in any organization is to oversee the employee **performance review** process. In health care, employee performance is critical because it affects patient care and satisfaction. Employee

performance review a process that allows managers and employees to identify strengths and weaknesses in their job performance.

performance reviews can be used to identify the organization's best employees, as well as those who need improvement. For the top-performing employees, the review process is an opportunity to reward good work through financial incentives or promotions. For lower-performing employees, it is an opportunity to reevaluate the goals of their position in the organization and identify possible training gaps. Performance reviews also allow employees to know how their manager views their work, and it may motivate the employee to address any performance weaknesses.

Employee performance reviews are important for documentation that may be used for litigation purposes, specifically in cases of demotions, layoffs, and terminations. These topics will be discussed later in this chapter.

Most employee performance reviews are conducted annually, although there is a growing trend of organizations moving toward more frequent reviews. Some organizations may choose to do a midyear review in addition to an annual review. Other organizations may conduct reviews on the anniversary date of when the employee started working for the organization. Many health care organizations also do reviews after an initial "probationary period" when employees are first hired. Probationary periods are usually about 3 months in length. During this time, if a manager determines that the employee's work has been unsatisfactory, they may opt to extend the probationary period and have another review in 3 to 6 months or decide to terminate the employee. In the probationary period, it is important for the manager to identify specific areas for improvement and indicate if there is a possibility of termination.

In most cases, the employee's manager conducts the employee performance review. However, relying on the opinions of one person may lead to bias and an inaccurate assessment. Some organizations have employees do a self-assessment as part of the review process. This is beneficial because the employee has to think about his or her own strengths and weaknesses. It also encourages employees to think about and plan for their future with the organization, including possible promotions or different jobs they would like to consider.

Another form of employee performance review is from peer or team ratings, which can be one of the most reliable sources of information. Peer reviews are useful because different people see different aspects of the employee's work, such as whether the employee is reliable and collaborative. However, peer reviews can also be biased if coworkers develop friendships or animosity toward the employee being evaluated. Another source of review is to use customer or patient reviews, such as surveys. However, these types of performance reviews generally reflect the performance of the organization as a whole and thus are difficult to attribute to individual employees. Organizations may also assess the performance of a manager using feedback from his or her employees. Lastly, employers may use multiple sources of feedback, sometimes called a *360° review*. A **360° review** is a holistic or more comprehensive feedback that comes from all directions in the organization. People who participate in an employee's 360° review usually include the employee's manager, peers, and direct reports. Occasionally, external consultants or vendors who work regularly with the employee are included as well.

Assessment

Performance reviews should always be applied consistently across the entire workforce, which is important in preventing discrimination and other forms of bias. Standard and appropriate assessment tools should also be used, regardless of how often the review is conducted or by whom. All assessment tools should focus on job-specific tasks, behaviors, and outcomes (Fig. 16.2).

There are several different approaches to performance assessment, including narrative methods that allow managers to provide qualitative feedback, and comparative methods

---

TAKE AWAY

Performance reviews document an employee's strengths and opportunities and may be used in litigation.

360° review a comprehensive feedback that comes from the employee's manager, peers, and direct reports.

TAKE AWAY

Performance reviews should always be applied consistently across the entire workforce.

FY 2018 Employee Evaluation – Criteria-Based Appraisal

Employee Name: Erin Rene Ory   **Position:** Coder
Supervisor: Tami JoAnne Davi   **Date: March 23, 2018**

Ratings scale to assess performance: **Exceeds (E=3 points)** – consistently performs at a level over and above standards; **Satisfies (S=2 points)** – consistently performs at the level defined by the standards; **Opportunity (O=1 point)** – generally meets more standards in the function, but needs improvement; **Unsatisfactory (U=0 points)** – Consistently performs at a level below the standards.

Job Functions	% Weight	Rating	Score=: Weight × Rating
1. **Job Function: Codes patient medical record information for diagnosis and procedures.** • Assigns ICD-10-CM codes accurately in accordance with coding guidelines, CMS regulations and hospital policies. • Assigns CPT-4 codes accurately in accordance with coding guidelines, CMS regulations, and hospital policies. • Assigns ED charges, as needed, in accordance with coding guidelines, CMS regulations and hospital policies.	40%	☐ E (3) ☐ S (2) ☐ O (1) ☐ U (0)	1.20
2. **Job Function: Maintains acceptable coding productivity for outpatient claims.** • Codes, charges, and abstracts an average of at least 110 ED charts per day. • Maintains a minimum 99% accuracy rate as determined by independent audit.	30%	☐ E (3) ☐ S (2) ☐ O (1) ☐ U (0)	.90
3. **Job Function: Employs full use of encoding software and abstracting system.** • Uses the encoder to ensure proper coding and sequencing. • Accurately abstracts all information in the abstracting system to reflect correct UB-04 data. • Correctly refers to the computer system when necessary for lab results, transcription, and older claims information.	15%	☐ E (3) ☐ S (2) ☐ O (1) ☐ U (0)	.45
4. **Job Function: Performs other financial and compliance duties as necessary.** • Assists patient financial services personnel with any claims issues to ensure that proper billing is facilitated. • Works with the registration department to ensure data integrity on patient information. • Complies with the standards set by department policy, CMS, and other regulatory agencies.	5%	☐ E (3) ☐ S (2) ☐ O (1) ☐ U (0)	.05
5. **Job Function: Continuing Education** • Maintains credentials through ongoing education. • If uncredentialed, seeks to obtain a coding credential, as appropriate. • Attends mandatory educational sessions for coding information.	10%	☐ E (3) ☐ S (2) ☐ O (1) ☐ U (0)	.20
		TOTAL	2.8 **Performance above standard**

Figure 16.2 Sample evaluation form. (From Davis N, LaCour M: *Foundations of health information management,* ed 4, St. Louis, 2017, Elsevier.)

narrative assessment in a performance review, qualitative feedback that is detailed and meaningful.

comparative assessment in a performance review, assignment of employee rank compared with other employees.

where managers compare employees to one another. The **narrative assessment** is useful because it provides meaningful and detailed feedback to employees and identifies training and career development opportunities for the employee. However, it has the disadvantage that it may be more time intensive for the manager, and managers are more likely to record negative events rather than positive events.

In **comparative assessments**, employee performance is assessed based on their colleagues' performances and ranked. This approach often increases the competitiveness of the work environment and may lead to improved employee performance. However, comparative assessments are unpopular with both managers and employees, and they provide little feedback to employees on how they can improve their "ranking."

Discussion

Once the employee's performance review has been completed, a meeting should be scheduled between the manager and the employee to review it. The meeting should focus on the strengths of the employee to inspire him or her toward further achievement. But the managers should come prepared to discuss both the strengths and weaknesses of the employee's performance. The manager should provide specific examples of positive and negative comments. Employees should also be encouraged to provide their own feedback on areas for improvement during the conversation. In general, employees should not be surprised with their performance review because any concerns or issues should have been brought up by the manager before the performance review. Thus it is important for the manager to address concerns earlier rather than later and wait until the performance review.

If areas for improvement have been identified, both parties should agree upon an action plan. The action plan should include milestone goals with a clear timeline and resources the employee may need to be successful. This may include additional training or development. If an employee's performance has been unsatisfactory and the manager feels a termination or demotion may be required, the manager needs to indicate this verbally and in writing to the employee and start detailed documentation of conversations and actions taken for the employee's personnel file.

TAKE AWAY

During a performance review, opportunities for improvement are supported with an action plan.

TERMINATIONS AND DISMISSALS

An effective performance review should include meaningful feedback and discipline when necessary to change employee performance. However, when employees continue to exhibit negative behaviors or do not improve their performance, they may face termination. In the health care setting, employee terminations most often occur due to poor performance or unethical behavior.

Out of all employment-related events, termination poses the greatest legal liability. Wrongful termination of employment can be due to reasons that are discriminatory or unlawful, but they may also happen when employers fail to follow their own written protocols for employee termination. Unacceptable behaviors, which may result in terminations, are defined by the health care organization's policies and procedures and overall employment law.

employment-at-will legal framework in which an employer or employee may terminate employment at any time and for any reason, as long as there is no legal employment contract.

Legal Framework

Most states follow **employment-at-will** laws. This means that unless an employee has a legal employment contract, the employer or the employee may terminate employment at any time and for any reason. However, employers should be cautious not to unintentionally "promise" an employee employment for a specific period, whether in writing, such as in an employee handbook or offer letter, or verbally. If such a promise is made, the employee's at-will status may no longer apply.

There are other circumstances in which employers lose their protection under the employment-at-will law. For example, employers can be held liable for breaches of implied contracts, breaches of implied covenants of good faith and fair dealing, or for terminations due to a refusal to do something illegal (known as the *public-policy exception*).

Breach of Implied Contract

Implied contracts occur when an employer implies or suggests that an employee's job is protected or guaranteed for a specific period. For example, if a manager tells an employee that he will never lose his job as long as he has good work performance, this would be an implied (or unwritten) contract.

> **implied contract** when an employer implies that an employee's job is protected or guaranteed for a specific period.

Breach of Covenant of Good Faith and Fair Dealings

Employers also lose protection under the at-will doctrine when they breach the **covenant of good faith and fair dealings**. Basically, employees enter into employment with an assumption that the employer will act fairly and in good faith. If a terminated employee can prove that he or she was fired without just cause and was terminated unfairly, then a court may decide in favor of the former employee. However, if employers maintain good documentation of an employee's performance or behavioral issues and progressive disciplinary action, the court may decide in favor of the employer.

> **covenant of good faith and fair dealings** legal framework in which employees enter into employment with the assumption that the employer will act fairly and in good faith.

Public-Policy Exception

A part of the at-will law is the **public-policy exception** where employers cannot fire employees for refusing to do something illegal or that would be against the best interest of the public. When an employee becomes a **whistle blower**, one who reports illegal activities within an organization to authorities, he or she cannot be fired in retaliation. In this way, the employee was acting in the best interest of the public.

Employers also cannot fire employees for:
- Filing a workers compensation claim
- Filing a discrimination or harassment suit
- Requesting leave under the Family and Medical Leave Act (FMLA)
- Requesting accommodations for a disability
- Other retaliatory reasons

> **public-policy exception** exception to the at-will doctrine that says employers cannot fire employees for refusing to do something illegal or that would be against the best interest of the public.

> **whistle blower** one who reports illegal activities occurring within an organization to law enforcement authorities.

Discrimination

When employers terminate employees due their belonging to a "protected class," this is called *discrimination* and it is illegal. **Title VII of the Civil Rights Act** prohibits employers from terminating employees based on their belonging to a "protected class" such as race, color, religion, national origin, sex, pregnancy, age, disability, or citizenship. Employees are also protected under the Americans with Disabilities Act (ADA) and the Age Discrimination in Employment Act (ADEA), as well as state and local employment laws.

> **Title VII of the Civil Rights Act** legislation that prohibits employers from discriminating against employees based on gender, race, national origin, or religion for purposes of hiring, terminating, or determining wages/salary.

Disciplinary Process

From a liability standpoint it is critical that employers have a systematic disciplinary process and procedures in place. In the event that a terminated employee should sue a company, the courts will review the case to determine if the disciplinary process was uniformly and appropriately applied to all employees, that there was sufficient documentation of poor performance, that the employee had notification of his or her performance issues, and that the employee understood job expectations. A well-designed disciplinary system can be used to support and document these factors.

TAKE AWAY

A systematic, uniformly applied disciplinary process is legally sound.

Employers need to ensure that the disciplinary process and the potential consequences are clearly communicated to all employees. The most common disciplinary system is progressive and includes the following steps:

1. Identifying poor performance or behavior, or rule violation
2. Providing the employee with a verbal warning
3. Investigating any violation
4. Determining appropriate disciplinary action(s)
5. Providing the employee with a written warning
6. Providing the employee with a final written warning
7. Terminating the employee
8. Providing the employee with an exit interview

It is important to ensure that all managers receive training on the disciplinary process to ensure all proper steps are taken when disciplining or terminating an employee.

Ending Employment

Termination of an employee may be either voluntary or involuntary. *Voluntary termination* may be initiated solely by the employee, also called *resignation*, may be due to retirement; or may be due to job abandonment, which is when an employee is absent from work for 3 consecutive workdays and fails to contact his or her supervisor. *Involuntary termination* is initiated by the management of the employee's organization. Examples of involuntary termination are the employee is unable to perform the essential functions of his or her job, misconduct, tardiness, absenteeism, and layoffs. Oftentimes, involuntary termination is the result of progressive disciplinary action to correct a performance problem. However, certain types of employee misconduct are so severe that one incident of misconduct will result in immediate termination without prior use of progressive disciplinary action.

Of all parts of the disciplinary process, the termination stage may be the most complex. As with the previous employee–manager meeting, the termination meeting should be held in a private and comfortable setting at the end of a work shift or workweek. If there is a possibility of litigation, the manager may want to have a representative from the human resources department attend the meeting as a witness and as a resource for questions. The manager should come to the meeting prepared with necessary written documents, most importantly the termination notice. The termination letter should not be emailed to the employee before the meeting. The termination letter should include the reasons for termination. If there are multiple reasons for the employee's termination, each one should be detailed in the letter. The manager will ask the employee to sign the termination letter to indicate he or she has received it. If the employee refuses, ask the witness to sign it.

An important step when employees depart from an employer is to ensure that the employees do not take any property or confidential information with them. This is especially critical for health care organizations where employees have access to patient information. The best approach is to create an employee property inventory during employee onboarding after first being hired. Thus, when employees leave the organization, security or the manager can review the property being removed. Health care organizations should take special precautions to ensure that computer and electronic medical record data are protected in order to be compliant with HIPAA requirements.

Exit Interview

When an employee is terminated, whether voluntarily or involuntarily, an exit interview should be conducted with the departing employee before he or she leaves. The purpose of exit interviews is to learn reasons for the employee's departure and then use

TAKE AWAY ●· · · · · · · ·

Termination of an employee may be either voluntary or involuntary.

this feedback for organizational improvement. Effective exit interviews should yield useful information about the organization to assess and improve all aspects of the working environment, culture, processes and systems, and management and leadership. Exit interviews are also an opportunity for the organization to transfer knowledge, experience, and job responsibilities from the departing employee to a successor or replacement. Exit interviews can be invaluable to an organization because it gives it a unique opportunity to survey and evaluate the opinions of departing employees, who generally are more forthcoming, constructive, and objective than employees still in their jobs. An exit interview is also an opportunity for the organization to provide additional information to the terminated employee regarding 401(k), COBRA, payouts, and last day of pay.

For the departing employees, the exit interview provides them a chance to give some constructive feedback and to leave on a positive note. It is important to end on mutual respect because the departing employee may need a referral or recommendation, may wish to return to the organization in the future, or career paths may cross again in different positions at different organizations. For the involuntarily terminated employee, an exit survey may not always be conducted or may not follow the same format because the organization has already documented the reasons for the termination. Commonly asked questions in an exit interview include:

- Did you feel the organization provided you with sufficient training and opportunities for advancement?
- Do you have any suggestions for ways the organization or your department might enable the work environment to be more pleasant and productive?
- What do you value about the company?
- What did you dislike about the company?
- What could your supervisor do to improve his or her management style and skill?
- Were your job responsibilities characterized correctly during the interview process and orientation?
- Did you receive adequate feedback about your day-to-day performance and in the performance development planning process?

An exit interview should not be confused with the meeting at which notice of termination is given. Exit interviews are conducted after the termination decision. Managers should be trained to keep information regarding employee exit interviews confidential and not discuss them with other colleagues or employees to avoid any possible litigation for defamation.

Employee Turnover and Retention

Whether employees leave an organization voluntarily or involuntarily, health care organizations must evaluate the impact of employee turnover and retention. Workforce shortages in health care have dire consequences compared with in other industries because this negatively affects the quality of patient care and patient health outcomes. Employee turnover rates in health care are higher than in other industries for a number of reasons. One of the most significant reasons is the changing demographics of the health care workforce. The baby boomer generation is beginning to age out of the workforce, but the new-graduate pool has been declining. With fewer individuals entering the health care workforce, especially in areas such as nursing, and more individuals aging out of the workforce over the next few years, employers must focus resources on retaining their current health care professionals.

With high demand and low supply, many highly qualified employees may continue to job hunt even when they are employed. Adding to this increased competitiveness in job switching, technology has made job hunting easier than ever.

TAKE AWAY

When an employee is terminated, an exit interview should be conducted before he or she leaves.

TAKE AWAY

High demand and low supply make turnover a problem in the health care industry.

Turnover Costs

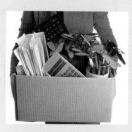

Each year employee turnover costs the United States' economy billions of dollars. Typical direct replacement expenses may include the costs of termination; staff time for exit interviews; recruiting, advertising, and search fees; staff time to interview prospective employees; referral fees; employment testing; reference-checking fees; pre-employment medical reviews; relocation and moving expenses; staff paid time for orientation; training staff pay; training materials; supervisor "coaching" time; and even possible unemployment taxes as turnover increases unemployment benefits.

Additionally, indirect costs result from an employee leaving an organization. Patient satisfaction and continuity of care may be affected, and employees who are left behind to assume the former duties of the departing employee may feel disgruntled and even rejected. There may be missed project deadlines, decreased customer service, delays in care, added overtime costs, and negative impacts on organizational performance, especially in areas of safety and productivity. Lastly, indirect costs are associated with new hires, including the possibility of learning curve errors, which may lead to medical errors.

The first logical question in analyzing employee turnover in any organization is to figure out why employees leave, both voluntarily and involuntarily. When considering those who are involuntarily terminated for poor performance, policy violations, or other reasons, organizations should carefully evaluate the hiring, selection, and training processes in the organization. High rates of terminations may suggest that the organization's hiring process needs some reevaluating. For those who voluntarily leave, the best source of information will likely be from questions asked during an exit interview. Using information from departing employees, organizations may be able to improve key aspects that improve the work environment to prevent further turnover and improve overall employee retention.

Improving Employee Retention

This section of the chapter will focus on improving employee engagement and performance and preventing absenteeism. We will also discuss strategies to combat some of the main drivers of turnover: inadequate compensation and/or benefits, too few opportunities for career growth, poor management, overall inadequate organizational culture, and lack of job autonomy and flexibility.

Improving Employee Engagement

High turnover rates are often due to the lack of employee engagement. Engaged employees are those who put in extra effort, are actively involved, and are fully invested in their jobs (Fig. 16.3). Employees who are engaged are focused on the success of the employer, and they are also less likely to experience burnout. Disengaged employees, on the other hand, are those who work the minimum amount required, remain apathetic, and are only influenced by their paychecks.

Employers should develop their own retention strategies and tailor them with a focus on employee engagement. The following are some approaches that different organizations have found successful in improving employee engagement:

- Create and clearly communicate the organizational vision to employees.
- Establish behavior expectations and consistently apply standards to all employees.

TAKE AWAY

Engaged employees are those who put in extra effort, are actively involved, and are fully invested in their jobs.

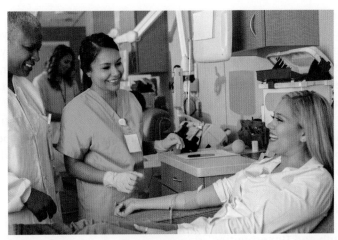

Figure 16.3 Engaged employees are actively involved and fully invested in their jobs. They are less likely to change their place of work.

- Provide resources in support of expectations and organizational priorities.
- Design systems that hold employees accountable.
- Allow employees autonomy, task variety, and task significance in their job responsibilities.
- Institute work policies that are respectful.
- Encourage managers to demonstrate both transformational leadership and sincere caring for the welfare of individual staff members.
- Create flexible work hours and scheduling.
- Ensure employees receive feedback and coaching for career development to improve engagement and performance and to establish a positive organizational work culture.

Reducing Absenteeism

One way employees separate themselves from an organization is by leaving it, but another is through absenteeism. Disengaged employees are less likely to report for work or complete a full work shift and leave early. In actuality, it is usually only a few employees who account for the total absenteeism within the organization.

Absenteeism is a particular problem area in the health care field. When employees "call in sick" or take an unscheduled leave of absence, additional workers will have to be called in to cover. Additionally, if there is no staff member to cover the work shift, patient care and safety may be compromised due to the understaffing, which may lead to patient dissatisfaction.

Most employee absenteeism is voluntary and avoidable. Policies on absenteeism should be clearly described in the employee handbook and other organizational documents and be enforced consistently. Different strategies to reduce absenteeism are:

- **Use of discipline process**: verbal warning, followed by written warning, suspension, and possible termination.
- **Positive rewards**: giving employees cash, gift cards, "buying back" unused sick leave, recognition, additional time off, or other rewards for meeting attendance goals.
- **Paid time off accounts**: employees receive a set amount of paid days off work, which can be used for vacation, holidays, or sick leave. When the employee runs out of days, then they have to take unpaid leave. This approach has been proven to reduce 1-day absences, but it increases the probability of employees using the totality of their account hours, as employees will use the remaining unused days for vacation days.

TAKE AWAY ● · · · · · · · ·

Most employee absenteeism is voluntary and avoidable.

Compensation and Benefits

Higher compensation remains a key driver in employee retention. Employers may opt to use signing bonuses, relocation reimbursement, premium or differential pay, forgiveness loans, and extensive benefits to reward and retain employees. However, employers should understand that in addition to being satisfied with compensation, employees want to be satisfied with how pay is determined.

Although compensation is one of the most important factors in attracting new talent, it is not always enough to hold on to employees. Employees may be swayed by having competitive benefits, such as health insurance, tuition assistance, and retirement. Additional benefits and perks that contribute to employee retention are paid lunches, flexible scheduling, or having special facilities onsite, such as childcare, exercise clubs, hair salons, post offices, or dry cleaners.

Career Growth and Opportunities

Employers need to be creative in developing training, coaching, and mentoring programs to retain qualified employees and capitalize on their skills. For flatter or horizontal organizations or those with few or no levels of middle management between staff and executives, these organizations need to consider career ladders that provide alternatives to managerial promotions. Employers may consider tuition-aid programs and continuing education programs that provide employees with additional professional certifications and licenses.

Although some organizations may fear that developing employees' skills makes them more attractive to other employers, they need to recognize that career development also improves retention. Employers need to identify ways to use employees' newly gained knowledge and skill within the organization. Then employees will be encouraged to pursue new career opportunities within the organization rather than leaving.

Supportive Managers

Another significant determinant of employee retention is the management style of the employee's direct supervisor. Most studies find that employees leave poor managers, not jobs. Employees want to have healthy relationships in the workplace, both with managers and coworkers. They want fair and nondiscriminatory treatment and support from their managers. Employees need to feel valued, and it is important to show them how their work contributes to the overall success of the organization. It is also important for employees to know that their managers are really listening and responding to employee input.

Organizations with healthy turnover rates assess the training of their top managers. So one of the best strategies in employee retention is leadership development. Employers and managers need to develop strong relationships with employees from the start to build trust. Employees have to believe that upper management is competent and that the organization will be successful. An employer has to be able to inspire this confidence and make decisions that reinforce it. An employer cannot say one thing and do another. For example, employers should not reprimand employees for missing deadlines when they constantly miss their own deadlines. In addition, employers need to engage and inspire employees by enacting policies that show they trust them, such as not practicing micromanagement or an authoritarian style of management.

Organizational Culture

Several studies have found that the overall work environment and organizational commitment to employees significantly affect employees' decision to leave an employer. Successful health care organizational cultures are those that are results oriented, well managed, promote job security and continuity, emphasize strong values, have a strategic

TAKE AWAY ●·········
Career development makes employees attractive to other enterprises, but also improves retention.

TAKE AWAY ●·········
To keep high-performing employees, organizations have to create environments where people want to stay and grow.

vision, and aim to support patient-centered care. To keep high-performing employees, organizations have to create environments where people want to stay and grow.

An important component is to match work–life benefits to the needs of employees. This could be in the form of offering nontraditional work schedules, such as a compressed workweek, telecommuting, flextime, or providing extra holidays. When work–life balance is structured properly, both the employee and employer benefit. For example, employees will be more productive because they will be less stressed, healthier, and enjoy the work they do. Employers should also encourage employees to set personal and life goals, such as spending more time with their families. This communicates that the employer really does want the employees to have a life outside of work and achieve a healthy work–life balance.

LEARNING CHECKPOINT 16.3
Performance Reviews and Termination and Dismissal

1. Which type of performance review includes feedback from peers?

   a. Narrative assessment
   b. Comparative assessment
   c. 360° review
   d. a and b only

2. Which occurs when an employer implies or suggests that an employee's job is protected or guaranteed for a specific period?

   a. Public-policy exception
   b. Implied contract
   c. Covenant of good faith and fair dealings
   d. Employment-at-will

3. In the disciplinary process, which comes first?

   a. Verbal warning
   b. Written warning
   c. Termination
   d. Exit interview

EMPLOYMENT LAWS

Many aspects of human resources are subject to federal legal and regulatory requirements. This section will discuss the top 10 employment laws that every manager should know, specifically in regard to prohibiting discrimination; family and military leave; overtime pay and wages; gender-pay differences; and workplace safety (Box 16.1). Additionally, the topic of sexual harassment will be discussed with strategies to ensure that managers are proactive in preventing such harassment in their organizations.

Discrimination

Many employment laws are aimed at prohibiting discrimination among different "protected classes," including but not limited to:

- Race
- Religion

**BOX
16.1**   **TOP 10 EMPLOYMENT LAWS EVERY HEALTH SERVICES ADMINISTRATOR
SHOULD KNOW**

1. Title VII of the Civil Rights Act
2. Age Discrimination in Employment Act (ADEA)/Older Workers Benefit Protection Act (OWBPA)
3. Americans with Disabilities Act (ADA)
4. Genetic Information Nondiscrimination Act (GINA)
5. Pregnancy Discrimination Act (PDA)
6. Family and Medical Leave Act (FMLA)
7. Uniformed Services Employment and Reemployment Rights Act (USERRA)/National Defense Authorization Act (NDAA)
8. Fair Labor and Standards Act (FLSA)
9. Equal Pay Act (EPA)
10. Occupational Safety and Health Act (OSH Act)

- Sex
- National origin
- Age
- Disability
- Genetic information
- Pregnancy

Civil Rights

Title VII of the Civil Rights Act of 1964 prohibits employers from discriminating against employees based on race, religion, sex, or national origin for purposes of hiring, terminating, or determining wages and salary. The Civil Rights Act established the first definition of "protected classes." It also created the EEOC to enforce the Civil Rights Act. In addition, this act enacted laws to prohibit employers from retaliating against an employee who files a complaint about discrimination and requires employers to reasonably accommodate employees' religious practices.

The Civil Rights Act prohibits discrimination related to all types of employment actions, including but not limited to recruitment, job advertisements, testing, hiring, training, compensation, benefits, promotions, terminations, layoffs, and other terms and conditions of employment.

It is worth noting that even if an organization has no intent to discriminate, hiring practices may have the adverse impact of doing so in practice. Adverse impact, also known as **disparate impact**, is when hiring practices result in decisions that disproportionately affect a protected class.

The EEOC, which enforces federal employment discrimination laws in the United States, published the **Uniform Guidelines on Employee Selection Procedures (UGESP)** to assist employers in determining whether a hiring or promotion process has a disparate impact on any race, sex, or ethnic group. The UGESP establishes a "rule of thumb" that if the selection rate for any protected class is less than 80% that of another class, then there may be evidence of disparate impact. For example, if 50% of non-Hispanic applicants pass a particular preemployment test, but only 20% of Hispanic applicants pass, the ratio would be 20/50, or 40%, which would violate the 80% rule.

The **Age Discrimination in Employment Act (ADEA)** prohibits employers from discriminating against employees or job applicants over age 40 because of their age. Most cases of age discrimination are due to wrongful discharge or mandatory retirement policies. However, ADEA applies to any adverse employment action, including denying promotions or training opportunities.

TAKE AWAY ●·········

The Civil Rights Act prohibits discrimination against protected classes.

---

disparate impact hiring practices resulting in decisions that disproportionately affect a protected class.

Uniform Guidelines on Employee Selection Procedures (UGESP) EEOC guidance to assist employers in determining whether a hiring or promotions process has a disparate impact on any race, sex, or ethnic group.

Age Discrimination in Employment Act (ADEA) legislation that prohibits employers from discriminating against employees or job applicants over age 40 because of their age.

Employers may, however, have grounds for their employment actions if the employee was terminated for poor performance, misconduct, or other just cause or reason of business necessity. Employers may demonstrate that the employee's age met the requirements of a bona fide occupational qualification. In other words, a worker is unable to perform the job due to age. An example would be if an applicant over age 65 was applying for a job modeling clothes for teenagers.

Additionally, as the cost of health care continues to climb, employers have been faced with interpreting how the ADEA applies to employee health benefits. As a response, the ADEA was amended by the **Older Workers Benefit Protection Act of 1990 (OWBPA)**. This amendment prohibits employers from denying benefits to older employees.

> ● **Older Workers Benefit Protection Act (OWBPA)** legislation that prohibits employers from denying benefits to older workers.

Disabilities

The ADA prohibits employers from discriminating against employees based on disability. The law defines a disability as any physical or mental impairment that "substantially limits" one or more major "life activities." Major life activities may include but are not limited to walking, standing, breathing, learning, seeing, hearing, concentrating, thinking, eating, sleeping, communicating, and/or working. This also includes operations of major bodily functions, which include but are not limited to the immune, digestive, or respiratory system; and includes protection for individuals with chronic conditions such as diabetes. The law does not include coverage of impairments that last fewer than 6 months.

Employers should pay particular attention to job descriptions to prevent disability discrimination. Job descriptions must be accurate and up to date to determine essential job functions, as stipulated in Box 16.2. For example, if a job description states that lifting objects over 25 pounds is an essential function, then employers should ask applicants whether they would be able to lift objects over 25 pounds.

Qualified individuals are entitled to "reasonable accommodations" under the ADA. **Reasonable accommodations** are modifications that enable disabled individuals to perform essential job functions successfully in a work environment. The ADA states that reasonable accommodations are those that do not create an "undue hardship" on the organization, such as an adjustment or modification that is too expensive or difficult for the organization to provide. The EEOC has issued guidance on specific industries, including health care, and provides suggestions on how to accommodate many disabilities at the Job Accommodation Network site: www.askjan.org/soar. Box 16.3 provides some examples of reasonable accommodations.

In addition to making accommodations for physical disabilities, accommodations may be necessary for employees with psychiatric disabilities such as depression because

> **TAKE AWAY** ●············
>
> Employers should pay attention to job descriptions to prevent disability discrimination.

> ● **reasonable accommodations** modifications that provide disabled individuals with a work environment or work process to allow them to perform essential job functions successfully.

BOX 16.2	WHICH PARTS OF AN EMPLOYEE'S DUTIES ARE ESSENTIAL JOB FUNCTIONS?

- Employee spends most of his or her work time doing the function.
- Consequences of work not being done would be dire (such as poor patient care).
- Previous employees in the role would describe the function as essential.

- The job was created specifically for the function to be performed.
- Only a limited number of organizational employees can do the job, so everyone has to "pitch in" when needed (such as answering phones).

> ### BOX 16.3   EXAMPLES OF REASONABLE ACCOMMODATIONS
>
> - Modifying restrooms to be accessible
> - Installing ramps at building entrances
> - Rearranging office furniture
> - Job restructuring that reallocates functions that are not primary to the position to another position within the organization

it is the leading cause of disability globally according to the World Health Organization. The EEOC provides specific rules on the types of adjustments needed to accommodate individuals with psychiatric disabilities. Some examples of adjustments are:

- Making changes to the way employees receive feedback, such as feedback that is more detailed, structured, positive, or provided more frequently
- Adjusting schedules, such as offering flextime, job sharing, or part-time hours
- Flexible leave policies, such as allowing individuals more unpaid leave
- Modifying workspaces, such as adding cubical dividers to reduce noise
- Changing organizational policies, such as more frequent breaks or allowing food or drink to mitigate side effects of medications
- Increasing natural lighting

Organizations should also pay attention to how employees with psychiatric disabilities are perceived or treated by coworkers. An organization is responsible for the behavior of its employees. All employees should be trained on anti-harassment policies as they relate to people with disabilities, including psychiatric disabilities. To prevent harassment, organizations should also keep information about all disabilities, physical or mental, confidential. However, it should be noted that if an employee becomes a threat to himself or herself or other employees, the employee is not protected under the ADA.

Substance Addiction

Although the ADA was created with broad goals of protecting the disabled, the ADA did recognize that some disabilities could pose safety risks, including drug and alcohol addiction. Individuals with alcoholism or a history of drug addiction may be considered disabled based on the ADA's guidelines. Just as with other disabilities, an employee is only covered by the ADA if they have an addiction severe enough to substantially affect a major life activity. However, it is worth noting here that the courts have frequently supported employers in establishing workplace rules, including not coming to work under the influence of alcohol or other drugs. The best approach for employers is to set workplace behavior policies that require employees to be sober and not under the influence of any substances while on the job and to do their job competently. The employer needs to ensure that they apply these rules and policies consistently and keep records of any disciplinary actions related to the policy.

Discrimination Based on Genetic Information

The **Genetic Information Nondiscrimination Act (GINA)** protects employees from discrimination based on genetic information. Genetic information, as defined by the EEOC, includes information from genetic tests and diseases or health conditions for an individual and his or her family. The objective of this law is to prevent employers from discriminating against an employee based on the probability that he or she, or his or her family, may develop a disease or condition in the future. GINA prohibits discrimination as it relates to any personnel action, including hiring, changes in pay, job assignments, promotions, layoffs, or terminations.

TAKE AWAY ●·········

An organization is responsible for the behavior of its employees.

○ **Genetic Information Nondiscrimination Act (GINA)** legislation that protects employees from discrimination based on genetic information.

Discrimination Based on Pregnancy

Pregnancy discrimination continues to be an issue in the United States. The **Pregnancy Discrimination Act (PDA)** is an amendment to Title VII of the Civil Rights Act, and it prohibits employers from discriminating against an employee based on pregnancy. The PDA requires employers to treat employees who are or may be affected by pregnancy-related conditions in the same manner as other employees with similar circumstances regarding their ability to work. Other laws, such as the ADA and the FMLA, may also apply.

The PDA applies to any aspect of employment, including pay, job assignments, benefits, promotions, training, terminations, and layoffs. Employers cannot deny a woman a position or promotion solely on the fact that she is pregnant or had an abortion. Nor can a woman be fired or forced to take leave on such a basis as long as she is capable of performing her job. Employers must treat pregnant employees the same as they would treat other employees.

Employers cannot require pregnant employees to take leave if they are able to perform the essential job duties. Pregnant employees may be required to use vacation benefits before collecting sick or disability pay, but only if it also applies to other employees for other types of disabilities or illnesses. Employers cannot prohibit an employee from returning to work for a specific length of time after the birth of a child. Also, new parents have the option to use leave under the FMLA, which will be discussed later in this chapter.

If an employee is unable to work due to pregnancy-related conditions, the organization must treat her in the same way in which it treats all temporarily disabled employees. Relatedly, impairments due to a pregnancy may be considered a disability under the ADA. Pregnancy on its own is not a disability under the ADA. The ADA applies to pregnancy-related conditions that qualify as a disability, such as preeclampsia, because they impair a major life activity, even if the condition is temporary.

Organizations must apply the same personnel processes for pregnant employees as they would for any other types of disabilities or illnesses. This includes providing reasonable accommodations, such as reassigned work, modified work schedules, or the same options for taking leave. The PDA also prohibits employers from requiring pregnant employees to follow any medical clearance processes that would not also be applied to other disabilities or illnesses, such as requiring a physician's statement regarding the employee's ability to work before granting leave.

The PDA also has provisions regarding health insurance. Employer-sponsored health insurance must include pregnancy-related services and cover them in the same manner that other medical services are covered. In addition, the PDA prevents employers from excluding single women from maternity benefits under their health insurance. Additionally, employers cannot require a pregnant employee with a single-coverage health insurance policy to switch to family health coverage when she becomes pregnant. However, she must be allowed to make the change after the birth so that the child is covered.

Family Leave

The **Family and Medical Leave Act (FMLA)** allows employees with at least 1 year of service to take up to 12 weeks of unpaid leave each year for the birth or adoption of a child or to care for themselves or a sick child, spouse, or parent with a serious health condition (Fig. 16.4). "Parent" is broadly defined as the biological, adoptive, step, or foster parent of an employee or an individual who stood *in loco parentis* to the employee when the employee was a son or daughter. However, FMLA does not cover domestic partners, siblings, grandparents, or in-laws. The FMLA protects employees from losing their jobs during the 12 weeks of medical leave.

Pregnancy Discrimination Act (PDA) legislation that prohibits employers from discriminating against a woman who is or may become pregnant.

TAKE AWAY

Pregnancy on its own is not a disability under the ADA, but pregnancy-related conditions that impair life activities are qualifying disabilities.

Family and Medical Leave Act (FMLA) legislation that allows employees with at least 1 year of service to take up to 12 weeks of unpaid leave each year for the birth or adoption of a child or to care for themselves or a sick child, spouse, or parent with a serious health condition.

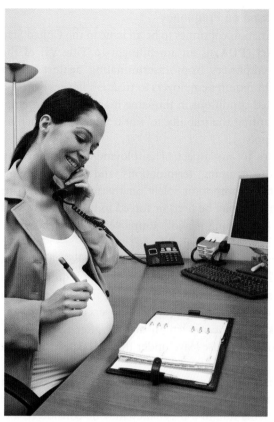

Figure 16.4 The FMLA allows employees with at least 1 year of service to take up to 12 weeks of unpaid leave each year for the birth of a child.

The FMLA defines a "serious health condition" as an illness, impairment, or condition (physical or mental) that includes a "period of incapacity" for one of the following reasons:

- Treatment in an inpatient setting
- Treatment requiring three missed calendar days of work, school, or daily activities
- Care for pregnancy or prenatal care
- Treatment for a serious chronic condition
- Care for conditions where treatment has been ineffective and the incapacity is permanent or long term

To be eligible, employees must have worked for the same employer for at least 12 months. It does not need to be 12 months of continuous service. Organizations may count any time the employee worked over the past 7 years. Employees may take up to 12 weeks of unpaid leave during a set 12-month period. Employers are required to determine how the period of 12 months will be measured for all employees. Several states and private companies also have more generous maternity and family leave than what is outlined in the FMLA.

It should also be noted that when an employee returns from FMLA leave, they are entitled to be reinstated into the same position they held before taking leave or to a position with equivalent benefits and pay. If an employer places the employee in a new position, the job must also require the same level of skill and responsibility as the previous position. Employers are also required to allow the employee time to "catch up" on any skills or work that were missed during his or her leave of absence.

Military Leave

The **Uniformed Services Employment and Reemployment Rights Act (USERRA)** prohibits employers from discriminating against any employee who volunteers or is called for military service. When reservists return from any active duty tour of less than 5 years, the organization must reemploy them either in their old position or in an equivalent position if they meet the following criteria:

1. Military service was five years or less and was in a civilian position.
2. The employee was not released from service for misconduct.
3. The employer received notice from the employee before leaving for military service.
4. The employee returned to the civilian job and applied for reemployment.

Individuals serving in the military, and their families, were also granted new leave rights under the **National Defense Authorization Act of 2008 (NDAA)**. The NDAA allows employees to take 12 weeks of unpaid leave for "any qualifying exigency" that results from a call to service or active military service of a spouse, child, or parent. Qualifying exigencies are preparation activities or postdeployment activities that are necessary as a result of one's military service, including legal and financial preparations, counseling, and/or rest and recovery.

It is important to point out that the 26 weeks of military leave under the NDAA is not in addition to the FMLA. The two types of leave occur simultaneously. So, if an employee uses 12 weeks of nonmilitary, FMLA leave, the most NDAA leave that can be taken is 14 weeks.

Wages

The **Fair Labor Standards Act (FLSA)** protects employees from compensation discrimination. Specifically, it sets the federal minimum wage and requires that employers pay time-and-a-half for any overtime for hourly employees who work more than 40 hours per week. FLSA also regulates the number of hours and types of work that minors (individuals under age 18) can perform.

To ensure FLSA compliance, organizations need to understand the definition of "hours of work." Hours of work are any hours when the employee is "on duty." Thus the only excluded time would be that used for personal activities. Meal breaks lasting 30 minutes or more do not need to be counted if the employee is "off duty."

Some hourly employees may be eligible for payment for travel time. Examples include when travel is a regular part of the job; 1-day travel assignments, except for meal times and customary work commute time; and travel during normal working hours. Typical commuting from home to work and vice versa does not count as paid time unless the employee is actually working during the commute. Also, if employees are required to wait for an assignment or other work, they are entitled to paid time.

There are also circumstances when an employee attends training that he or she may be entitled to paid time. This does not include instances where attendance is beyond normal work hours, the employee does not perform any productive work during the training, training does not directly apply to the job, and/or the training is voluntary.

The FLSA also establishes the **federal minimum wage**, which is the lowest amount that can be paid for hourly work. The minimum wage as of January 2017 is $7.25 per hour. This wage has not increased since 2009. The minimum wage may vary in some states or even in some cities and counties.

Gender-Pay Differences

The **Equal Pay Act (EPA)** requires that employers pay men and women "equal pay for equal work." Two jobs do not have to be identical to violate the EPA, but they must be

Uniformed Services Employment and Reemployment Rights Act (USERRA) prohibits employers from discriminating against an employee who volunteers or is called for military service.

National Defense Authorization Act (NDAA) legislation that allows employees to take 12 weeks of unpaid leave for "any qualifying exigency" that results from a call to service or active military service of a spouse, child, or parent.

Fair Labor Standards Act (FLSA) legislation that protects employees from compensation discrimination. Specifically, it sets the federal minimum wage and requires that employers pay time-and-a-half for any overtime for hourly employees who work more than 40 hours per week.

federal minimum wage the lowest amount that an employee can legally be paid for hourly work.

Equal Pay Act (EPA) legislation that requires employers to pay men and women equal pay for substantially equal work.

"substantially equal." Whether or not two jobs are substantially equal does not depend on the job titles, but it is the job content that matters. Specifically, do the jobs require the same skills, efforts, and responsibilities? Although the gender-pay gap has significantly narrowed since the 1950s in the United States, a pay gap still exists. In 2015, female full-time workers made only 80 cents for every dollar earned by men—a gender wage gap of 20%. In health care, male physicians are paid almost 9% more than their female counterparts.

Workplace Safety

○ **Occupational Safety and Health Act (OSH Act)** federal legislation that promotes work safety and requires employers to ensure workplaces are free of hazards.

The **Occupational Safety and Health Act (OSH Act)** promotes work safety and requires employers to ensure workplaces are free of hazards. The health care industry has the highest incidence of occupational injury and illness. Health care workers may, for example, be exposed to infectious diseases and needle injuries.

As discussed in Chapter 11, the OSH Act imposes many requirements upon organizations to ensure the workplace is free from recognized hazards and complies with the federal standards under the law. The OSH Act also created the Occupational Safety and Health Administration (OSHA) for federal enforcement of the law. This federal agency may inspect work sites for compliance with OSHA standards. Inspections are often performed when there is fair certainty of danger of death or physical harm; a work-related fatality, hospitalization, or amputation has occurred; or at the request of an employee who suspects a hazard that could cause harm. Employees may file an OSHA complaint anonymously online at: www.osha.gov/workers.

Sexual Harassment

The Civil Rights Act of 1964 prohibited sexual harassment against females in the workplace. The law was later expanded in 1991 to include males.

The Supreme Court has defined two types of sexual harassment that are prohibited by the Civil Rights Act:
1. *Quid pro quo:* Types of harassment where job security, promotion, and benefits are tied to sexual favors.
2. **Hostile work environment:** Types of harassment where the behavior is so severe that it affects the productivity of others indirectly. In hostile work environment cases, harassment may not be directed at the person filing the complaint. Any individual who observes and is offended by sexual material and has difficulty doing his or her job as a result is a victim of sexual harassment.

TAKE AWAY ●·········

Quid pro quo and hostile work environment are the two types of sexual harassment defined by the Supreme Court.

Unfortunately, sexual harassment is not rare in the health care industry. Sexual harassment does not just include supervisors and/or coworkers, but also a customer or patient. For example, a health care organization may be liable if an employee is continually being sexually harassed by a patient. It is also worth noting that harassment does not have to occur within the workplace. If there is a link to the workplace, harassment outside of the workplace may also be illegal.

Victims of sexual harassment must report every incident to the employer. That way, if an employer has already given the harasser a warning, they will have documentation that the harassment has occurred again and that more severe action is necessary. If victims are uncomfortable talking to their supervisor, they may consider talking to a union representative, a person in the human resources department, or a lawyer before filing a complaint. Employees also have the option of filing a complaint with the state fair-employment agency or the federal EEOC and/or filing a civil suit for damages. It is important to note that federal and most state laws require that a complaint be filed within 180 days of the act of sexual harassment.

LEARNING CHECKPOINT 16.4
Employment Laws

1. True or False. Disparate impact is when hiring practices result in decisions that disproportionately affect a protected class.

2. True or False. The Age Discrimination in Employment Act (ADEA) prohibits employers from discriminating against employees based on disability.

3. True or False. A medical coder is asked to move her desk to another office, but because of a back problem she is unable to. Her manager cites this as a reason she did not get a raise in her yearly review. This is a violation of the ADA.

4. True or False. A laboratory technician, who was hired 6 months ago, wants to take 2 weeks of unpaid leave because his wife just had a baby. His employer denies the request, but offers 2 long weekends with 3 working days in between. This is a violation of the FMLA.

5. True or False. Title VII of the Civil Rights Act established the federal minimum wage.

● CASE STUDY

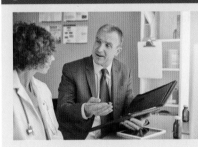

Dr. Smith calls Molly into his office and asks her about how the implementation of the new EHR software is going. "Have you or the team had any challenges? Do we need to make some changes or improvements?" In this way, Dr. Smith focuses on the project task, rather than on Molly's weaknesses. Molly responds that she has been really stressed about it and is glad that Dr. Smith asked about it. By the end of the conversation, Dr. Smith and Molly mutually agreed that it would be helpful to the team to get additional training on the system. Dr. Smith also decided to schedule weekly team meetings with Molly and Bob to collaborate on any other challenges that may require further training.

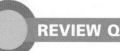

REVIEW QUESTIONS

1. Why is human resources increasingly important in the health care industry?

2. What are the benefits of internal recruitment, and what are the disadvantages? What are the benefits and disadvantages of external recruitment methods?

3. Outline the key steps in the hiring process.

4. What is the difference between training and development?

5. Why is diversity training important?

6. What is the purpose of the performance review process?

7. In most states, employment is at-will, meaning that an employer can terminate an employee at any time for any reason. If that is the case, what stops an employer from firing a person who performs well and has no disciplinary problems?

8. How can health care organizations improve and manage employee retention?

9. What are the two types of sexual harassment prohibited by the Civil Rights Act of 1964?

10. How do the Family Medical Leave Act (FMLA) and the National Defense Authorization Act of 2008 (NDAA) protect families and military personnel, respectively?

CHAPTER 17

LEADERSHIP, MOTIVATION AND CONFLICT MANAGEMENT

Carol Colvin

CHAPTER OUTLINE

INTRODUCTION
FUNCTIONS OF MANAGEMENT
  Planning
    Policies and Procedures
  Organizing
  Leading
  Controlling

MOTIVATION
  Internal and External Motivation
CONFLICT MANAGEMENT
  The Value of Conflict
    Communication

Thinking Win-Win
Role of the Health Services
  Administrator

VOCABULARY

chain of command
emotional intelligence (EI)
empathy
facilitator
goal

mission statement
motivation
objective
policy
procedure

productivity
span of control
strategic planning
stretch goal
unity of command

CHAPTER OBJECTIVES

After completing this chapter, the student should be able to do the following:

1. List and explain the four functions of management.
2. Discuss the motivation of employees.
3. Discuss strategies for managing conflict in the workplace.

INTRODUCTION

So far in this textbook, we have learned about the operations and the many processes of a health care organization. We have also discussed the multifaceted role of the health services administrator in the oversight of these operations—from supervising office workflow and documentation, to managing supplies, to budgeting, quality assurance, and compliance. This chapter examines aspects of leadership and organizational management in health services administration, including strategies for motivation and conflict resolution. Specifically, two aspects will be discussed—management and leadership—and their importance in the health services administrator's role.

The *management* function in health services administration focuses on the execution and implementation of the day-to-day tasks and processes of the health care organization, such as planning, organizing, leading, and controlling. It also includes decision making, managing changes, and communication. In contrast, a health services administrator's *leadership* is what inspires others to perform, facilitates change, and guides the organization toward its long-term goals and vision. Peter Drucker, an educator, author, and management theorist, summed up the difference as: "Management is doing things right; leadership is doing the right things."

CASE STUDY

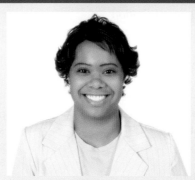

Fifth Street Medical is a local walk-in clinic that has suffered from a high rate of employee turnover. Although its patient load increased by 45% over the past three years, profits have been low due to reduced margins from employee turnover and the costs associated with hiring and training new employees. Additionally, the increase in patients and having to train new employees have resulted in an increased workload on current employees, resulting in increased office tension, staff exhaustion, and low morale. Fifth Street Medical has turned to Nicole, who is a consultant in health services administration, to address these issues.

During her first visit, Nicole observes the clinic for a few hours, taking notes of the daily workflow. She meets the office manager, Ms. Johnson, and a few other members of the team, including the front office staff, the medical assistants, and the nurse practitioner, Ms. Simpson. The medical assistant staff seems to be an area of concern, as most of them have been with the clinic for less than 6 months. There are currently 7 staff members in this area, but more than 15 people have transitioned through these roles in the past year.

After speaking with most of the staff members, Nicole briefly meets with Dr. Bamford, who joined the practice just a few years ago. Dr. Bamford's professional reputation and medical expertise were main factors in the increase in patient load. She is genuinely glad to be serving the community and makes an effort to speak to each patient who comes in rather than delegating all patient consultation to Ms. Simpson, the nurse practitioner. She expresses concern with the high employee turnover rate, but has little insight as to what might be the causes other than the high patient traffic in the office and the increased workload, which may be a little overwhelming at times. Dr. Bamford encouraged Nicole to spend time with Ms. Simpson who really "runs the place."

Ms. Simpson does seem to control the office, and, after speaking with her, Nicole understands the root of the employee turnover problem. Before Dr. Bamford was hired, most patients saw Ms. Simpson, with few ever seeing the physician on staff. When asked what she considers to be the cause in staffing turnover, Ms. Simpson

CASE STUDY—cont'd

stated that there was confusion in the workload now. The staff did not know where to direct patients even though they were instructed by her that all patients needed to see her before being cleared to see Dr. Bamford. Later that day, Nicole observed a medical assistant explain to Ms. Simpson that a patient was growing angry because he had been waiting for more than an hour for Dr. Bamford.

Clearly, Fifth Street Medical is having challenges with conflict management and organization. As you read through the chapter, think about this situation. What can Nicole do to help reduce employee turnover and increase morale at the clinic?

FUNCTIONS OF MANAGEMENT

Organizational management generally addresses these main functions: *planning, organizing, leading,* and *controlling.* The health services administrator must possess or develop skills for these specific functions to be an effective manager.

Planning

The first function of management is planning, which is developing steps and actions to take that will accomplish the goals of the organization. Some planning is short term and requires only a few weeks or months to achieve its goals. In comparison, **strategic planning** is a long-term endeavor and sets goals for usually 5 years or more. Oftentimes, strategic planning is the responsibility of the organization's top executives, although the health services administrator may contribute to the plan. The health services administrator's role in strategic planning varies based on the size of the organization. In small medical offices and organizations, the health services administrator may be responsible for spearheading the strategic plan. Strategic planning in larger organizations is usually the responsibility of a committee that includes the board of directors and chief executives, with the health services administrator providing information and other data to assist the committee in making decisions.

> **Strategic planning** The executive function of setting long-term goals for an organization and developing steps to achieve those goals.

In most organizations, strategic planning begins with the creation of a **mission statement**, which is a written declaration of the organization's purpose and values. Often, the mission statement reflects a company's *culture*, which guides the behavior of its employees. For example, a mission statement for a diagnostic imaging center might be:

> **Mission statement** A written declaration of the organization's purpose and values.

To become the largest and most respected medical imaging provider in the region by consistently demonstrating quality, compassion, and accessible care using the most advanced technology.

Using this mission statement as a guide, the company's strategic plan to grow in size may include moving into a larger office space, merging with another imaging provider, or beginning a joint venture with another organization. It might also include investing in a new marketing campaign or offering a new service.

An organization's **goals** are its statements of general purpose and of desired outcomes. There are two main types of organizational goals: *official* and *operative.* An organization's official goals are often communicated in the organization's mission statement and are often qualitative in nature, meaning they are subjective and harder to measure. In the example earlier with the diagnostic imaging center, the official organizational goal is its mission statement.

> **Goal** A statement of general purpose and desired outcome.

An organization's operative goals are often detailed in its strategic plan and describe the actions the organization will take to achieve its purpose. Compared with official goals, operative goals are more quantitative or measurable and based on metrics. For example, one of the operative goals for the diagnostic imaging center may be: "To grow patient cases by 14% by this time next year by expanding new services."

Goals provide the organization or individual departments with a focus to achieve a task or action, often within an allotted period. For example, the health services administrator may be given an operative goal to increase revenue by 5% by the end of the year and to reduce the claims rejection rate to less than 10% in the next 3 months. The health services administrator would then develop specific business processes or an action plan on how he or she would meet these goals.

In setting and communicating goals, it is necessary that goals be realistic and concise. Setting **stretch goals**—those beyond current capabilities—should be done carefully, as failure to meet goals may lead to employee dissatisfaction and low morale, which in turn may decrease productivity. Employee skill and ability level should be congruent with the set goals to ensure that they are attainable. It is also important to provide feedback as the employee moves toward the goal. Feedback allows for adjustments to be made as necessary to the course of action and will allow for quick detection if a goal is out of reach or the deadline needs to be modified.

Objectives are individual, defined, and measurable actions to achieve short- or medium-term goals. Objectives are necessary to support the strategic plan, which ultimately aims to meet the organization's mission. Some examples of objectives are:

- "Keep patient wait times to an average of 30 minutes or less."
- "Respond to any inquiries from the patient portal within 24 hours."
- "Review patient survey results at the staff meeting each Monday."

Goals and objectives provide employees specific targets and activities, with every task designed to achieve the organization's mission. The health services administrator formulates these activities through *operational planning,* which links the strategic plan with the activities the employees will deliver and the resources required to deliver them. Specifically, the operational planning process details the "who, what, when, and how" of the daily operations. It defines how human, financial, and physical resources will be allocated to achieve short-term goals that support the organization's objectives.

Policies and Procedures

Central to operational planning are policies and procedures that guide the day-to-day business behaviors of the organization's staff. A **policy** is a statement that guides decision making in the health care organization. Many policies in the health care organization will relate to human resources, such as the employee dress code, break periods, sick leave, absence, tardiness, and conduct. Other policies may speak to employee use of supplies and equipment, computers, the Internet, and social media. Policies may have broader implications and may address the organization's operations, such as the protection of patient confidentiality and maintaining sanitary work spaces.

A **procedure** is a description of the way tasks are to be completed or the way in which a policy is carried out. A procedure typically specifies:

- The person responsible for performing an action
- When the action should be performed
- How the action is to be performed

Oftentimes, a step-by-step procedure is written to support each of the organization's policies. An example of a policy and procedures for a medical office is provided in Fig. 17.1.

Organizing

The second function of management is organizing. Organizing is about allocating and coordinating the organization's human resources, specifically employees and their time,

---

Stretch goal A goal beyond what is currently possible.

Objective An individual, defined, and measurable statement of an action that will achieve short- or medium-term goals.

Policy A statement that guides decision-making.

Procedure A description of the way tasks are to be completed or the way in which a policy is carried out.

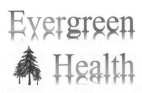

Policy No. 4.02

Security and Confidentiality

Effective: 01/30/2016

Reviewed: 01/2018

Approved by: Jim Smalls, Heath Care Administrator

Policy:
Evergreen Health will verify the identity of all patients before seeing the provider.

Procedure:
1. Upon presenting to the facility, patients will be directed to the check-in kiosk.

2. The front-desk receptionist will request the patient's insurance card and photo identification.

3. The receptionist will verify the patient's information and compare the individual to the patient image in the EHR.

4. The patient will be asked to provide his or her date of birth.

Figure 17.1 Sample policy and procedure in a medical office.

to accomplish certain functions and to ensure activities and tasks are completed. The coordination of tasks and activities is designed to ensure a smooth workflow and that they are done in a logical order to maximize productivity. **Productivity** is the measure of efficiency of work, or the rate at which work is produced balanced with the time and resources spent. Time management is also an important part of a health services administrator's organization function. Box 17.1 discusses time management in more detail.

Organizing is also managing who does what. Which staff member should send referrals to other providers? Who is responsible for collecting and opening the mail, distributing new inventory, or fulfilling patient requests for medical records? In addition to assigning tasks, organizing means deciding who reports to whom. Should the medical assistants report to the nurse or the health services administrator? Referring back to the organizational chart in Fig. 2.7, notice how each position is organized and the lines of authority and responsibility. According to the organizational chart, both the medical assistant and licensed practical nurse should report directly to the registered nurse, who reports directly to the health services administrator. This is called **unity of command**, meaning that these positions report to only one person.

In comparison, **span of control** is a term that approaches organization from the opposite direction, referring to the number of employees or departments that report to an individual. In the organizational chart, the registered nurse's scope of authority includes the medical assistants and the licensed practical nurses. However, the health services administrator's scope of authority is broader because it includes all five departments listed below that position. The organizational chart also explains the **chain of command** in the organization, with those at the top of the chart having the most authority and decision-making power. Deciding how the work is distributed and delegated is all part of the function of organizational management.

Productivity The measure of efficiency of work, or the rate at which work is produced balanced with the time and resources spent.

Unity of command The quality of a position reporting to only one supervisor.

span of control the number of employees or departments that report to an individual.

chain of command the authority of an individual within an organization.

Leading

The management function of leading consists of staffing, scheduling employees to work at certain times, delegating tasks, motivating employees, and providing constructive

BOX 17.1   TIME MANAGEMENT

As a health services administrator, you are responsible for managing that most important resource: the physician's time. With time management, planning and prioritizing are key. The main goal is to allocate time to the most important activities for that day. One way to start improving time management is to keep a time log. For one day, you will need to write down what you have done in 15-minute time periods. Once you see how you have spent your time on paper, you may be convinced of the need for time management techniques and tools to help prioritize.

One of the first strategies in time management is to organize your day's tasks and activities. It could be as simple as a notebook or a digital assistant, which may be synced to your smartphone so that you can access your schedule when not close to a computer or out of the office. Another strategy that may be used as a supplement is using a whiteboard calendar that can be color coded and serve as a reminder of when and what you need to do.

Look at your recurring activities—meetings, bill paying, ordering supplies, and quality assurance audits—and place them in a monthly grid that shows those time slots as blocked out or unavailable. Although your workdays will most likely be 8 hours, consider your own work patterns and habits. Are you most aware in the morning or the afternoon? Schedule your most difficult activities, such as personnel reviews and staff meetings, for the times when you are the sharpest. Specific times should be allocated to checking and answer emails, texts, and voicemails because this can be an enormous drain of time.

Another important strategy is to delegate tasks. As your staff learns to handle some of the more routine tasks, you will then be able to focus on tasks that may be unexpected, complex, or require your immediate attention.

Last but not least, plan for the unexpected. Just as scheduling patient appointments must allow for the occasional walk-in, you need to be prepared for the unexpected interruption that may demand immediate attention. Although some activities may not suffer for being delayed a day or two, your schedule will likely have you doubling up on tasks and rushing to finish when you do finally have time. Try to make your schedule flexible each day or week to include a "flex-time" slot for those unforeseen activities.

Created by Betsy J. Shiland

feedback. In addition, part of leading is the mentoring, training, and developing of employees, which prepares them for success in their current job and potentially for career advancement. When there is effective leadership, it inspires others to maintain productivity and keeps employees focused on assigned tasks.

The next section of this chapter discusses motivation and conflict management, each of which are central to effective leadership. Box 17.2 contains a list of leadership behaviors all successful managers need to display.

Controlling

Controlling refers to the process of monitoring the performance and operations of the organization to ensure desired results. It helps ensure that objectives and accomplishments are consistent with one another throughout an organization. It also helps maintain compliance with essential organizational rules and policies. How are the employees performing? What is the quality of the work being done? Are objectives being met? Is the organization working toward the goals set in the planning function?

The function of controlling is how a manager knows what is working and what is not, and what changes need to be made to achieve the goals, objectives, and mission of the organization. Organizational control typically involves four steps: (1) establish standards; (2) measure performance; (3) compare performance to standards; and (4) take corrective action as needed. Standards can be developed from policies and procedures, the objectives and goals, or action plan. An action plan, for example, should have a method to measure that objectives have been met and performance has improved. This can be done by collecting data and information for tracking daily operations and overall organizational performance, including progress related to strategic objectives and action plans. If goals and objectives are not being met, what changes must be made to the action plan to ensure success in the future? When used appropriately, organizational controls can lead to better performance by enabling the organization to execute its strategy more effectively.

BOX 17.2 — LEADERSHIP HABITS OF SUCCESSFUL MANAGERS

Set expectations. Employees who do not know what they are supposed to do or how to behave in specific situations will have a difficult time accomplishing objectives. It should be clear to each staff member what needs to be done, how it should be done, and by what time or date.

Provide regular feedback. Employees need to know when they have done well and when there is an opportunity for improvement. Praise and recognition are important motivational tools that let employees know their work is appreciated, and coaching is necessary when an employee misses the mark.

Delegate. Some managers are tempted to take on tasks themselves because they think they can do the job best or want to ensure it is done correctly. However, delegating and assigning work tasks to staff are crucial for productivity and efficiency for several reasons. First, the manager is a busy person with many different responsibilities, and there simply are not enough hours in the day for him or her to do every task in the workplace. Second, delegating a work assignment to employees *empowers* them to do the job and to do it well. It communicates to employees that the manager trusts them and has confidence in their abilities. Delegation grants to the employee a sense of ownership in that specific assignment and gives him or her a stake in the organization as a whole.

Remove obstacles. Managers must make sure that employees have a clear path to achieving their assignments. Do the employees have the resources they need to do their jobs in a timely manner? If the fax machine is continually malfunctioning and it is taking the administrative staff 30 minutes to send each referral, it is important to fix or replace the fax machine. Are staff doing any extra or unnecessary tasks that are taking up too much of their time? A good manager is always on the lookout for ways to streamline workflow to eliminate wasteful practices.

Be available and open. A good leader has a strong presence in the workplace and makes himself or herself available to hear employee concerns. Listening to a problem can often lead to a solution that can make the health care organization a better place to work. Oftentimes, the best improvements to the operation come from the suggestions of the staff who perform those tasks on a daily basis.

Be exemplary. A good manager does not ask employees to behave any differently than he or she does. Show up on time, follow office policies, and act as you wish your employees to act.

LEARNING CHECKPOINT 17.1
Functions of Management

1. In most organizations, strategic planning begins with the creation of a(n) _____.

2. A statement that guides decision making is a(n) _____.

3. _____ means that the medical assistant reports only to the registered nurse.

MOTIVATION

As stated earlier, motivation is central to the leading function of management. **Motivation** is a process that evokes, guides, and sustains a behavior. Not only does it encourage the action or movement of an individual or group; motivation also determines the extent to which the response occurs and how long it persists.

Motivation can be compared with energy. When you need to move a stationary object, you must apply force, which requires energy. The amount of energy applied determines the movement or speed at which the reaction occurs. Movement will cease when energy is removed. It is the same with motivation. It is the energy that causes a reaction, determines the force of that action, guides the action, and causes it to continue.

motivation a process that evokes, guides, and sustains a behavior.

Regardless of the type of work environment, it is important to know how to motivate employees and colleagues. It would be difficult for a health care organization to operate efficiently and meet goals without being able to motivate its employees and maximize their potential. Motivated employees not only produce more work, they also produce a better quality of work. Put simply, motivation increases productivity, making it a critical factor in an organization's success.

Internal and External Motivation

In the workplace, motivation should be applied in a consistent and sustained manner and not only on occasions when an increase in production or performance is needed. When motivation is used as a trigger for an immediate reaction, employees may not consistently perform at a high level and may do so only when there is an immediate demand.

Sustained performance requires both external and internal motivators (Table 17.1). With external motivation, a person does something to receive a reward, like compensation or praise. External motivators include the office environment, such as cubicle space versus office space, money, employee benefits, and service discounts. These motivators can create spikes in productivity, but their effects usually decrease after a period of time. Internal motivation comes from within oneself wherein a person behaves in a certain way because it is enjoyable to them. For example, a medical coder tries to complete all her charts before lunch because she feels good about having a clean desk when she takes her break. Internal motivators elicit and control behaviors, which causes these behaviors to persist. These motivators originate in a culture that is responsive to the needs of the employees, such as one that sets achievable goals, offers a compensation structure that is merit or performance based, and improves employee satisfaction. Internal motivators sustain behavior.

However, both internal and external motivators must be present to encourage successful behavior and performance that continues for the long term. For example, external motivators, such as offering a retirement savings plan and a health insurance plan, will also contribute to intrinsic motivators, such as the feeling of job stability and security.

Additionally, employees are motivated by equity or the perception of fairness. The higher an employee's perception of equity, the more motivated the employee will be. This has an inverse relationship as well. The lower an employee's perception of equality in the workplace, the less productive he or she will be. If an employee feels that another colleague is getting higher pay for the same or less amount of work or more recognition or praise, he or she will feel dissatisfied. From a management perspective, if inequality exists, the scale can be balanced using subtle management techniques. For example, if an employee feels he is working harder than his colleagues and is not being recognized for it, and offering a raise is not a possibility, a simple thank you can make the employee feel appreciated.

TABLE 17.1	
EXTERNAL VS. INTERNAL MOTIVATORS	
External Motivators	**Internal Motivators**
Pay or compensation	Autonomy in daily work activities
Location of job	Growth potential
Cubicle vs. office space	Ability to help others
Extra employee benefits such as service discounts	Challenging tasks vs. repetitive tasks

CONFLICT MANAGEMENT

Conflict is an unavoidable part of almost any job and workplace. Conflicts in a health care setting can range from everyday disagreements to major controversies that can lead to litigation or, in rare cases, even violence in the workplace. They can arise between physicians, between physicians and staff, and between the staff and the patient or the patient's family. Whatever the nature of the conflicts, they almost invariably have an adverse effect on productivity, efficiency, and patient care and can lead to miscommunication, poor morale, and high rate of staff turnover.

Conflict is between opposing sides created by incompatible needs, drives, or interests, and it is inevitable when working with others. It is often the result of differences from varying perspectives. For example, a health care professional reacts to a situation or conflict based on his or her training and life experience. He or she may also manage daily situations from the standpoint of office policy or precedents set by previous situations. When employees face the same problems in different ways, conflict often results.

CURRENT TRENDS IN HEALTH CARE

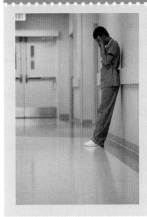

A 2015 study reported by *Marie Claire* stated that more than 85% of all nurses have been the victim of bullying in the workplace. This may reduce the quality of care and put patients at risk as personal agendas and vendettas interfere with job duties. Additionally, some nurses have quit their places of work, and sometimes the profession altogether. As a result, many nursing programs, such as American Sentinel, are realizing the importance of conflict resolution skills in professionals and are including them in their training and curriculum.

http://www.marieclaire.com/culture/news/a14211/mean-girls-of-the-er/

The Value of Conflict

In health care, as in any other industry, conflict can be valuable when managed properly. Despite being viewed as negative and something to be avoided at all costs, conflict can produce multiple positive outcomes in the workplace. Diverse attitudes and backgrounds can produce creative approaches to solve problems and reach goals in an organization. Additionally, conflict can often trigger critical thinking as a team effort to seek resolution. An effective health services administrator should be able to manage conflict in a way that produces positive outcomes and steers the team toward the goals that support the mission of the business.

If conflict is well managed, it can improve team effectiveness and cohesiveness. Meaningful conflict can also produce the following results:

- **Employee engagement.** Employees who feel free to disagree or offer different viewpoints are more likely to engage in workplace problem solving and discussions.
- **Increased understanding.** When a team learns to resolve conflict, it often helps them to better understand their goals, both individually and as a team.
- **Team focus.** Conflict focuses team members on the task at hand and allows them to stay zoned in and moving toward the goal.

- **Team cohesiveness.** Stronger relationships between employees can develop when honesty is promoted and divergent perspectives are respected.
- **Employee morale.** When employees feel free to speak in a professional manner, without fear of repercussions or retaliation, they are more likely to feel like a respected and valued part of a team.

Effectively managing conflict allows a team to identify problems and seek solutions. A team that learns to embrace conflict by respecting the ideas of others can increase efficiency, effectiveness, and employee satisfaction.

Communication

Conflict management in the health care industry is commonly associated with the management of information both before and after patient care takes place. Communication is vital in providing effective services to patients in an efficient and effective manner. When unresolved conflict exists in a health care setting, communication becomes the unfortunate victim, which has a direct effect on patient care, employee satisfaction, and customer loyalty.

When it comes to conflict, communication is both the cause and the resolution. Thus the health services administrator should take steps to address conflict and improve communication. For example, a common method is establishing a professional code of conduct that includes all health care providers and staff. Clearly written, established rules make it easier for all employees to follow rules and guidelines while taking personality out of the equation, which is often at the root of conflicts. The health services administrator should also include conflict management and resolution training as a part of the staff's continuing education.

With communication at the center of both conflict and conflict resolution, it is important to develop a business culture conducive to teamwork and collaboration. Being able to reduce the frequency and intensity of workplace conflicts and empower employees with skills to address conflict has multiple benefits to the health care organization, including:

- Employees who understand how to communicate internally are more likely to communicate effectively externally, leading to fewer customer complaints.
- Decreased employee turnover, which leads to decreased training costs. Additionally, long-term employees tend to produce more work in shorter time frames with fewer errors compared with new employees.
- Increased patient loyalty, which means fewer marketing costs associated with recruiting new patients. Generally, it is cheaper to keep a customer than to attract a new customer.
- Lower rates of medical errors mean lowered costs in follow-up treatments, lowered costs of compensation to patients in cases where there are losses due to medical errors, and lowered administrative costs due to legal fees and marketing costs to repair market share and patient base.
- Creating breakthrough ideas. Allowing team members to work through conflict in a professional, respectful manner can lead to breakthrough ideas as everyone works toward a common goal through honest feedback without fear of negative repercussion. Conflict often produces ingenuity.

Thinking Win-Win

In his book *The 7 Habits of Highly Effective People*, Stephen Covey describes his fourth habit of effectiveness as "think win-win." This is based on a teamwork concept where both parties can win and dispels the myth that in order for one party to have a successful outcome, or win, the other party or parties must lose.

In most competitions, there can only be one winner. This way of thinking is referred to as the *scarcity mentality*. There is one pie, and each piece someone take means less for me. When conflict arises, the resolution is expected to have one winner and one or more losers. However, Covey proposed a paradigm shift where there did not have to be a loser, but everyone could win through collaboration and teamwork. Covey called this the *abundance mentality*, where the mind-set views life as a welding together of cooperative efforts in which outcomes can be mutually beneficial to all involved. In this way of thinking, there is an unlimited amount of pie. Everyone can have some because there is plenty to go around. When we view resources and talent as unlimited or unrestricted, we open up ourselves and our businesses to previously unrecognized potential. When conflict arises and we use the abundance mentality, a resolution can be found where all parties win.

Three characteristics will be exhibited when a business, including a health care organization, thinks with a win-win mentality:

1. **Integrity**. The business has a system of values and morals that it adheres to.
2. **Maturity**. The leaders and employees within the organization are able to express their ideas and feelings in a way that takes into consideration the ideas and feelings of others, but are able to do so with confidence.
3. **Abundance mentality**. There is a shared opinion within the organization that there is enough for everyone. Teamwork is more prevalent than competition.

To embody these characteristics in an organization, all managers, including the health services administrator, must be empathetic and confident at the same time. Effective leadership with a win-win mindset also requires the ability to articulate the benefit to all parties involved.

Take Learning to the Next Level

The key to thinking win-win is to understand needs before determining a solution. Consider the example of two friends, Susan and Jane, who both want the last orange. What is your suggestion?

Was it to split the orange in half?

This is the most common response when we think about compromise. But what if we started by looking at why each person needed the orange?

Susan wants to use the juice from the orange to make a smoothie, but it will require the entire orange. Jane, however, is making a cake that requires the rind of the entire orange to flavor the mix.

Now knowing their needs, does the solution change? If the orange had simply been split in half, both friends would have lost. However, knowing what the needs are of each friend, Jane took the orange peel and gave Susan the fruit. Both parties won.

Do you approach your friendships and relationships with a win-win mentality, always trying to understand the needs of the other individual? Think about situations in your life where you can implement this strategy.

Role of the Health Services Administrator

As a health care administrator, recognize that some staff members may be used to thinking in a certain way and may not be able to readily accept that there is an option for everyone to benefit from the outcome of a decision. Thus the manager needs to have the ability to point out and communicate how a problem or conflict is being resolved with everyone as a winner. This is extremely important when it comes to shifting the culture of your organization. Showing results that promote the interests of all and still manage to resolve conflicts can lead to changed employee perceptions and foster team building.

In Covey's development of the conflict resolution process of win-win, there are four steps that the health services administrator should take to achieve the optimal solution to a problem:

1. **Be empathetic**. Allow the other side to express its needs and concerns, and seek to understand the other's point of view.
2. **Identify the key issues and concerns involved**. In doing so, you must separate people from the problem.
3. **Define acceptable results**. What results are necessary for each side? What compromise can be reached? Although the solution will most likely not be what each party began hoping for, it is important to emphasize that the goal is to come to a resolution that will be mutually beneficial to all involved.
4. **Identify the option that will allow you to achieve those acceptable results that you have defined**.

As the health services administrator, you will most likely find yourself in the role of peacekeeper at some point because conflict is inevitable. In this role, the health services administrator functions as a **facilitator**, or someone who works with a group of people to help them understand their common goals and then to devise a plan to achieve them. The facilitator does not take sides, but acts as a neutral party whose role is to encourage understanding and engagement to bring about an outcome. This task is accomplished through coordinating and managing the communication between the parties. When communication lines are open, the flow of new ideas can develop that accomplish the goals of the group.

Management of conflict through facilitation requires that the health care administrator have a significant amount of **emotional intelligence (EI)**. EI refers to the ability of the manager to recognize his or her own emotions and the emotions of others, to control and differentiate between those emotions, and to act upon those emotions accordingly to solve problems or make decisions. EI is generally classified as having four quadrants (Fig. 17.2). These are:

- Social awareness: having empathy and situational and organizational awareness
- Self-awareness: being aware of one's own emotions, and being able to assess those emotions accurately and apply them to other situations

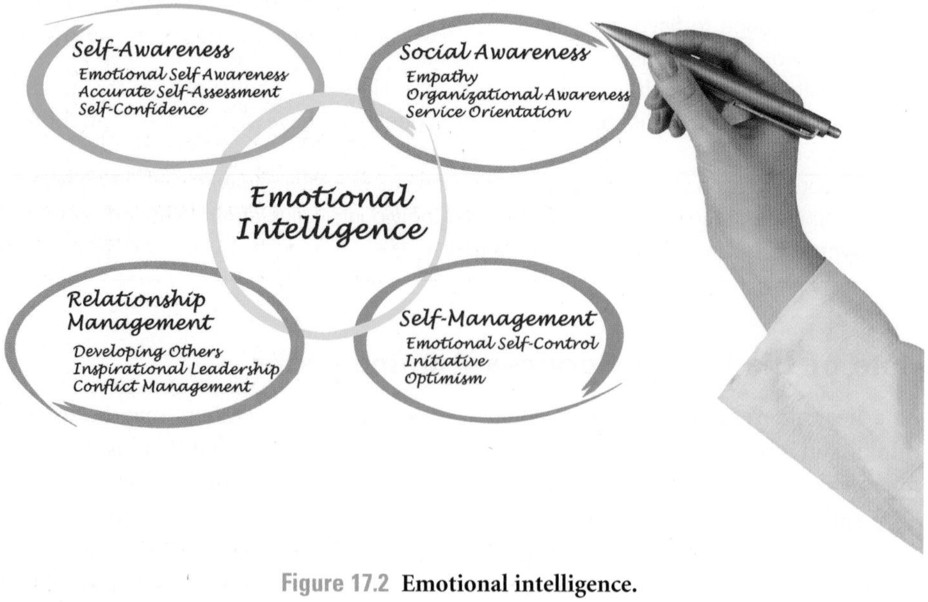

facilitator someone who works with a group of people to help them understand their common goals and then to devise a plan to achieve them.

emotional intelligence (EI) the ability of the manager to recognize his or her own emotions and the emotions of others, to control and differentiate between those emotions, and to act upon those emotions accordingly to solve problems or make decisions.

Figure 17.2 **Emotional intelligence.**

- Relationship management: being able to communicate with others and influence the emotions of others to encourage teamwork and collaboration
- Self-management: having behavioral self-control, resilience, personal agility, and stress management skills

EI is important because it allows a manager to effectively approach the conflict resolution process, taking into account the emotions involved among the parties concerned, and separate and focus those emotional components into finding a solution. Lack of EI in management can escalate conflict and cause further divide among the team members. Emotional decision making in the absence of EI can widen the communication gap between opposing opinions and can damage the self-esteem of the individuals and the cohesiveness of the team.

In addition to facilitating conflict resolution, there are "Three Golden Rules of Engagement" that should guide the manager's actions and address both the egos and the practical needs of both parties. The "Three Golden Rules of Engagement" are:

1. Practice empathy in listening and responding.
2. Keep all parties involved in the discussion by asking for opinions, ideas, and thoughts.
3. Establish and support self-esteem.[1]

In using these three rules, it is important to understand that if either party feels as if his or her needs are not taken into consideration or being respected, it will be difficult for the health services administrator to come to a solution where there is a "win" for both sides. Thus the first rule involves practicing **empathy**, or the ability to understand and share the feelings of others. If you listen for understanding and respond with understanding, each party will feel as if his or her individual needs are being acknowledged and considered in the resolution process. This sets the stage for the open communication needed for problem solving, which brings us to the second rule. It is vital that both sides are able to contribute to the discussion and share ideas so they are an integral part of the solution and have some ownership in the resolution. Both rule one and two support rule three, which establishes an environment where all parties are valued and considered necessary to goal achievement in a business. These three rules support and can be used with Covey's four-step process, discussed earlier, to help the health services administrator in conflict resolution.

> **empathy** the ability to understand and share the feelings of others.

---

[1]Steinbrecher, S. (2013, October 29) "Resolving conflict: six simple steps to keeping the peace." http://www.huffingtonpost.com/susan-steinbrecher/resolving-conflict-six-si_b_4171635.html.

▪ LEARNING CHECKPOINT 17.2
▪ Conflict Management

1. What does it mean when a team embraces a "win-win" strategy?

    a. They focus on common goals.
    b. They try to outdo previous successful outcomes.
    c. A winner does not mean there must be a loser.
    d. Everyone on the team thinks positively to achieve goals.

2. An individual who works with a group of people to help them understand their common goals is a:

    a. facilitator
    b. team player
    c. communicator
    d. resolver

Continued

LEARNING CHECKPOINT 17.2—cont'd
Conflict Management

3. Which defines emotional intelligence?

    a. The ability to understand and share the feelings of others
    b. The ability to recognize emotions in others and act on them to solve problems
    c. The ability to devise a plan to help people achieve common goals
    d. A shared opinion within the organization that there is enough for everyone

4. What are the four quadrants of emotional intelligence?

    a. Patience, negotiation skills, unbiased ideas, diversity
    b. Social awareness, self-awareness, relationship management, self-management
    c. Physiological needs, safety, belonging, self-actualization
    d. Head, heart, mind, hands

CASE STUDY

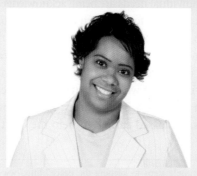

After observing the facility, Nicole recognized that much of the low morale and turnover may be attributed to interactions with Ms. Simpson and the medical staff. She scheduled a sit-down with Ms. Simpson to provide her feedback on her behavior and the way it is affecting the staff. Ms. Simpson said she felt the staff does not respect her expertise when they allow patients to see Dr. Bamford instead of her and expressed worry that her patient load would decrease if everyone is encouraged to see the physician instead of her. Ms. Simpson added that she knows what is best for the business because she is the only employee who has been working there since it opened. She does not think anyone else fully understands the needs of the community and how the clinic has grown over the past 15 years.

Nicole offered that patient wait times during heavy traffic flow can exceed 1 hour. If Dr. Bamford is available to see patients to reduce wait time, staff members do not feel that they should be restricted from utilizing her. Moreover, if Dr. Bamford is available when a patient specifically requests to see her, the patient should be allowed to do so without first having to be cleared by Ms. Simpson. Ms. Simpson agreed that these were reasonable rules that would help the clinic meet its objective to see patients in 30 minutes or less.

Nicole explained that communication often helps resolve conflicts in the workplace. She suggested that Ms. Simpson write up an official policy for the Policy and Procedures Manual so the staff have clear instructions for directing patients. She also recommended that Ms. Simpson provide staff with regular feedback in a formalized, documented process. This helps keep the lines of communication open and lets staff know what is expected of them. Lastly, she recommended that conflict resolution training be made a part of all new orientations.

1. What are the four functions of management, and how are they related?

2. How do internal and external motivators compare?

3. Conflict in the workplace can be positive if managed well. What does the text say is at the center of conflict and conflict resolution? Why do you think this is the case? How can this produce positive results?

PROJECT MANAGEMENT

Carol Colvin

CHAPTER OUTLINE

INTRODUCTION
PROJECTS
   The Project
      Manager

PROJECT MANAGEMENT LIFE
   CYCLE
   Initiation
   Planning

Execution
Monitoring and Controlling
Closing
METHODOLOGIES

VOCABULARY

agile methodology
critical path methodology
deliverable
project

project execution plan
project management
project manager
scope of work (SOW)

stakeholder
waterfall (traditional) methodology

CHAPTER OBJECTIVES

After completing this chapter, the student should be able to do the following:

1. Understand the characteristics of a project and the function of a project manager.
2. Outline the five phases of the project management life cycle.
3. Become familiar with various project management methodologies.

INTRODUCTION

A health care organization must not only meet patient medical needs, but it must also do so in a manner that is both cost and time efficient to generate enough profit to remain in business. Balancing customer expectations and needs with business factors, such as time and costs, can be a challenge. As a result, health care organizations must have a stable business model that supports the mission of the business, produces a profit, and is focused on customer needs and expectations.

Additionally, a health care organization must have in place regular operations and procedures that can adapt to changes to the business environment (such as new regulations or updates in technology) streamline processes, or reduce costs and expenditures. These changes to the business model or the business operation require a project and an individual to carry out the project. The health services administrator may be tasked with managing or leading this project and thus must be prepared to complete the project on time and within budget. This chapter will provide an overview on project management, which includes the initiating, planning, executing, controlling, and closing of projects to achieve specific goals.

CASE STUDY

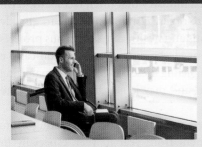

Stars Valley is in need of a community health care facility that can service walk-in patients. Currently, only two local physician's offices are located in the community of 30,000 people. Both physicians are no longer accepting new patients, leaving many of the residents without health care or having to drive to the neighboring town almost 30 minutes away. Adam has been hired by a franchise walk-in clinic to determine the staffing needs the new facility to be built and opened in the coming year. As the project manager, Adam begins by gathering some market data:

- Population of region: 30,201
- Estimated annual salary requirements for general practitioner medical doctors in the region: $210,000
- Estimated annual salary requirements for nurse practitioners in the region: $130,000
- Average time doctor or nurse practitioner spends with each patient: 20 minutes
- The franchise has an annual primary health care provider budget for the new facility of $700,000.
- The clinic will be open 12 hours each day, from 8 AM to 8 PM, 7 days a week.

As you read through this chapter, follow along with Adam in the project management process. What phase has he completed so far? What steps should he take next in preparation for the clinic?

PROJECTS

The initiatives or need to improve a business or its operation are called **projects**. Most projects are a one-time endeavor that produces a unique product, service, or process. For example, in a health care organization, these projects may be realigning of staff to reduce costs or adding a new wing to a facility. Projects also have definite deadlines and defined scope and resources.

Once a need has been identified, the project must be defined. When defining the project, the health care organization should outline what needs to be achieved by the

> **project** a temporary endeavor that produces a unique product, service, or process.

project. An unclear or undefined project is a recipe for disaster. Consider a health care organization that wants to improve customer service levels. Without a clear plan to increase customer service levels and what objectives are to be met, employees will not know what to do, what actions to take and may find it difficult to achieve the goal. Thus a project must have planned objectives and measurable outcomes, often requiring specific **deliverables**. This creates the ability to successfully track and monitor the project's completion.

Regardless of what the project is, it must be completed on time and on budget. To do this, the steps and processes in project management must be understood. **Project management** is the application of processes, methods, knowledge, skills, and experience utilized together to meet the project requirements. It is important to point out that a project may include several smaller projects underneath a larger project. For example, consider the case study in this chapter. Although the main project is staffing, it can be divided into smaller projects, such as determining state licensing requirements and staffing qualifications, processing the requisition, recruitment, hiring, and training. These smaller projects can be designated to other teams, managers, or departments, such as regulatory compliance, human resources, and facilities. Project management must occur to ensure that both the main and smaller projects and their objectives are defined and are successfully completed.

Being able to successfully manage a project is crucial in any business, including in health care. In fact, health care is a highly regulated industry that often faces long-term risks and financial consequences if the health care organization is not able to quickly and successfully comply with changes in regulations and health care laws. Thus projects involving process changes, information storage, or electronic communication can be urgent for a health care organization. Delays in completing these projects or mismanaging them can be costly, may result in noncompliance, and may jeopardize the health care organization's ability to do business.

For example, the health care industry has been showing trends of investing more resources and expenditures in project management from year to year, especially in health information technology (HIT) (Fig. 18.1). Widespread use and adoption of HIT within the health care industry will improve the quality of health care, prevent medical errors, increase administrative efficiencies, and decrease paperwork. In addition to these benefits, the Department of Health and Human Services enacted the Health Information Technology for Economic and Clinical Health Act in 2009 that required the adoption and use of HIT. Health care providers and organizations would be offered financial incentives for transitioning to an electronic health record (EHR) system by 2011, but would be levied penalties for failing to demonstrate such use by 2015. Although

deliverable the product or outcome of a project management development process.

project management the application of processes, methods, knowledge, skills, and experience packaged together to realize project objectives.

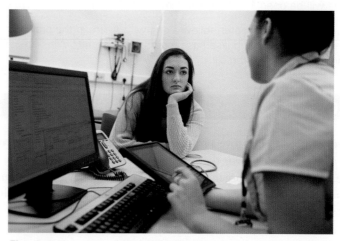

Figure 18.1 A nurse shows the patient her test results on a tablet.

implementing a full-featured EHR system proved to be a difficult transition for many health care organizations, the implementation process would not have been possible without project management support.

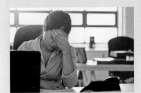
The Project Manager

In any project, the individual in charge of overseeing or managing the project from start to finish is the **project manager**. Project managers facilitate the project from the beginning phases of defining the goals and objectives to the end phases where it is determined if the project was successful or not. The project manager is the key strategic role in a project and holds the responsibility of planning, coordinating, and procuring resources as needed, executing the project plan within the designated time and budget constraints, and overseeing the implementation of the project into the regular business workflow.

> **project manager** a person who facilitates the project from beginning to end phases and coordinates all aspects in between.

In addition to the project manager, there are **stakeholders** of the business or organization. Stakeholders may be an individual, a group, or an organization that may affect and/or be affected by the decision, activity, or outcome of the project. They are often involved with defining the goals or purpose of the project. One of the most important activities a project manager needs to undertake is effectively engaging stakeholders. The project manager needs to communicate and work with stakeholders to meet their needs and expectations and address issues as they occur. All the project deliverables and outcomes can be undermined if there are areas of an organization with poor stakeholder commitment.

> **stakeholder** any individual with an interest in the business or project, including but not limited to business owners, investors, employees, and customers.

Stakeholders may be most involved at the start of the project and, as the project progresses, their involvement and influence begin to reduce. Regardless, it is important for the project manager to develop and maintain stakeholder engagement throughout the life cycle and phases of the project. For example, the project manager should notify stakeholders of any project updates and may be required to provide project reports and presentations.

Regardless of the industry or project, there are five important characteristics all successful project managers should embody (Fig. 18.2). Project managers should be:
- **Organized**. When managing a project of any size, the project manager needs to be organized. Every project has a multitude of details that a project manager must

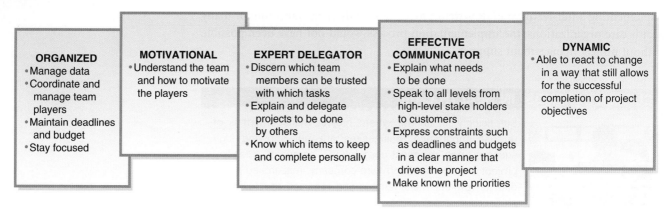

Figure 18.2 Characteristics of the project manager.

oversee, including team members, budgets, deadlines, resource planning, data collection and storage, and performance measurements. To be successful in each of these areas, there must be a designated process in which information is tracked, collected, and stored. Objectives should be clearly stated in a way that all stakeholders understand what the deliverables should be and when they should be accomplished.

- **Motivational.** A project manager must be able to motivate the team members. The ability to motivate employees to accomplish tasks and to achieve goals is a key factor in being able to manage deadlines and meet budgets. Within a team, multiple types of personalities and characteristics may exist. A good project manager should recognize this and be able to manage the different types of personalities in a way that challenges the team and encourages them to realize their full potential.

- **Knowledgeable about when to delegate or own.** Under most projects, there may be several smaller projects and most likely even more tasks. It is vital that a project manager know when to own a task and when to delegate. This is where many projects fail, when the project manager tries to do it all himself or herself. For example, a business may appoint a high-performing employee as the project manager. However, this may not always be the best decision because a highly proficient employee may not always be the best manager. The employee may be very successful in completing many tasks, but most likely will not be able to perform them all. It is not feasible for the project manager to complete each of the tasks within the project. An effective project manager must understand the skill sets of the team and be able to trust each team member to complete assigned tasks. Project managers who are unable to delegate will most likely find themselves missing deadlines, suffer from burnout, or see decreased team morale when team members are not allowed to use their skills to help move toward the goal.

- **Effective communicators.** A project manager must be able to communicate to the team the necessary tasks to be completed, the resources available to complete the tasks, and what the deadlines are. The project manager must also report the progress and any related data to all stakeholders throughout the project's lifespan. For example, it is the responsibility of the project manager to explain to stakeholders the reasons and rationale behind certain actions or decisions being made related to the project. This will require a full understanding of the project, as well being able to use technical speech and verbiage, depending on the needs of the stakeholder being addressed.

- **Dynamic.** A good project manager is dynamic, meaning that he or she can handle situations that are constantly changing. Adjustments to a project may be due to changes in resources, budget shortages, time overruns, or changes to deadlines from unexpected items or tasks. The project manager should be able to adapt to a changing situation and keep the team focused with positive attitudes to ensure completion of the project.

Take Learning to the Next Level······················

Now that we have looked at some of the major characteristics that contribute to the success of a project manager, consider your own project management skills. Are you organized? Do you communicate effectively? How well do you handle change?

Follow the link provided and take the project manager self-assessment. Do you think it is accurate? Do you agree or disagree with your rating?

https://www.mindtools.com/pages/article/newPPM_60.htm

LEARNING CHECKPOINT 18.1
Projects

1. True or False. Each project may encompass several smaller projects.

2. True or False. All projects are temporary.

3. True or False. People outside the organization can be stakeholders.

PROJECT MANAGEMENT LIFE CYCLE

As discussed earlier, every project has a defined beginning and ending. This is the project management life cycle, and it has five main phases (Fig. 18.3). The project begins with *initiation,* and then it goes through *planning*. Next, there is the *execution* of the project, the *monitoring and control,* and, finally, the end or *closing* of the project. We will discuss each individual phase for a better understanding.

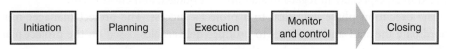

Initiation → Planning → Execution → Monitor and control → Closing

Figure 18.3 The project management life cycle.

Initiation

Projects begin or are initiated as a result of a variety of reasons or issues. Projects may be needed due to new business opportunities, technology, resources, or leadership. Or they may be the result of negative reviews, business losses, or compliance issues. Whatever the reason, projects begin as an idea that is intended to produce a positive outcome. In the initiation phase, the project begins with a proposed idea that addresses the issue, which is the objective(s). In this first phase, the following activities may take place:
- Present the need for the project.
- Conduct a feasibility study.
- Create a project proposal or project charter.
- Set up a project command center.

During the initiation phase, the scope of the project is expressed in written format, called the **scope of work (SOW)**. The SOW should contain any milestones, reports, deliverables, and end products that are expected to be provided by the performing party. The SOW should also contain a timeline for all deliverables. The SOW gives the project its necessary parameters and states what work will be done in association with the project to produce the project objectives or deliverables.

○ **scope of work (SOW)** a written document defining the parameters of a project and what work will be completed as part of the project.

Planning

After the initiation phase, the planning phase, also called the *design phase*, provides the road map for the project. In this phase, the project manager and the team work together to create a plan for execution, which would include allocating resources, developing timelines, and creating budgets. The plan should be clear and provide the appropriate amount of detail to guide the project manager and the team to completion. During the planning phase, the following activities may take place:

- Allocation of financial resources for budgetary reasons
- Designation of employee talent and labor, as well as other resources for project needs
- Definition of deliverables
- Schedule creation for project and deliverables
- Risk planning
- Planning for communication

project execution plan a written document that defines how the work will be accomplished for project completion.

The **project execution plan** is also developed in this phase and is the plan to achieve the project objectives. Whereas the SOW explains what work will be done during the project, the project execution plan explains how this work will be accomplished. The project execution plan sets out the strategy for managing the project and describes the policies, procedures, and priorities that will be adopted. It may also define strategies in relation to items outside of the SOW. The progress of the project should be routinely assessed against the project execution plan throughout the project's life cycle, and the project execution plan should be amended and developed as necessary.

Execution

During the execution phase, the project is officially underway and the plan is carried out. Sometimes referred to as the *construction phase,* the execution phase is the actual performing of the work planned and approved during planning phase. This phase is considered the "getting the work done" part of the project and typically is where the greatest amount of resources, especially in regard to staff and the budget, and effort occur.

The execution phase is critical to a project's success. The project manager must coordinate the staff and resources to produce deliverables based on the project plan. While the project manager works with the team to perform the work of the project as planned, the progress of the team must be continually monitored and controlled.

Monitoring and Controlling

This phase takes place at the same time as the execution phase. While the project plan is being carried out, the project manager must be able to monitor the plan's progress to determine if the project is on track and will meet the deadline. During this phase, the main activities of the project are tracked, reviewed, and revised at regular intervals to ensure the desired results are delivered. The monitor and control phase should take into consideration the risks that were identified in the planning phase.

The purpose of this process and phase is to determine and assess any risks to the project that may cause setbacks or failure and what steps and actions must be taken to minimize them. Any problems or issues should be addressed and resolved as they occur in this phase. In addition, the project manager must be dynamic and be able to adjust the plan or reallocate resources as necessary, or make any corrective actions to keep the project moving forward to ensure that the objectives defined during the initiation phase are met.

During this phase, the project manager must also be able to communicate effectively with the stakeholders to provide progress updates on the project, which may include any missed activity dates, adjustments in timelines and deadlines, and any tasks that need to be added to the plan. Thus it is important to continually monitor the plan to make sure that objectives are being met and are consistent with the project's budget and timelines.

Closing

The closing phase ends the project by confirming completion of project deliverables and communicating to the stakeholders the level of success in meeting the project's objectives. Success is determined in many ways, including completion of the work and that the deliverables have been accepted, as outlined in the initiation phase. This means the project is 100% completed. However, it is possible that a project was able to stay on track as far as budget and timelines but did not meet stakeholder expectations. It is also possible that the project accomplished the end objectives, satisfying the customer and stakeholders, but was not completed within the designated time frame or within budget.

Additionally, the project may be closed due to the project being canceled or suspended by the project's sponsor or stakeholder. If the project has been canceled or suspended, the project manager should document the reasons for cancellation or suspension and note if there are any plans to reactivate the project in the future.

Regardless, it is important for the project manager to confirm completion of the project, usually by completing a project closure report. This report should include if the project's objectives met the needs or goals determined in the initiation phase, recap the success and failures of the project, and note any work that will be required for future projects. Additionally, another best practice is to capture what lessons the project manager and the team learned from the project to allow for better planning in future projects.

■ LEARNING CHECKPOINT 18.2
■ Project Management Life Cycle

1. Which phase includes the development of the SOW?

   a. Initiation
   b. Planning
   c. Monitoring
   d. Closing

2. When is the project execution plan developed?

   a. Initiation
   b. Planning
   c. Monitoring
   d. Closing

3. Which stage takes place concurrently with execution?

   a. Initiation
   b. Planning
   c. Monitoring
   d. Closing

METHODOLOGIES

In project management, multiple methodologies provide a procedure or model for the project. Following are several of the most common types of project management methodologies currently being used.

The **waterfall (traditional) methodology** is one of the most common project management methodologies used across all industries, especially in health care (Fig. 18.4). The waterfall methodology is used when there is a need for thorough planning, in addition to controlled and predictable processes throughout the project. In this methodology, phases of the project are sequential. One deliverable is designed, produced or implemented, tested, and completed before the next step of the project begins. This offers stability to the project by making sure that each of the pieces is sound before moving on and stacking other plans and activities on top of a faulty foundation.

○ **waterfall (traditional) methodology** a project management method that is sequential and completes one phase, including designing, producing, testing, and adjusting, before moving to the next phase.

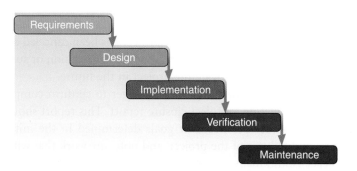

Figure 18.4 Waterfall model.

An example of when the waterfall model could have been used to more effectively execute a project is the launching of the healthcare.gov website in 2013. After passage of the Affordable Care Act, the Department of Health and Human Services planned to register millions of Americans for health care coverage on the federal government's website. In preparation for this, a large-scale software project was developed to manage the enrollment. However, due to a premature deadline set by stakeholders, who did not fully grasp the level of detail and time required to build a software program of that magnitude, no time was allotted to test each phase before moving on to the next phase. Instead, all website components were rolled out at the same time.

The federal government's goal was to enroll more than 39,000 people each day. However, due to the faulty software and other website glitches, only 6 people were able to sign up on day one, followed by 248 people on the second day.[2] In addition to the website and software issues, which forced the technical support team to fix all issues concurrently on the live date, unrealistic deadlines set during the planning phases compounded the project launch's failure, preventing the team from producing the required deliverables.

The **agile methodology** is used for projects that include short-term deliverables in an environment that requires a great deal of flexibility. The agile methodology is characterized by short sprints of productivity that produce deliverables in short intervals. Unlike more traditional methodologies, such as the waterfall method, where outcomes and deliverables are defined in the initiation phase, the agile methodology has no clearly

○ **agile methodology** a project management method that is characterized by extreme flexibility and short sprints of productivity with deliverables produced in short intervals.

[2]Larsen, M. (2013, November 4). "Is poor project management to blame for the launch of the Obamacare site?" http://www.projectmanagers.net/i/is-poor-project-management-to-blame-for-the-launch-of-the-obamacare-site/

defined deliverable at the beginning. Instead, although there is still a disciplined prioritization process, this type of methodology provides for flexibility and constant change, which is part of the process. The type of project that may be ideal for the agile methodology is often found in innovative areas where feedback from multiple stakeholders is key to the success of the project. It allows for quick adjustments and constant communication, which drives the end deliverable.

The **critical path methodology** is a project management methodology where each phase is interdependent. It allows for completion of projects on time by focusing on key tasks. For example, in the planning phase, all activities are laid out, including the time it will take to complete each step and the relationships between the activities. This helps determine if a project will be able to meet expected timelines and allows the project manager to determine which activities are critical to the progression of the project and to make adjustments when needed. By defining the length of time that it will take to complete each task, which tasks are critical to the project, and which tasks can be delayed without delaying the entire project, it is possible for the project manager to determine the path and time to completion and the earliest and latest times that each activity can start. The critical path methodology allows for predetermined flexibility between each task and increases the probability of completing the project on time.

○ **critical path methodology**
a project management method where each phase is interdependent and all activities are laid out, with critical and noncritical tasks determined in the planning phase. The length of time to complete each task and its relationship to the next task is defined in the planning phases and allows for the project manager to maintain control and keep the project on track.

○ CASE STUDY

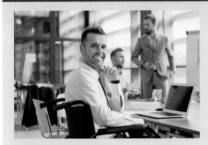

Adam, who is responsible for recommending the staffing model at a new Stars Valley walk-in clinic, is in the initiation phase. His project began with an idea for a business opportunity and he is now collecting information. Within the project, his deliverable would be detailed in the SOW—it should be a report listing a set of staff who will meet the needs of the new clinic. The SOW will also contain the timeline for his delivery. In the planning phase, Adam will decide whether he needs to hire others to help him complete these deliverables and will set up a timeline of what tasks need to be done and when. For example, to decide the staffing levels of the clinic, it would be helpful to know how long potential patients are willing to wait for services.

During the planning phase, Adam budgets time and money to conduct a survey of residents, asking what their maximum expected wait time might be at a walk-in clinic. He also asks for what kinds of services people in the area might come to the clinic.

In the execution phase Adam delivers his survey via a mailer. After several weeks the response is lower than planned—only 5% of those surveyed returned responses. In the monitor and control phase, Adam decides to extend the survey period for 3 weeks and issues a second set of mailers. He communicates with his stakeholders to inform them of the adjusted deadline.

After the extended survey period, Adam has enough responses to compile his results and perform statistical calculations. As a deliverable, he prepares the following information:

- Population of region being seen at other facilities within a 30-mile radius each day: 87
- Expected daily patient load upon opening: 100
- Survey responses from potential customers in the area suggested that the acceptable expected wait time to be treated at a community health care facility is 30 minutes.

Continued

● CASE STUDY—cont'd

- More than 95% of all patients who visit a community health care facility can be seen and treated by a nurse practitioner, with no need to see the residing physician.

When making his recommendations, Adam considers the cost of several combinations of practitioners. A nurse practitioner is the most efficient way to offer care, but must be supervised by a residing physician. Adam knows that one or even two physicians could not see 100 patients in one day when the average time spent with each patient is 20 minutes. At most, one provider could see three patients an hour, or about 24 patients in a 9-hour day with a short break. Adam does some math to find that he would need the coverage of four providers to handle a single day's patient load. Since physicians and practitioners cannot work 12 hours a day, 7 days a week, he will need a mix of full- and part-time providers. Two physicians can split duties to be on site during all operating hours, but that would use $420,000 of the proposed $700,000 budget, and the clinic will need at least three nurse practitioners every day. He concludes, therefore, that the franchise must plan to spend at least $940,000 each year to properly staff the clinic and recommends the stakeholders reexamine their budget using his findings at closing phase.

REVIEW QUESTIONS

1. Project management is important in any industry because projects are driven by a need for improvement. In the health care industry, what additional parameters must a project consider other than the traditional project management considerations of time, finances, and resources?

2. What are the top five characteristics of an effective project manager?

3. What are the five phases of the project management life cycle?

4. Explain the difference between the waterfall methodology of project management and the agile methodology.

ANSWER KEY

CHAPTER 1

Learning Checkpoint 1-1. What Is Health Services Administration?

1. Patient registration personnel are part of the <u>administrative</u> staff in a medical office.
2. Another name for a physician, physician's assistant, or nurse practitioner is a <u>provider</u>.
3. A <u>claim</u> is a statement of services sent to a health insurer for payment to the provider.

Learning Checkpoint 1-2. A Career in Health Services Administration

1. Health services administrators, medical billers, and medical coders are all types of <u>allied</u> health professionals.
2. To be <u>certified</u>, a candidate must complete an accredited educational program and pass an examination.
3. Which credential is offered by PAHCOM? <u>Certified Medical Manager (CMM)</u>

Review Questions

1. True or False: A health services administrator plans, coordinates, and supervises the operations for an entire facility.
   True.
2. List three duties of a health services administrator in a smaller facility.
   Answers will vary, but can include managing patient relations; assisting in billing, hiring, and training staff members; and managing inventory.
3. List three types of facilities that employ a health services administrator.
   Answers will vary, but should include physician's offices, urgent care centers, hospitals, clinics located within hospitals, retail care centers, surgery centers, imaging centers, nursing homes, and assisted living facilities.
4. What is the difference between a credential and a certification?
   Credentials are usually based on education and training earned from a university or agency and provide verification of knowledge in an area, whereas certifications are issued by a third-party agency and offer verification that a base-level understanding of a job or skill has been acquired.
5. List two professional credentials available to health services administrators.
   The American Academy of Professional Coders (AAPC) Certified Physician Practice Manager (CPPM) credential.
   The Professional Association of Healthcare Office Management (PAHCOM) Certified Medical Manager (CMM) credential.
6. Why is the health care field growing?
   Answers should include an aging US population, longer lifespans, and a new focus on preventative care.

CHAPTER 2

Learning Checkpoint 2-1. Health Care Professionals

1. What do the credentials DO stand for? <u>Doctor of Osteopathy</u>
2. Which member of the health care team creates the care plan? <u>The physician</u>
3. Which credential allows the nurse to deliver primary care? <u>Advance practice registered nurse (APRN)</u>
4. A PA and an APRN will have earned at least a(n) <u>master's</u> degree.
5. The abbreviation MA stands for which member of the health care team? <u>Medical assistant</u>
6. Medical billers and coders submit a(n) <u>claim</u> to the insurance company.
7. A(n) <u>radiographer</u> is an allied health professional who produces x-rays, computed tomography (CT) scans, magnetic resonance images (MRIs), and other types of anatomical images.

Learning Checkpoint 2-2. Ambulatory Care Settings

1. What do the initials PCP stand for? <u>Primary care provider</u> or <u>primary care physician</u>
2. A(n) <u>diagnostic</u> facility offers imaging studies like x-rays and MRIs.
3. A(n) <u>urgent care clinic</u> provides services for patients who need immediate medical care but whose injuries or illnesses are not serious enough to be seen in an emergency department.
4. A(n) <u>retail care clinic</u> offers care for mild ailments in a department store or drug store chain.

Review Questions

1. What is the difference between certification and licensing?

    The difference is that licenses are legal requirements, whereas certifications are not legally required for employment. However, some employers may prefer or even require certification.

2. What is a scope of practice?

    The scope of practice is defined as the types of procedures a health care professional is permitted to perform in accordance with their licensure.

3. How are physician assistants (PAs) and advance practice registered nurses (APRNs) similar to physicians? How are they different?

    PAs and APRNs are similar to physicians in that they may diagnose and treat patients, along with offering patient education and documentation of the treatment. They all prescribe medicine and deliver primary care. PAs and APRNs work under the supervision of a physician, who completes more schooling than the PA or APRN.

4. List three clinical roles of the medical assistant (MA) in the medical office.

    Answers will vary. Medical assistants take vital signs, record patient information, take patient history, administer medications and injections, and collect and prepare specimens for laboratory testing. They instruct patients about medications and special diets, authorize drug refills as directed, telephone prescriptions to a pharmacy, draw blood, prepare patients for x-rays, take electrocardiograms, remove sutures, and change dressings. They also facilitate communication between the patient and other health care professionals.

5. What do medical billers and coders do, and who offers their certification?

    Medical billers and coders perform the important task of translating patient medical information into numeric or alphanumeric codes to submit a claim to insurance companies for them to determine the appropriate charge for the patient visit. Through this process of billing, the medical biller and coder ensure that the health care provider and the medical facility are paid or reimbursed for the services they provided to the patient. The American Health Information Management Association (AHIMA) and the American Association of Professional Coders (AAPC) each offer multiple certifications.

6. Besides physicians nurses, and MAs, what other clinical health care professionals help deliver patient care? List three and briefly describe what they do.

   See Table 2.2.

7. What is the difference between ambulatory care and acute care?

   Ambulatory care patients are outpatients whose treatment is intended to occur in a single visit. In acute care, the patient is admitted to the facility as an inpatient and will stay overnight for at least one night. Costs are generally lower in ambulatory settings, in part because patients in acute care settings have a medical condition or source of trauma that requires immediate or around-the-clock care for a severe episode of illness or injury.

8. List and describe three different ambulatory care settings.

   See Table 2.3.

9. List and describe three different inpatient care settings.

   Answers may include the following:
   - *Hospital: provides medical services to the general population in the form of emergency care, critical care, intensive care, and various types of patient care requiring inpatient treatment.*
   - *Long-term care facility (LTC): provides care on an inpatient basis to patients who are chronically ill and need extended services or treatments from a few weeks to a few months.*
   - *Skilled nursing facility (SNF): a type of long-term care facility where medical professionals provide subacute care to patients, often to those who have been discharged from a hospital but still require medical care.*
   - *Intermediate care facility (ICF): provides long-term care most often to developmentally disabled patients who do not require the degree of medical care given at a hospital or subacute health care facility.*
   - *Assisted living facility: provides housing and support services, such as personal care, housekeeping, and coordinated recreational activities.*

10. Describe the function of hospice care. What services does it provide?

    Hospice care is medical care for terminally ill patients and their families. Treatment is palliative, aiming to provide relief from the symptoms of the illness and to relieve or reduce pain, and care for the emotional needs of the terminally ill patient and family.

CHAPTER 3

Learning Checkpoint 3-1. History of Health Care in the United States

1. In 1910 the <u>Flexner</u> Report critiqued the lack of standardization and quality control of medical education.

2. A premium is a fixed amount paid each month for an insurance policy.
   a. deductible
   b. reimbursement
   c. claim
   d. *premium*

3. <u>Medicaid</u> is an entitlement program created in 1965 to provide health care to the poor.
4. Which legislation changed CMS reimbursement to a prospective payment system?
   a. Consolidated Omnibus Reconciliation Act (COBRA)
   b. Emergency Medical Treatment and Active Labor Act (EMTALA)
   c. *Tax Equity and Fiscal Responsibility Act of 1982 (TEFRA)*
   d. Employee Retirement Income and Security Act (ERISA) of 1974
5. In what year did the Affordable Care Act (ACA) become law?
   a. 1910
   b. 1965
   c. 1973
   d. *2010*

Learning Checkpoint 3-2. Legal and Regulatory Oversight

1. The Centers for Medicare and Medicaid Services (CMS) is an agency under:
   a. *Department of Health and Human Services (DHHS)*
   b. Department of Health, Education, and Welfare (HEW)
   c. The Joint Commission
   d. The Professional Association of Health Care Office Managers (PAHCOM)
2. Whereas licensure is mandatory, <u>accreditation</u> is voluntary.
3. Which organization accredits hospice care organizations?
   a. Commission on Accreditation of Rehabilitation Facilities (CARF)
   b. *Community Health Accreditation Partner (CHAP)*
   c. The Compliance Team (TCT)
   d. The Joint Commission

Learning Checkpoint 3-3. Paying for Health Care

1. Regarding the insurance of a minor, the parent or legal guardian is responsible for payment and is the <u>guarantor</u>.
2. Anita's hospital bill was $7199.00, and she owed $720.00 after insurance. Her insurance policy stipulates that she pay a 10% <u>coinsurance</u> for hospitalization services.
3. A preferred provider organization is a type of <u>managed</u> care.
4. Under the Affordable Care Act (ACA), children can remain on their parent's insurance policies until the age of <u>26</u>.
5. Which component of Medicare helps pay for outpatient services?
   a. Part A
   b. *Part B*
   c. Part C
   d. Part D

Review Questions

1. How is the HMO model different from other types of insurance? What are the benefits to patients and insurers?

   The goal of HMOs was to decrease the cost of health care delivery through these lowered payments and preventive medical services, such as wellness screenings. Health care providers are not independent under an HMO, but instead work for a hospital or corporation. Additionally, health care providers are not paid for services rendered, but receive an overall payment based on diagnosis, creating a strong incentive to reduce costs. This allows insurers to offer policies to subscribers (patients) at lower rates.

2. What is the function of the Medicare Conditions of Participation (CoP)?

CoP are terms that a facility or provider must follow in order to receive reimbursement from the Centers for Medicare and Medicaid Services. These standards address the quality of providers, dictate certain policies and procedures for patient care and safety, and set requirements for facility administration and governance.

3. What is the difference between Medicare and Medicaid?

Although these are both entitlement programs, Medicare serves those aged 65 years and older, along with individuals who have certain chronic diseases. Medicaid is for the medically indigent, or those in poverty who cannot afford to pay for health care. Medicare is administered at the federal level, whereas Medicaid is run jointly at the national and state levels.

4. List and explain three reasons for rising health care costs.

Answers may include:

- *Lack of competition and inability or unwillingness to compare prices. Because care is almost always paid for by a third party, such as employers or the state or federal government, many people may not care to make cost-saving decisions or find the task too laborious. In addition, some patients may look at the price of services and assume that higher cost means higher quality—they would purposely avoid the lowest-priced care. These factors work together to eliminate the downward pressure on prices that would normally arise from comparing prices and choosing the lowest-cost service.*

- *Overtreatment. Because physicians are paid for each service provided, there is an incentive to perform a service even if it is not necessary. In addition, some health care providers practice defensive medicine, where the provider recommends or performs treatments and procedures not because he or she believes the patient requires it, but in order to safeguard against malpractice and litigation.*

- *The lack of coordination between providers may result in test duplication, medication mismanagement, and unnecessary treatments. Poor continuum of care may also result in complications for the patient and more hospital stays, resulting in even more cost.*

- *Advances in medicine have saved millions of lives, but the technology to treat many conditions costs money.*

- *Pharmaceutical companies will invest in specialty medicines and injectable drugs that are expensive to develop and costly when they reach the market.*

- *Health care fraud wastes tax dollars and drives up health care costs.*

CHAPTER 4

Learning Checkpoint 4-1. Workflow

1. Which type of scheduling allows walk-ins?
   a. wave scheduling
   b. modified wave scheduling
   c. *open access scheduling*
   d. cluster scheduling

2. The _____ is the primary reason for the patient's visit.
   a. workflow
   b. triage
   c. *chief complaint*
   d. SOAP note

3. Which happens first?
   a. *staff make a copy of the patient's insurance card*
   b. staff take the patient's vital signs
   c. the provider establishes a diagnosis
   d. the patient schedules a follow-up appointment
4. Submitting a claim to the patient's payer is part of the _____ process.
   a. check-in
   b. clinical assessment
   c. check-out
   d. *revenue cycle*

Learning Checkpoint 4-2. The Facility

Circle the correct answer.

T or *F*   1. The maintenance of the medical office is usually monitored by the property owner.
T or F   2. Vacuuming usually takes place at night when the office is closed.
T or F   3. Used needles are referred to as sharps.
T or F   4. The reception area, as well as the rest of the office, should be open enough to accommodate a wheelchair.

Review Questions

Match the term with its definition.

D	1. stream scheduling	A. a tabular map of the times each provider is available
F	2. buffer time	B. a graphic display of the steps in a process
A	3. scheduling matrix	C. a web-based tool that allows the medical office and its patients to communicate securely
B	4. workflow map	D. a method of assigning a set appointment time to each individual patient.
E	5. open access scheduling	E. a method that has no appointments at all and allows for patients to be seen as they arrive at the facility
C	6. patient portal	F. a section of the schedule that is open for walk-ins or patients who need to see the physician urgently
G	7. triage	G. a method of sorting patients by the urgency of their needs

8. Which parts of the facility must be regularly inspected or serviced?
   Answers will vary, but may include fire alarms, extinguishers, and sprinklers; equipment like exam tables and copy machines; the heating and cooling system; lights and light bulbs; the parking lot and landscaping.

CHAPTER 5

Learning Checkpoint 5-1. The Medical Record

1. The patient's name is a type of:
   a. *demographic data*
   b. legal data
   c. financial data
   d. clinical data

2. The group number on the patient's insurance card is a type of:
   a. demographic data
   b. legal data
   c. *financial data*
   d. clinical data
3. The operative report is a type of:
   a. demographic data
   b. legal data
   c. financial data
   d. *clinical data*
4. A(n) _____ specifies who will make medical decisions for the patient and under what type of circumstances.
   a. master patient index
   b. advance beneficiary notice (ABN)
   c. advance directive
   d. *medical proxy*
5. A(n) _____ details the types and limits of care in the event that a patient is unable to communicate his or her wishes.
   a. advance beneficiary notice (ABN)
   b. *advance directive*
   c. discharge summary
   d. informed consent

Learning Checkpoint 5-2. Uses of Documentation

1. The term <u>continuum of care</u> refers to a patient's medical care over time.
2. <u>Litigation</u> is the dispute of a matter in a court of law.
3. The term <u>incidence</u> refers to the number of new cases of a disease.

Review Questions

1. What are the four categories of information kept in medical documentation? What are examples of each type?
   See Table 5.1.
2. What is the statute of limitations for medical documentation in your state? Why do some states have different medical records retention requirements for minors as opposed to adults?
   The statute of limitations is often extended for minors to begin at the age of consent, usually 18 or 21. This is to legally protect individuals until they become adults. Otherwise, if a child was treated at age 5 and the statute of limitations was the same 6 years as it is for adults in that state, the patient's records could be discarded when the patient is age 11.
3. Besides medical records, what other types of documentation are kept by ambulatory facilities?
   These records include the master patient index, appointment schedules, maintenance records for the facility and any equipment owned or leased by the facility, financial records, and continuing medical education verification.
4. List three uses for medical documentation.
   Answers may include patient care, support of litigation, reimbursement, support of licensing and credentialing, administrative decision making, and research.

5. Why do health care professionals use codes to record information?

Codes allow health care professionals to communicate in a standardized, precise manner. They classify information into a distinct, specific, universal vocabulary describing the patient's condition and the treatment and services the patient received.

CHAPTER 6

Learning Checkpoint 6-1. Electronic Health Records

1. Which function of the EHR allows a provider to order an x-ray?
   a. the patient portal
   b. health information exchange (HIE)
   c. *computerized physician order entry (CPOE)*
   d. clinical decision support (CDS)
2. A structured path of decision making is called a(n) _____.
   a. *algorithm*
   b. contraindication
   c. audit trail
   d. patient portal
3. The directed exchange and the consumer-mediated exchange are each types of _____.
   a. EHRs
   b. medical records
   c. *HIEs*
   d. patient portals
4. Which is a function of the patient portal?
   a. e-prescribing
   b. ordering labs
   c. viewing the audit trail
   d. *viewing lab results*
5. A query-based exchange allows one provider to search the patient database of another.

Learning Checkpoint 6-2. Challenges and Incentives

1. Which program provided financial incentives for providers who use health information technologies?
   a. *meaningful use*
   b. HITECH
   c. ARRA
   d. Medicaid
2. The Office of the National Coordinator for Health Information Technology (ONC) was created under which president?
   a. Ronald Reagan
   b. William Jefferson Clinton
   c. *George W. Bush*
   d. Barack Obama
3. Which legislation was commonly known as the Recovery Act?
   a. *ARRA*
   b. HITECH
   c. HIPAA
   d. none of these

Review Questions

1. What are three features of an electronic health record (EHR)?
   See Box 6.1.
2. List three ways EHR technology improves the delivery of health care.
   Answers will vary. Students should note that health care professionals can view and update patient information in real time and that the patient's record can be viewed without regard to physical location. The accuracy of information collected is also improved. In addition, clinicians can be warned of contraindications and advised on treatment plans. The security of health information is also enhanced.
3. What is a health information exchange (HIE)?
   An HIE is a group of providers whose computer systems are networked to form a secure, accessible database of patient records.
4. What are the challenges and barriers to the implementation of EHRs?
   See Box 6.2.
5. Why did the federal government develop programs to hasten the implementation of EHRs?
   The benefits of a fully functional, secure, and interoperable EHR system has the potential to improve safety, quality, efficiency, and costs in the delivery of health care, but initial costs are a barrier to implementation. Much of federal government involvement comes in the form of financial incentives to offset those costs.
6. How is practice management software (PMS) different from the EHR?
   Whereas the EHR centers on patient clinical data, the PMS facilitates functions to keep the practice operating smoothly. PMS does store demographic and financial information for each patient treated by the office, but this is used for billing and scheduling purposes.

CHAPTER 7

Learning Checkpoint 7-1. Managing Inventory

1. The medical office runs out of diabetic test strips. This is called a(n) <u>stock-out.</u>
2. The clinic never wants to run out of hydrogen peroxide, so it sets a(n) <u>par level</u> of twelve 1-liter bottles.
3. *True* or False. Sterile gauze has an expiration date.
4. True or *False*. The amount of time an item may be stored before use is called shrinkage.

Learning Checkpoint 7-2. Ordering

1. The medical office relies on business relationships with <u>vendors</u> to provide the materials, equipment, and outsourced services that make it possible to conduct business.
2. A vendor can deliver human rabies immunoglobulin within 2 days of an order. Two days refers to:
   a. *lead time*
   b. shelf life
   c. expiration date
   d. par level
3. *True* or False. A purchase order lists the prices of the items ordered.

Review Questions

1. What are some ways the medical office manager knows how much of an item to order?

    To determine the amount of individual items needed, the medical office manager can generally use the recent history of the item. If the medical office begins to offer any new services, this may mean an increase in the supplies needed.

2. How is inventory tracked in a medical office?

    A common approach is to use a spreadsheet that lists all of the supplies needed in the health care facility, how many are on hand, and how many need to be ordered. Larger health care facilities may use automated software to keep track of supplies.

3. List some reasons employees may steal from the organization.

    Employees may steal because they have personal financial pressures, because they feel like they are treated unfairly, or just because the opportunity is present.

4. List three qualities to look for when selecting a vendor.

    Answers will vary. Managers should compare prices, of course, but also the vendor's lead time and return policies. It is also important to check reviews and references of the vendor and its products.

5. Why do medical offices use purchase order forms when ordering supplies?

    The completed PO offers both the medical office and the vendor a written document of the supplies being requested, the amounts, the price, and the person who authorized the order.

6. How does a bar code reader streamline inventory management?

    As supplies are delivered, staff scan the items with a bar code reader, which inputs the updated quantity into the system automatically. This allows staff to know exactly how much of the item the facility has on hand.

7. What are three goals when managing inventory?

    Reduce the amount of funds tied up in inventory, establish a relationship with vendors, ensure continuity of supply, and reduce real cost.

CHAPTER 8

Learning Checkpoint 8-1. Financial Statements

1. A resource owned by a company is an <u>asset</u>.
2. The decrease in value of a fixed asset over time is called <u>depreciation</u>.
3. What balance sheet item reflects money owed to the company? *Accounts receivable*
4. <u>Net</u> income is the income for the company after subtracting costs of goods sold, operating expenses, taxes, shareholder distributions, and other expenses.

Learning Checkpoint 8-2. Budgeting

1. The retail clinic pays $18 each month for a firm to remove, shred, and recycle its paper waste securely. In May, the cost per month will rise to $25. Is this a fixed cost or a variable cost?
2. A new all-in-one printer/copier/scanner/fax machine will cost $10,900, but it is expected to save $300 a month in staff time. What is the payback period for the item?
3. Henri's salary (including benefits) is $31,200, and he received a 3 on his performance review, meaning his work "Meets Expectations." He will receive a 3% raise in May. Dixon makes the same amount per year, but her score of 1, "Meets and Frequently Exceeds Expectations" will earn her a 5% raise. What is the payroll budget for these two employees for May?

Review Questions

1. What is the difference between long- and short-term liabilities?

   Short-term liabilities are due within 1 year; long term liabilities are due over a period of more than a year.

2. In a health care facility, more than one revenue stream may be reported. What is a revenue stream, and why do you think a medical office would report separate revenue streams? Give an example of a revenue stream that you might find in a medical office.

   A revenue stream is a source of income for a company that may be reported separately for tracking the profitability of that one product or service offering. Examples in health care include a pharmacy in a clinic, a weight loss offering within a medical office, and product offerings such as medical supplies at a doctor's office.

3. Which accounting method reports cash as it comes in?

   Cash basis accounting

4. Which type of income reports revenue after COGS?

   Gross income

5. What are some questions that a health services administrator should ask before making a capital expenditure?

   What are the immediate and long-term costs? How will income be affected? How will the balance sheet be affected? What is the payback period?

CHAPTER 9

Learning Checkpoint 9-1. Health Insurance Basics

1. The _____ is the person responsible for payment of health services.
   a. subscriber
   b. *guarantor*
   c. employer
   d. beneficiary

2. The charges for Moshe's magnetic resonance imaging (MRI) were $3199, and his policy stipulates a 10% coinsurance for this service. He has already met his deductible for the year. How much will Moshe have to pay out-of-pocket?

   $0, because he has met the deductible.

3. The processing of health information to obtain payment for health care services provided is called the _____.
   a. reimbursement cycle
   b. management of care
   c. billing cycle
   d. *revenue cycle*

4. Which feature of some health insurance policies was made illegal under the Affordable Care Act (ACA)?
   a. out-of-pocket maximums
   b. out-of-pocket minimums
   c. *lifetime maximums*
   d. lifetime minimums

5. Copayments and coinsurance are _____ for in-network providers than they are for out-of-network providers.
   a. higher
   b. *lower*

Learning Checkpoint 9-2. Reimbursement Methodologies

1. Which reimbursement methodology establishes the payment amount before the patient receives medical services?
   a. fee-for-service
   b. self-pay
   c. episode-of-care reimbursement
   d. *prospective payment system*

2. A _____ is the amount of money the provider submits on a claim.
   a. UCR rate
   b. fee schedule
   c. *charge*
   d. DRG

3. Which is a component of the resource-based relative value scale (RBRVS)?
   a. malpractice costs
   b. geographical price differences
   c. the cost of running the physician's practice
   d. *all of these*

4. Which system groups services into Ambulatory Payment Classifications (APCs)?
   a. ambulance fee schedule
   b. *outpatient prospective payment system (OPPS)*
   c. resource-based relative value scale (RBRVS)
   d. Home Health Prospective Payment System (HHPPS)

5. _____ is a flat-rate reimbursement that a health care provider receives per patient for providing medical care.
   a. fee-for-service
   b. *capitation*
   c. prospective payment
   d. UCR rate

Learning Checkpoint 9-3. Revenue Cycle Management

1. During the _____ process, administrative staff makes certain the patient's insurance is active.
   a. scheduling
   b. preauthorization
   c. *verification*
   d. coding

2. A _____ is a health care provider's request for reimbursement.
   a. *claim*
   b. appeal
   c. denial
   d. query

3. Which coding system is used solely for outpatient procedural health care claims?
   a. *CPT*
   b. HCPCS
   c. ICD-10-CM
   d. ICD-10-PCS

4. At the urgent care center, 910 of 1056 submitted claims are clean. What is the facility's clean claims rate?
   a. *86%*
   b. 13.8%
   c. 910
   d. 146

Review Questions

1. What features of health insurance plans attempt to share costs between the insurer and the subscriber?

   Policies generally have three different types of cost-sharing charges: a deductible, copayments, and coinsurance, although not all plans include each of these three types of cost sharing. Premiums paid by the subscriber are not a type of cost-sharing charge.

2. Differentiate between the OPPS and the RBRVS.

   The OPPS is the prospective payment system for hospital outpatient services for Medicare. Health care facilities are paid based on APCs, which are determined by HCPCS codes. The RBRVS is the prospective payment system for physician services. It is based on the relative value unit, geographic adjustment, and the conversion factor.

3. Explain why documentation is so important to the revenue cycle.

   The documentation must support the code assigned. Poor documentation can result in denials and lost revenue.

4. Explain when a query is appropriate.

   A query is appropriate when the documentation is incomplete, contradictory, or illogical.

5. Who should write a denial letter?

   It depends on the reason for the denial. If it is due to medical necessity or other clinical issue, then the physician should write it. If the denial is coding related, then the health information management professional can write it.

6. How do A/R days indicate the effectiveness of a medical office's revenue cycle?

   Shorter average A/R days (<2 weeks) mean that claims are being paid promptly and therefore that the claims submitted are relatively clean. If the average A/R days of the medical office's patients are several months or longer, it indicates there is a problem with claims submission.

CHAPTER 10

Learning Checkpoint 10-1. Quality.

1. Which of CMS's quality reporting measures came first?
   a. *Physician Quality Reporting System (PQRS)*
   b. Quality Payment Program (QPP)
   c. Merit-based Incentive Payment System (MIPS)
   d. Advanced Alternative Payment Model (APM)

2. Who administers the Healthcare Effectiveness Data and Information Set (HEDIS)?
   a. the Centers for Medicare and Medicaid Services
   b. *the National Committee for Quality Assurance (NCQA)*
   c. The Joint Commission
   d. the RAND Corporation

3. A TJC site survey is an example of an
   a. internal audit
   b. *external audit*

4. _____ charges are services and/or procedures that have been performed by the health care providers or organization but were never billed to the insurer and/or the patient.
   a. Unclaimed
   b. Undocumented
   c. *Unbilled*
   d. Retrospective

Learning Checkpoint 10-2. Performance Improvement

1. A(n) <u>sentinel event</u> is any unanticipated event in a health care setting resulting in death or serious physical or psychological injury to a patient or patients, not related to the natural course of the patient's illness.
2. The <u>lean</u> PI methodology focuses on removing wastefulness.
3. <u>Benchmarking</u> is a PI method used by the health care organization to compare performance of its processes with the same processes at another organization or with its own previous results.
4. A(n) <u>flowchart</u> is a data presentation tool that illustrates workflow.
5. A(n) <u>decision matrix</u> is used when the PI team must narrow its focus or choose among several categories or issues.

Learning Checkpoint 10-3. Risk Management and Disaster Management

1. True or *False*. The incident report is part of the patient's medical record.
2. *True* or False. The person in charge of risk management at the facility should also be on the safety committee.
3. *True* or False. All facilities must have a disaster plan in place regardless of facility size.
4. True or *False*. The risk manager executes the disaster plan in the event of an emergency.

Review Questions

1. How can each of the six domains of quality improve patient care in an ambulatory care facility? Give an example for each domain.
   Answers will vary:
   - *Safe care avoids injuries to patients. An example is assisting patients who have difficulty walking.*
   - *Effective care provides services based on scientific knowledge to all who could benefit and refrains from providing services to those not likely to benefit. For example, a practitioner refrains from prescribing antibiotics to patients with a cold or the flu because these infections are viral and the medication will not help them.*
   - *Patient-centered care is respectful of individual patient preferences, needs, and values and ensures that patient values guide all clinical decisions. Examples include acknowledging the patient's needs and working to meet them; some patients, for instance, prefer to see a practitioner of the same gender.*
   - *Timely care reduces waiting time for both those who receive and those who give care. Examples include answering the phone and patient portal messages promptly, reducing time in the waiting room and exam room, returning laboratory results quickly, and making sure providers are not waiting to see patients.*
   - *Efficient care avoids waste, including waste of equipment, supplies, ideas, and energy. For example, wasting supplies increases overall care costs.*
   - *Equitable care provides care that does not vary in quality because of personal characteristics such as gender, ethnicity, geographic location, and socioeconomic status. For example, health care professionals should treat every patient the same regardless of who they are, what they look like, and their ability to pay for services.*

2. At the retail clinic, you must reduce patient wait times. Using the PDCA method, what would you do in each step?
   Answers will vary, but students should follow the steps in Table 10.1.

Match the data presentation tool with its use/description.

3. __D__ Cause-and-effect (fishbone) chart
4. __F__ Line graph
5. __E__ Bar chart (or graph)
6. __A__ Pie chart
7. __G__ Control chart
8. __B__ Scatter diagram
9. __C__ Flowchart

A. Displays the percentage each variable contributes to the whole
B. Displays relationships between variables, shows trends
C. Displays the process, identifies stakeholders, shows hand-offs in workflow
D. Displays multiple root causes of a problem and opportunities for improvement
E. Compares categories of data during a single point in time
F. Shows data trends, usually over a period of time
G. Displays variation in data points over time. A process is flawed when data points regularly stray outside the control limits

10. How does the risk manager improve quality in the health care facility?
    The risk manager actively monitors PCEs, leads or is involved with the safety committee, and works to ensure a safe environment for patients and employees through training, education, and facility improvements.

11. Discuss the need for disaster management and the considerations in disaster planning.
    Health care facilities must develop and maintain a disaster plan and have a duty to protect patient records. The disaster plan names a chief or coordinator and lists the responsibilities of other individuals. It also dictates specific procedures in the event of a disaster and contains a list of community resources.

CHAPTER 11

Learning Checkpoint 11-1. Overview of the Law

1. Once the provider has accepted the patient, a(n) <u>implied</u> contract exists.
2. An intentional act of contact with another that causes harm or offends the individual being touched or injured is called <u>battery</u>.
3. Tort law is a type of <u>civil</u> law.
4. When a provider ceases a patient's medical care without proper notice, it is called <u>abandonment</u>.

Learning Checkpoint 11-2. Consent for Treatment

1. What is a guardian ad litem?
   a. an emancipated minor
   b. a grandparent
   c. a parent
   d. *a guardian appointed by the court*
2. If a provider treats a patient without consent, what is the crime?
   a. *battery*
   b. assault
   c. malfeasance
   d. malpractice

3. Who provides information to the patient about the procedure?
   a. the health services administrator
   b. the medical assistant
   c. patient access staff
   d. *the provider*

Learning Checkpoint 11-3. Medical Liability or Malpractice

1. The physician's assistant (PA) at the retail clinic failed to recognize signs that Carey had Lyme disease. Carey sued once the disease progressed, and the jury awarded $100,000 in <u>compensatory</u> damages to make up for lost wages.
2. The type of negligence committed by the PA is <u>nonfeasance</u>.
3. The discharge instructions state that the physician ordered the patient to report to an emergency department if she experienced shortness of breath. The patient committed <u>contributory</u> negligence.

Learning Checkpoint 11-4. Medical Professional Lawsuit

1. During which stage of trial is a deposition given?
   a. arbitration
   b. *discovery*
   c. mediation
   d. verdict
2. Which type of trial does not use a jury?
   a. bench trial
   b. mediation
   c. arbitration
   d. *all of these*
3. What order demands that medical records be brought to court?
   a. *subpoena duces tecum*
   b. interrogatory
   c. burden of proof
   d. all of these

Learning Checkpoint 11-5. Laws Affecting the Health Care Facility

1. Which set of laws protects disabled persons?
   a. *ADA*
   b. OSHA
   c. HITECH
   d. CLIA
2. Which physical findings may mean a patient is a victim of child abuse?
   a. scrape on knee
   b. bruise on the arm
   c. *bruise on the back*
   d. cut on the face
3. A(n) _____ makes health decisions for the patient if he or she is unable to do so.
   a. *health care proxy*
   b. provider
   c. adult child
   d. spouse

4. What information is found on a materials safety data sheet?
   a. *the physical properties of the hazardous substance*
   b. the radiation hazards at the facility
   c. the location of sharps containers
   d. all of these

Learning Checkpoint 11-6. Health Care Fraud and Abuse

1. The <u>Stark Law</u> was passed to control provider conflicts of interest and to prevent using patient referrals for the provider's personal financial gain.
2. The <u>Sunshine Act</u> shows relationships between physicians, hospitals, and manufacturers to help prevent inappropriate influence on research, education, and clinical decision making.
3. Filing duplicate claims for the same service is a violation of the <u>Federal False Claims</u> Act.

Review Questions

1. Compare criminal, civil, and contract law. What are their differences? Why is it important to understand their application in the health care environment?

   Criminal law governs violations of the law punishable as offenses against the state or the federal government. Such offenses involve the welfare and safety of the public as a whole rather than one individual. A health services administrator can be prosecuted for criminal acts such as assault and battery, fraud, and abuse. Criminal offenses are classified into three basic categories: misdemeanors, felonies, and treason. Civil law is concerned with acts that are not criminal in nature but involve relationships with other individuals, organizations, or government agencies. Many types of civil law exist to address numerous issues. The three that most directly affect the medical profession include tort law, contract law, and administrative law. A valid legal contract has four essential elements: mutual understanding and agreement on the intent of the contract; the contract must involve something that is legal; both parties must be legally competent; and consideration, such as an exchange of something valuable, must be involved.

2. What are the essential components of consent for treatment?

   A provider must have consent to treat a patient, even though this consent usually is implied by the patient's appearance at the facility for treatment. However, the health care employee should always ask the patient's permission to perform procedures. More complex procedures require the patient's informed consent. A provider who fails to secure consent could be charged with the crime of battery. A case for battery can be established if an individual is physically harmed or injured or if an illness occurs because of the contact. Battery may also occur if there is no physical harm but an act is considered offensive or insulting to the victim, such as touching a person without consent. If the patient refuses to consent to treatment—and the treatment is performed anyway—then the patient can sue for battery. Informed consent involves a full explanation of the plan for treatment, including the potential for complications and the possible risks or side effects.

3. Describe negligence and liability.

   Negligence is defined as the performance of an act that falls below the standards of behavior established by law or the failure to perform an act that a reasonable and prudent provider would do in a similar situation. Professional negligence in medicine falls into one of three general classifications: malfeasance, which is intentionally doing something either morally or legally wrong; misfeasance, meaning performing an act that is legal but not properly performed; and nonfeasance, which is a failure to perform an act that should have been performed. Negligence is proven if all four of the parts exist: duty; dereliction or failure to perform duty; direct cause, meaning that the provider was aware of potential risks but did not inform the patient; and damages can be collected if negligence is proven. Medical professional liability, commonly called medical malpractice, is governed by the law of torts. Medical malpractice occurs when a provider treats a patient in a way that does not meet the expected medical standard of care and because of this the patient suffers harm. The "medical standard of care" is considered the type and level of care that a reasonably competent health care professional—in the same field and with similar training—would have provided in the same situation.

4. What are the elements of a medical professional liability lawsuit?

A malpractice case begins with the gathering of information via interrogatories, which are a list of questions from each party to the other in the lawsuit. Next, a deposition is given, which is an oral testimony of a party or witness in a civil or criminal proceeding taken before trial. Depositions are a discovery tool. Discovery is the pretrial disclosure of pertinent facts or documents by one or both parties to a legal action or proceeding. The patient record is often part of discovery requests. A subpoena is a document issued by a court that requires a person to be present at a specific time and place to testify as a witness in a lawsuit, either in a court proceeding or in a deposition. A subpoena duces tecum is a court order to produce identified documents or records. In a criminal court, the government brings the case and is represented by a prosecutor. In civil court, the person or group bringing the case to court is called the plaintiff (or complainant in some court systems), and the opposite party is called the defendant or respondent. A judge presides over the case, giving instructions concerning the law to the jury, if a jury is present. If no jury is present, the judge decides the case; this is called a bench trial. In a criminal case the burden of proof is on the prosecution, which must prove guilt beyond any reasonable doubt. Reasonable doubt is defined as the level of certainty a juror must have to find a defendant guilty of a crime. Civil cases must be proven by a preponderance of the evidence.

5. Identify and explain a minimum of four laws that affect a health care facility.

Answers may include a description of:

- *The Consumer Bill of Rights and Responsibilities, more commonly known as the Patients' Bill of Rights, which outlines the relationship patients should have with their insurers, health plans, and care providers.*

- *The Americans with Disabilities Act (ADA) was signed into law with the intent of eliminating discrimination against individuals with disabilities. The act addressed many areas in which a person might experience discrimination, including telecommunications, housing, public transportation, air carrier access, voting accessibility, education, and rehabilitation.*

- *The Health Insurance Portability and Accountability Act (HIPAA) is a federal law that sets national standards for how health care plans, health care clearinghouses, and health care providers protect the privacy of a patient's health information. The law has two provisions: Title I (Insurance Reform) and Title II (Administration Simplification). HIPAA's primary purpose is to limit the administrative costs of health care, protect patient privacy, and prevent medical fraud and abuse in the Medicare and Medicaid systems.*

- *The Health Information Technology for Economic and Clinical Health Act (HITECH) promotes the adoption and meaningful use of health information technology. The law encourages providers and health care entities to comply with HIPAA regulations by enacting stiff penalties for noncompliance. According to this law, providers who do not adopt electronic health records in their practices will be penalized in Medicare payments. The HITECH Act also requires that patients be notified if there is a breach that exposes their personal health information (PHI).*

- *The provider is charged with safeguarding patient confidences within the constraints of the law, but according to state laws, which vary somewhat across the nation, certain disclosures must be made. Births and deaths must be reported. In some states, detailed information about stillbirths is required. Public health statutes also require compliance with wounds of violence reporting, including gunshot wounds, knife injuries, or poisonings. Any death from accidental, suspicious, or unexplained causes must also be reported. In some states, occupational diseases and injuries must be reported within specific time limits. Every state has its own list of reportable diseases.*

- *The Child Abuse Prevention and Treatment Act states that all threats to a child's physical and/or mental welfare must be reported. This means that every teacher, health care worker, and social worker—in fact, every citizen—who suspects that a child is being neglected or abused must report this to the proper authority. The agency must record the report, and after three similar reports the agency must investigate.*

- *Another legal issue is the possibility of elder abuse. Mistreatment of aging people occurs at all social, racial, and economic levels. The abuse may be physical, mental, sexual, material, or financial; it may involve neglect or failure to provide adequate care, or it may involve self-neglect when aging people are unable or refuse to care for themselves. Abuse of elders by their caregivers may be difficult to identify. The aging victim could feel embarrassed, guilty, or afraid to report the abuse.*

- *The Patient Self-Determination Act brought the term "advance directives" to the forefront of medical care. This act requires health care facilities to develop and maintain written procedures that ensure that all adult patients receive information about advance directives and medical durable powers of attorney. Advance directives are legal documents that allow individuals to make decisions about end-of-life care ahead of time. They are a way for patients to communicate their wishes to family, friends, and health care professionals so that there is no confusion about what type of care they would like to receive—or not receive—when they are terminal. Advance directives specify which treatments the patient wants if he or she is dying or permanently unconscious.*

- *The Stark Law was passed to control provider conflicts of interest and to prevent using patient referrals for financial gain. It was originally enacted to prevent providers from ordering unneeded clinical laboratory tests as a way of increasing profits but now covers an extensive list of testing and treatment facilities. However, providers can legally refer patients to testing facilities within a managed care organization.*

- *The False Claims Act (FCA) allows for recovery of money from anyone who knowingly submits a fraudulent claim for reimbursement of services to the government. Administrative specialists must be very careful when billing any governmental body (such as Medicare/Medicaid) for provider services because the claim doesn't have to be entirely fraudulent to violate the FCA. Any false statement or document that supports a false claim can be considered breaking the FCA rules.*

- *The Sunshine Act, or the Physician Payments Act, is designed to make available to the public data that shows the financial relationship between physicians; teaching hospitals; and manufacturers of drugs, medical devices, and biologics. Manufacturers must submit yearly reports to the Centers for Medicare and Medicaid Services (CMS) that itemize the payments and transfers of value made to health care providers. The purpose of the law is to make sure the public is aware of money and benefits given to providers for prescribing drugs and medical devices produced by sponsoring manufacturers.*

- *The Emergency Medical Treatment and Labor Act (EMTALA) was passed by Congress in 1986 to make sure that everyone has access to emergency services regardless of their ability to pay. Medicare/Medicaid-participating hospitals that offer emergency services must provide screening and treatment for all emergency medical conditions, including a woman in active labor, regardless of the individual's ability to pay. The admitting hospital must then stabilize the patient, and if the patient cannot be stabilized in that institution then he or she must be transferred to an appropriate institution for continued care.*

6. How can ethical behavior influence patient care?

   Ethics are the thoughts, judgments, and actions on issues that have implications of moral right and wrong. Ethics are different from legal issues mainly because something that is legal is not necessarily ethical. Ethics is considered a higher authority than legality. The American Medical Association's Council on Ethical and Judicial Affairs (CEJA) clarifies the relationship between law and ethics as follows: Ethical values and legal principles are usually closely related, but ethical obligations typically exceed legal duties. In some cases, the law mandates unethical conduct. In general, when health care professionals believe a law is unjust, they should work to change the law. In exceptional circumstances of unjust laws, ethical responsibilities should supersede legal obligations. Ethics and morals are more closely related, although ethics often are attributed to professional interactions, whereas morals and values are usually personal in nature. Health care professionals not only must have a strong knowledge base about ethical issues they might face throughout their careers; they also must come to terms with some of the deeply rooted value systems that have been a part of their lives since youth. To treat all persons ethically requires us to examine our own values, beliefs, and actions; you cannot treat all patients with care and respect until you first recognize and evaluate personal biases.

CHAPTER 12

Learning Checkpoint 12-1. Privacy Rule

1. What is a business associate?

   An entity that provides a service to a health care provider and uses PHI, which is therefore subject to HIPAA compliance.

2. Name five types of unique patient identifiers.

   Phone number, Social Security number, fax number, email address, driver's license number, relative information, account numbers, etc. A full list is in Box 12.1.

3. A covered entity must obtain an individual's written authorization for use of disclosure of protected health information in which scenario?

   a. A coder must review a patient's chart to code a recent hospital stay.

   b. *A consulting physician needs to access a patient's record to inform his or her opinion.*

   c. A hospital administrator needs to access patient data to create a report about how many patients were treated for diabetes in the last 6 months.

   d. None of the above.

Learning Checkpoint 12-2. Security Rule

1. A(n) <u>privacy officer</u> is an individual designated to enforce HIPAA compliance in the facility.

2. None of the patient access staff have access to the progress note section of the patient's medical record. This is an example of a(n) <u>administrative</u> safeguard.

3. The housekeeping staff does not have a key to the file room. This is an example of a(n) <u>physical</u> safeguard.

Review Questions

1. When HIPAA was introduced to Congress, one of its primary goals was to increase the availability of health care to Americans, especially those in transition or between jobs. Which section of the HIPAA regulation is meant to ensure that workers are safeguarded when transitioning between jobs when it comes to the availability of health care insurance?

   Portability guidelines safeguard the availability of health care insurance to workers in transition.

2. A superbill in the respiratory therapy center lists the patient's name and medical record number, and the CPT code is circled. Is this PHI?

   Yes, because the superbill contains both identifying information and health data.

3. Under the HIPAA Security Rule, what is the difference between physical and technical safeguards? Give examples of both.

   Physical safeguards refer to the physical security of information, whereas technical safeguards refer to the transmission, storage, or access to data through technology. An example of a physical safeguard is a locked cabinet located in a locked room with controlled access. An example of technical safeguarding is a thumb scan system to access electronic data.

4. What are the three tiers of HIPAA violations? Provide an example of each.

   Tier 1 – An accidental HIPAA violation. Example – A health care employee forgets to log off her computer and leaves patient information on the screen where it is visible to others.

   Tier 2 – The violation is done on purpose as a disregard of policies and procedures. Example – One employee uses another employee's password and accesses a patient's medical information even though it is not a part of the job responsibility.

   Tier 3 – This violation is done with malicious intent and with disregard of HIPAA standards. Example – Selling personal health information (PHI) to ambulance-chasing lawyers or to people running black market credit card scams.

CHAPTER 13

Learning Checkpoint 13-1. Compliance Program

1. *True* or False. The OIG recommends an anonymous program for the reporting of compliance violations.
2. The <u>Standards of Conduct</u> describe acceptable and unacceptable behavior.
3. The <u>compliance officer</u> is an individual whose role is to make sure the operations of an organization meet regulatory requirements.
4. An <u>action plan</u> is a formal document listing goals and the people and resources needed to reach it within a certain time frame.

Learning Checkpoint 13-2. Compliance Program

1. A provider sees and treats a patient for routine foot care, but bills Medicare for "nail avulsion," a more complicated and more expensive procedure. This is a violation of the
   a. *False Claims Act*
   b. Anti-Kickback Statute
   c. Stark Law
   d. Conditions of Participation

2. Oliver is an APRN at a retail care clinic and sees many patients who complain of having a sore throat. Generally he can treat his patients with over-the-counter or prescribed medicine, but occasionally he must refer his patients to an ear, nose, and throat (ENT) specialist (an otolaryngologist). He always sends his patients to Dr. Nickerson, who gives Oliver $50 for any new referrals. This is a violation of the:
   a. False Claims Act
   b. *Anti-Kickback Statute*
   c. Stark Law
   d. Conditions of Participation
3. Which action could result in a mandatory exclusion?
   a. Failure to provide quality care
   b. *Felony conviction related to health care fraud*
   c. Loss of a state license to practice
   d. Failure to repay health education loans

Review Questions

1. What is a compliance program, and why is it important?

   Answers will vary. A compliance program is a set of internal policies and procedures put into place to help the health care organization comply with laws, regulations, and industry-accepted best practices. The key is to understand that these rules enhance the operation of an organization, improve quality of care, and reduce overall costs. Ensuring compliance means better patient care and better business.

2. What is the role of the OIG in compliance?

   The OIG monitors the DHHS federal health care programs (such as Medicare and Medicaid) to protect these programs against fraud, abuse, and waste. Providers and health care organizations must be compliant with CMS rules and regulations in order to treat Medicare and Medicaid patients and receive reimbursement for those services, which make up more than one-third of all health care spending nationwide.

3. Who develops a compliance plan?

   Every health organization should designate a compliance officer and a compliance committee to develop, implement, and oversee the compliance program.

4. What are the potential consequences of compliance violations?

   Cases of noncompliance can be intentional or unintentional, but both may have damaging effects on a health care organization's business operation. The result of violations may lead to criminal, civil, and administrative discipline of individuals or organizations found guilty of any violation against federal law or health care statutes. A provider on the exclusion list may not treat any beneficiaries of federal programs.

5. Why is it important to self-report or self-disclose when noncompliance has been identified in a company? What happens if the company does not self-disclose?

   Voluntary disclosure to the appropriate regulating bodies can help mitigate the extent of damages, such as minimizing any financial penalties and/or preventing being on the OIG's exclusion list.

CHAPTER 14

Learning Checkpoint 14-1. Professionalism

1. Which aspect of professionalism is the focus of the patient-centered medical home model?
   a. Sensitivity
   b. Respect
   c. *Collaboration*
   d. Dependability

2. Why is dependability an important professional behavior?
   a. *It builds trust.*
   b. It safeguards patient privacy.
   c. It helps improve safety.
   d. It improves collaboration.

Learning Checkpoint 14-2. Effective Communication

1. A woman sees the physician in the parking lot and asks about how to care for her husband's cast. Why does the physician suggest they speak in the exam room?
   a. They may not be able to hear each other well.
   b. The location is not private.
   c. The woman may not understand the physician's body language.
   d. *a and b*
2. Because the practice is in a community with a large Hispanic population, the health services administrator, Sarah, makes sure she has a Spanish-speaking team member on staff during operating hours. This is an example of:
   a. nonverbal communication
   b. *cultural competency*
   c. communicating with a hard-to-reach population
   d. acting on a needs assessment
3. How can an organization reduce the number of billing calls?
   a. Insist that patients discuss the matter in person.
   b. *Provide an estimate before or when services are rendered.*
   c. Use a friendly tone.
   d. Refer the patient to their third-party payer.
4. Which is an example of nonverbal communication?
   a. Greeting the patient
   b. Asking the patient to "please hold"
   c. Discussing the weather
   d. *Smiling*
5. What is the last step before sending an email?
   a. Cc-ing or Bcc-ing
   b. *Proofreading*
   c. Closing
   d. Signature
6. Which type of communication is only used internally?
   a. *Memorandums (memos)*
   b. Business letters
   c. Emails
   d. Nonverbal communication

Review Questions

1. What is professionalism?
   Professionalism is defined as the skills, judgments, and behaviors that are expected in the workplace.
2. Why is effective communication especially critical in the health care industry?
   Answers will vary, but could include that better communication leads to better biological and functional health outcomes, increased patient satisfaction, greater patient safety, reduced patient anxiety, fewer medical errors and malpractice lawsuits, and increases in job satisfaction and overall quality of care. Being able to effectively communicate with patients, their families, and other health care professionals is critical because

unlike other fields, dysfunctional communication can harm people's lives. The inability to effectively communicate can lead to receiving inaccurate patient history (including medication history), which can lead to inappropriate therapeutic decisions. This contributes to patient confusion, disinterest, and possibly nonadherence to treatment regimens, whereas good communication can increase the likelihood of patients following medical recommendations, self-managing chronic conditions, and adopting preventive health behaviors.

3. Name two barriers to effective communication.

   Privacy concerns and time constraints can present challenges for effective communication. Patients are more likely to share important and personal health history details if they trust that the information is being kept confidential—thus improving overall communication. Another significant communication barrier for health care professionals is lack of time. Patients are often rushed when sharing their medical history or describing their symptoms and health care needs with health care professionals. Patients are less likely to offer additional information if they feel the health care professional doesn't have time to listen.

4. What are the communication challenges for special populations?

   Elderly patients often have more complex health care needs and may have hearing and vision problems. Patients in pain may not be able to concentrate on the information being shared and thus may need information repeated or in writing to refer to later. Health care professionals also need to demonstrate cultural sensitivity for individuals who do not understand or accept American cultural beliefs, including spiritual roles, use of medication and nutrition, how diseases are spread, and approaches to decision making. Lastly, certain populations may have unique attributes that make them hard to reach in terms of patient engagement and treatment adherence. This may include limited financial resources, transportation challenges, low literacy levels, low socioeconomic status, and inability to speak English. Health care professionals need to be aware of these differences and understand how to adjust their communication strategies accordingly.

5. What is verbal and nonverbal communication, and how are they different?

   Verbal communication is sharing information, thoughts, and feelings through speech. Nonverbal communication, on the other hand, is communication that occurs without language, such as body posture, gestures, facial expressions, gazes, eye contact, and tone of voice.

6. How are business letters and memorandums (memos) different?

   Business letters and memorandums (memos) are both forms of business writing with the intent to inform and make requests. However, there are several differences between letters and memos. Perhaps one of the most significant differences between a business letter and a memo is the audience. Business letters are written forms of communication for external parties, whereas memos are written for internal colleagues and staff. Memos are less formal and less structured than business letters and the tone is more conversational. Memos also include less background information than letters.

7. Name the seven parts of a business letter.

   A business letter includes the business's address, the date, the recipient's address, greeting, main body, closing, and signature.

8. What is typically included in a meeting agenda?

   A meeting agenda typically includes:
   * *Date and time of the meeting*
   * *Location of the meeting*
   * *List of meeting invitees and any materials they should bring*
   * *Topics to be discussed (old and new business)*
   * *List of any guest speakers*

- *Attachments (if there is background information that attendees need to read before the meeting)*

9. What is typically included in meeting minutes?

   Meeting minutes typically include:
   - *Who attended and participated in the meeting, as well as those who were absent*
   - *The date and time the meeting was called to order*
   - *Documentation that minutes from the previous meeting were approved and accepted, identifying any amendments made to those minutes*
   - *A summary record of issues that were discussed*
   - *A description of announcements and decisions that were made*
   - *The time the meeting adjourned*

CHAPTER 15

Learning Checkpoint 15-1. Marketing Needs of the Health Care Facility

1. The <u>cost–benefit</u> analysis weighs the benefits of attracting patients against the costs required.

2. What does the acronym SWOT stand for? *Strengths, weaknesses, opportunities, threats*

Learning Checkpoint 15-2. Marketing Tools

1. Which marketing tool is interactive?
   a. Internet review
   b. Social media
   c. Automated phone calls
   d. *a and b*

2. Which term is a list of all the links on a website?
   a. *Site map*
   b. Blog
   c. Marketing plan
   d. Home page

Review Questions

1. How does identifying a target market help patients?

   By definition, the target market is the group of people most likely to need the practice's services. Focusing marketing activities on the target market lets this group of people know what the business has to offer.

2. Conducting a SWOT analysis, the health services administrator at a vein center recognized that by the end of the year, many people have met the deductible of their health care plan and can pursue some health services at no out-of-pocket cost. Which part of the SWOT analysis is this?

   This is an opportunity. It could bring increased business due to external forces.

3. Choose one of the marketing tools discussed in this chapter and discuss its advantages and disadvantages.

   Answers will vary.

4. What are some ways a practice can overcome bad press?

   High-quality customer service is a strong first-line defense. Participation in the local community, an official apology, and hiring a PR consultant can help improve image.

5. How does the health services administrator help resolve issues with problem patients?
   The health services administrator may act as a liaison between the patient and the providers or medical staff when issues arise that are somewhat complicated or need more time to resolve.

6. What information should be included in the "Welcome to Our Office" packet?
   The packet should list the providers, staff and their backgrounds, and the office philosophy. It should also include:
   - *Missed appointments and cancellation policy*
   - *Financial policy*
   - *Instructions and information for using the patient portal*
   - *Instruction sheets for certain conditions*
   - *List of community resources*

CHAPTER 16

Learning Checkpoint 16-1. Recruitment and Hiring

1. <u>Passive</u> candidates are those who are not currently seeking a new position, but may be inclined to consider it if the conditions, such as compensation and benefits, are attractive enough.
2. In a job <u>analysis</u>, the hiring manager identifies the skills, responsibilities, tasks, activities, training, experience, certifications, or licenses that are necessary for the success of the individual in a position.
3. A <u>structured</u> interview is one in which an organization gives an interviewer detailed and defined questions to ask.

Learning Checkpoint 16-2. Training and Development

1. Which type of training is for new hires?
   a. Orientation
   b. Onboarding
   c. Development
   d. *a and b only*
2. Which is a part of diversity training?
   a. Learning the names of supervisors
   b. *Understanding cultural norms*
   c. Discussing dress code and codes of conduct
   d. Learning organizational values, mission, goals, and strategic objectives

Learning Checkpoint 16-3. Performance Reviews and Termination and Dismissal

1. Which type of performance review includes feedback from peers?
   a. Narrative assessment
   b. Comparative assessment
   c. *360° review*
   d. a and b only
2. Which occurs when an employer implies or suggests that an employee's job is protected or guaranteed for a specific period?
   a. Public-policy exception
   b. *Implied contract*
   c. Covenant of good faith and fair dealings
   d. Employment-at-will

3. In the disciplinary process, which comes first?
   a. *Verbal warning*
   b. Written warning
   c. Termination
   d. Exit interview

Learning Checkpoint 16-4. Employment Laws

1. *True* or False. Disparate impact is when hiring practices result in decisions that disproportionately affect a protected class.
2. True or *False*. The Age Discrimination in Employment Act (ADEA) prohibits employers from discriminating against employees based on disability.
3. *True* or False. A medical coder is asked to move her desk to another office, but because of a back problem, she is unable to. Her manager cites this as a reason she did not get a raise in her yearly review. This is a violation of the ADA.
4. True or *False*. A laboratory technician, who was hired 6 months ago, wants to take 2 weeks of unpaid leave because his wife just had a baby. His employer denies the request, but offers two long weekends with 3 working days in between. This is a violation of the FMLA.
5. True or *False*. Title VII of the Civil Rights Act established the federal minimum wage.

Review Questions

1. Why is human resources increasingly important in the health care industry?
   Answers should recognize that the health care industry is experiencing a labor shortage and that increased demand, as well as more choices of places to work, make human resources critical to the success of the medical practice.
2. What are the benefits of internal recruitment, and what are the disadvantages? What are the benefits and disadvantages of external recruitment methods?
   Typically, internal recruitment allows managers to have better insight into an individual employee's skills, experience, and job performance. In internal recruitment, managers have an opportunity to observe a potential candidate over time, and employees are less likely to leave an organization than first-time hires recruited externally. The cost of internal recruitment and the time investment are also significantly less than external recruitment options. However, if an organization is strategically trying to change its corporate culture or bring in new innovative ideas, hiring from within is usually not preferred. Hiring from outside can bring fresh talent and new ideas, but generally costs more.
3. Outline the key steps in the hiring process.
   - *The hiring manager will create a job analysis, which identifies the skills, responsibilities, tasks, activities, training, experience, certifications, or licenses that are necessary for the success of the individual in a position. This informs the job description.*
   - *A job announcement is created, inviting applicants.*
   - *Applicants are prescreened.*
   - *Interviews are conducted.*
   - *A candidate is selected and made an offer.*
4. What is the difference between training and development?
   Training focuses on short-term needs of the organization, teaching the individual the skills he or she needs to perform the job. Employee development is broader in scope and focuses on long-term enhancement of individual employees to advance their careers.

5. Why is diversity training important?

   By raising awareness, diversity training helps employees at all levels within a health care organization better understand and care for patients with different backgrounds. Diversity training also supports the inclusion of minorities and supports collaboration, which is critical in health care.

6. What is the purpose of the performance review process?

   Employee performance reviews can be used to identify the organization's best employees, as well as those who need improvement. For the top-performing employees, the review process is an opportunity to reward good work through financial incentives or promotions. For lower-performing employees, it is an opportunity to reevaluate the goals of their position in the organization and identify possible training gaps. Performance reviews also allow employees to know how their manager views their work, and it may motivate the employee to address any performance weaknesses. Employee performance reviews are important for documentation that may be used for litigation purposes, specifically in cases of demotions, layoffs, and terminations.

7. In most states, employment is at-will, meaning that an employer can terminate an employee at any time for any reason. If that is the case, what stops an employer from firing a person who performs well and has no disciplinary problems?

   The covenant of good faith and fair dealings means that employees enter into employment with an assumption that the employer will act fairly and in good faith. If a terminated employee can prove that he or she was fired without just cause and was terminated unfairly, then a state may decide in favor of the former employee. However, with good documentation of an employee's performance or behavioral issues and progressive disciplinary action, the state may decide in favor of the employer.

8. How can health care organizations improve and manage employee retention?

   Ways to improve retention include:
   - *Improving engagement*
   - *Reducing absenteeism*
   - *Offering good compensation and benefits*
   - *Offering career growth*
   - *Having supportive management*
   - *Creating a culture that emphasizes results and values and understands work–life balance*

9. What are the two types of sexual harassment prohibited by the Civil Rights Act of 1964?

   Quid pro quo: *Types of harassment where job security, promotion, and benefits are tied to sexual favors.*

   Hostile work environment: *Types of harassment where the behavior is so severe that it affects the productivity of others indirectly. In hostile work environment cases, harassment may not be directed at the person filing the complaint. Any individual who observes and is offended by sexual material and has difficulty doing his or her job as a result is a victim of sexual harassment.*

10. How do the Family Medical Leave Act and the National Defense Authorization Act of 2008 (NDAA) protect families and military personnel, respectively?

    Although the time away from work is unpaid, each of these laws protects a person's job with up to 12 weeks of leave.

CHAPTER 17

Learning Checkpoint 17-1. Functions of Management

1. In most organizations, strategic planning begins with the creation of a(n) <u>mission statement</u>.

2. A statement that guides decision making is a(n) <u>policy</u>.
3. <u>Unity of command</u> means that the medical assistant reports only to the registered nurse.

Learning Checkpoint 17-2. Conflict Management

1. What does it mean when a team embraces a "win-win" strategy?
    a. They focus on common goals.
    b. They try to outdo previous successful outcomes.
    c. *A winner does not mean there must be a loser.*
    d. Everyone on the team thinks positively to achieve goals.
2. An individual who works with a group of people to help them understand their common goals is a:
    a. *facilitator*
    b. team player
    c. communicator
    d. resolver
3. Which defines emotional intelligence?
    a. The ability to understand and share the feelings of others
    b. *The ability to recognize emotions in others and act on them to solve problems*
    c. The ability to devise a plan to help people achieve common goals
    d. A shared opinion within the organization that there is enough for everyone
4. What are the four quadrants of emotional intelligence?
    a. Patience, negotiation skills, unbiased ideas, diversity
    b. *Social awareness, self-awareness, relationship management, self-management*
    c. Physiological needs, safety, belonging, self-actualization
    d. Head, heart, mind, hands

Review Questions

1. What are the four functions of management, and how are they related?
    The first function of management is planning, which is developing steps and actions to take that will accomplish the goals of the organization. The second function is organizing, which is the allocation workflow to accomplish the goals created during the planning function. Leading staffs the organization with people to carry out these goals, motivates them, and provides feedback. Finally, controlling monitors the organization's work toward its goals and makes corrections.
2. How do internal and external motivators compare?
    With external motivation a person does something to receive a reward, like compensation or praise. Internal motivation comes from within oneself wherein a person behaves in a certain way because it is enjoyable to them. External motivators can create spikes in productivity, but their effects usually decrease after time, whereas internal motivators are sustainable.
3. Conflict in the workplace can be positive if managed well. What does the text say is at the center of conflict and conflict resolution? Why do you think this is the case? How can this produce a positive result?
    Communication is at the center of conflict and conflict resolution. The communication of diverse ideas, if managed well, can produce creative outcomes and solutions not present without conflict. The resolution of conflict can increase employee morale, increase an employee's sense of being heard, and decrease employee turnover.

CHAPTER 18

Learning Checkpoint 18-1. Projects

1. *True* or False. Each project may encompass several smaller projects.
2. *True* or False. All projects are temporary.
3. *True* or False. People outside the organization can be stakeholders.

Learning Checkpoint 18-2. Project Management Life Cycle

1. Which phase includes the development of the SOW?
   a. *Initiation*
   b. Planning
   c. Monitoring
   d. Closing
2. When is the project execution plan developed?
   a. Initiation
   b. *Planning*
   c. Monitoring
   d. Closing
3. Which stage takes place concurrently with execution?
   a. Initiation
   b. Planning
   c. *Monitoring*
   d. Closing

Review Questions

1. Project management is important in any industry because projects are driven by a need for improvement. In the health care industry, what additional parameters must a project consider other than the traditional project management considerations of time, finances, and resources?
   The health care industry is unique because of the added restrictions of local, state, and federal regulations as constraints and drivers in any project consideration, whereas some other industries may only face the constraints of time, resources, and finances.
2. What are the top five characteristics of an effective project manager?
   Organized, motivational, skilled at delegations, effective communicator, and dynamic
3. What are the five phases of the project management life cycle?
   Initiation, planning, execution, monitoring and control, and closing
4. Explain the difference between the waterfall methodology of project management and the agile methodology.
   The waterfall method follows a sequence, where one step is completed, tested, and adjusted before moving to the next step. In contrast, the agile method is flexible and allows for constant feedback to be implemented and adjustments to be made. It produces short-term deliverables.

GLOSSARY

360° review A comprehensive feedback that comes from the employee's manager, peers, and direct reports.

Abandonment To withdraw protection or support; in medicine, to discontinue medical care without proper notice after accepting a patient.

Accountable Care Organization (ACO) A network of diverse health care providers who are jointly responsible for the care and outcome of a bank of Medicare patients.

Accounts payable (AP) Money owed to vendors and other businesses.

Accounts receivable (AR) Monies owed to an organization.

Accreditation Voluntary compliance with a set of standards for operation developed by an independent, not-for-profit organization.

Accrual basis accounting A method of tracking finances in which transactions are recorded when goods or services are exchanged, rather than when cash is exchanged.

Act The formal action of a legislative body; a decision or determination of a sovereign state, a legislative council, or a court of justice.

Action plan A formal document listing goals and the people and resources needed to reach it within a certain time frame.

Acute care Inpatient health care for severe illnesses or injuries requiring a stay in a facility where the average stay is 30 days or less.

Administrative safeguards The policies and procedures documented in writing that show how a health care provider will comply with the Health Insurance Portability and Accountability Act (HIPAA).

Advance beneficiary notice (ABN) Notice to the patient of an amount, service, or procedure that may not be covered by the health insurance company or that the physician believes may not be medically necessary.

Advance directive Documentation that details the types and limits of care in the event that a patient is unable to communicate his or her wishes.

Advanced Alternative Payment Model (APM) A Centers for Medicare and Medicaid reimbursement program that rewards the use of technology during the care of certain clinical conditions and populations.

Advanced beneficiary notice (ABN) A written document notifying a Medicare patient that Medicare will not cover a service, usually because it is not determined to be medically necessary.

Advanced practice registered nurse (APRN) A clinical health care professional who provides primary care under the supervision of a physician.

Affordable Care Act (ACA) Legislation that set new guidelines for health insurers, mandated insurance coverage for all Americans, and reformed the way individuals who are not eligible for employer-sponsored coverage purchase insurance.

Age Discrimination in Employment Act (ADEA) Legislation that prohibits employers from discriminating against employees or job applicants over age 40 because of their age.

Agenda A list of what will take place during a meeting, often sent to meeting participants to prepare for before a meeting.

Agile methodology A project management method that is characterized by extreme flexibility and short sprints of productivity with deliverables produced in short intervals.

Algorithm A structured path of decision making.

Allied health professional A health care professional who provides a supporting function in health care delivery.

Allowable amount The full amount the insurer will reimburse a provider that is in its network of providers for a covered service.

Ambulatory care Outpatient health care provided to patients who arrive at the facility, receive treatment, and leave on the same day.

Ambulatory Payment Classification (APC) Grouping of procedures and services that are provided to Medicare patients through the hospital outpatient prospective payment system.

Ambulatory surgery center (ASC) A surgical facility that performs procedures on patients who are not admitted to a hospital for recovery.

American Recovery and Reinvestment Act (ARRA) The 2009 legislation providing federal funding in science, research, and infrastructure, including a portion called Health Information Technology for Economic and Clinical Health (HITECH) to promote health information technology.

Appeal The request for an insurer to reconsider their decision to deny a health care claim.

Arbitration A type of alternative dispute resolution that provides parties to a controversy with a choice other than going to court for resolution of a problem.

Assault An intentional attempt to cause bodily harm to another.

Asset Resources owned by an organization.

Assignment The amount of money Medicare will pay for medical services.

Assisted living facility Facility that provides housing and support services, such as personal care, housekeeping, and coordinated recreational activities.

Audit An examination of the documents, procedures, and processes of an organization to ascertain how it is doing business.

Audit trail A feature of the electronic health record that tracks users who accessed a patient record and when they did so.

Authentication The assumption of responsibility for the data collected.

Balance sheet A financial statement listing an organization's assets, liabilities, and net worth.

Battery An intentional act of contact with another that causes harm or offends the individual being touched or injured.

Benchmarking An improvement technique that compares one facility's process with that of another facility that has been noted to have superior performance.

Blind carbon copy (bcc) A sending option used in email in which the sender wants to include someone on the email for information only, but the individual's identity is not shared with other recipients.

Bloodborne pathogen Microorganism in the blood that can cause disease.

Brainstorming A data-gathering quality improvement tool used to generate information related to a topic.

Buffer time A section of the schedule that is open for walk-ins or patients who need to see the physician urgently.

Bundling Payment for multiple procedures or services under one combination code.

Business associate A business that provides a service to a covered entity and uses protected health information (PHI).

Business letter Written form of communication for external parties. Business letters are often more formal and structured and include more background information than do memorandums.

Capital expenditure Money set aside for large purchases over a certain dollar amount whose use will span multiple fiscal years.

Capitation A flat rate reimbursement that a health care provider receives per patient for providing care.

Carbon copy (cc) A sending option used in email in which the sender wants to include someone on the email for information only and is not expecting that individual to respond.

Care plan The assessment of problems and plan for treatment of a patient.

Cash basis accounting A method of tracking finances in which transactions are recorded at the time when cash is exchanged.

Centers for Medicare and Medicaid Services (CMS) A division of the Department of Health and Human Services responsible for overseeing Medicare, Medicaid, and Children's Health Insurance Program (CHIP).

Certification The verification that an individual or entity has met certain professional standards.

Chain of command The authority of an individual within an organization.

Chargemaster A list of services provided, the charges, and the associated codes.

Charges The amount of money that the health care provider submits for payment.

Chief complaint The primary reason for visit.

Civil money penalty (CMP) Fine levied on covered entities that violate Health Insurance Portability and Accountability Act (HIPAA) regulations.

Claim A statement of services sent to a health insurer for payment to the provider.

Clinic An ambulatory setting providing general or specialized care, sometimes on a walk-in basis and sometimes at a reduced cost for disadvantaged populations.

Clinical decision support (CDS) A function of the electronic health record that recommends approaches for diagnoses of specific diseases, guides selection of the correct diagnostic tests, and assists in the treatment and monitoring of patients.

Cluster scheduling A method of scheduling that assigns similar patients or medical care on the same days.

Coinsurance A cost-sharing provision in which the health care consumer pays a percentage of the total health care cost.

Comparative assessment In a performance review, assignment of employee rank compared with other employees.

Complementary and alternative medicine (CAM) Health and wellness therapies used along with (and complementary to) conventional medicine, focusing on the "whole person," including the physical, mental, and spiritual health of the individual.

Compliance officer An individual whose role is to make sure the operations of an organization meet regulatory requirements.

Compliance program A set of internal policies and procedures put into place by an organization to help the organization comply with laws and industry-accepted best practices.

Computer-assisted physician order entry (CPOE) An electronic system in which a provider enters patient care orders to communicate to other members of the care team, and which provides decision support and alerts.

Concurrent audit An audit performed before the bill is generated and submitted to the insurance carrier.

Conditions for Coverage (CfC) The terms that a facility or provider must follow in order to receive reimbursement from the Centers for Medicare and Medicaid Services.

Conditions of Participation (CoP) The terms that a facility or provider must follow in order to receive reimbursement from the Centers for Medicare and Medicaid Services.

Consumer-mediated exchange A type of health information exchange in which patients can request their information be sent to another provider.

Continuing education unit (CEU) A measure of the amount of education an individual has acquired, after a degree or credential, required to stay current in the field.

Continuing medical education (CME) unit A measure of the amount of education a medical professional has acquired, after a degree or credential, required to stay current in the field.

Continuity of care The communication and coordination of care among various health care professionals and facilities for the treatment of a patient's specific period of illness or across a patient's lifetime.

Continuum of care The provision of care for a patient over a period of time.

Contraindication A reason not to pursue a treatment.

Copay (copayment) A fixed amount the insured owes to the provider at the time of service.

Corporate integrity agreement (CIA) An enforcement tool used by the Office of the Inspector General (OIG) to promote compliance.

Countersignature Evidence of supervision of a subordinate's documentation.

Covenant of good faith and fair dealings Legal framework in which employees enter into employment with the assumption that the employer will act fairly and in good faith.

Covered entity An entity that must comply with Health Insurance Portability and Accountability Act (HIPAA) regulations. This includes health care providers that transmit protected health information (PHI) electronically, health plans, and health care clearinghouses.

Credential A professional qualification, represented by the abbreviation a qualified individual may list after their name.

Critical path methodology A project management method where each phase is interdependent and all activities are laid out, with critical and noncritical tasks determined in the planning phase. The length of time to complete each task and its relationship to the next task is defined in the planning phases and allows for the project manager to maintain control and keep the project on track.

Cultural competency The ability of providers and health care organizations to effectively deliver health care services that meet the social, cultural, and linguistic needs of patients.

Cultural sensitivity Knowledge and interpersonal skills that allow health care professionals to understand and work with individuals from diverse cultures.

Current Procedural Terminology (CPT) A coding system that documents and reports medical, surgical, radiology, laboratory, anesthesiology, and evaluation and management (E/M) services.

Damages Money that is awarded by a court to an individual who has been injured through the wrongful conduct of another party.

Day sheet A summary of the provider's charges and payments received in a single day.

Decision matrix A quality improvement tool used to narrow focus or choose between two or more related possible decisions.

Deductible The amount of money a subscriber must pay for medical services before an insurer will pay claims.

Deemed status The compliance of a health care entity with federal regulations through a survey by an accreditation agency.

Defendant A person required to answer in a legal action or suit; in criminal cases, the person accused of a crime.

Deliverable The product or outcome of a project management development process.

Denial A decision by the insurer to not reimburse the health care provider for the service(s) billed.

Department of Health and Human Services (DHHS) The agency of the United States government with oversight of health care.

Deposition An oral testimony of a party or witness in a civil or criminal proceeding taken before trial.

Depreciation The cost of an asset over time.

Development Long-term gains of skill for an individual employee.

Directed exchange A type of health information exchange with the ability for one provider to send information to another securely.

Discharge summary Documentation of a visit given to the patient at checkout.

Disclosure The voluntary self-reporting of an infraction.

Disparate impact Hiring practices resulting in decisions that disproportionately affect a protected class.

Diversity An appreciation and recognition of individual differences such as race, gender, age, religious beliefs, sexual orientation, and socioeconomic status.

Do not resuscitate (DNR) order A document specifying the lifesaving measures that should or should not be performed if a patient ceases cardiac or pulmonary function.

Double booking The scheduling of two patients to see the same provider at the same time.

Electronic health record (EHR) A system that maintains patient demographic and clinical information digitally and offers physician order entry, e-prescribing, and decision support.

Emancipated minor A person under the age of majority (usually 18) who has been legally separated from his or her parents by the courts and is responsible for their own care.

Emergency Medical Treatment and Active Labor Act (EMTALA) Legislation that requires health care providers to screen and treat anyone who presented to their emergency department with an "emergency medical condition."

Emotional intelligence (EI) The ability of the manager to recognize his or her own emotions and the emotions of others, to control and differentiate between those emotions, and to act upon those emotions accordingly to solve problems or make decisions.

Empathy The ability to understand and share the feelings of others.

Employee referral program A recruitment strategy that provides existing employees with financial incentives for referrals of potential job candidates.

Employment-at-will Legal framework in which an employer or employee may terminate employment at any time and for any reason, as long as there is no legal employment contract.

Encounter An episode of service to a patient in an outpatient setting. Also called a *visit*.

Entitlement program Government financial support based on an individual's age, condition, employment status, or other circumstances.

Epidemic A disease afflicting many people at the same time.

Equal Employment Opportunity Commission (EEOC) Federal agency created by the Civil Rights Act of 1964 to enforce the provisions of the Civil Rights Act.

Equal Pay Act (EPA) Legislation that requires employers to pay men and women equal pay for substantially equal work.

Evaluation and management (E/M) codes A subset of Current Procedural Terminology (CPT) coding that represents the amount of time and skill needed to treat the patient.

E-visit A patient interaction with a provider using telecommunications technology.

Exclusion Disciplinary action that excludes a health care facility or provider from participating in any type of federal health care program.

Expert witness One who provides testimony to a court as an expert in a certain field or subject to verify facts presented by one or both sides in a lawsuit.

Facilitator Someone who works with a group of people to help them understand their common goals and then to devise a plan to achieve them.

Fair Labor Standards Act (FLSA) Legislation that protects employees from compensation discrimination. Specifically, it sets the federal minimum wage and requires that employers pay time-and-a-half for any overtime for hourly employees who work more than 40 hours per week.

Family and Medical Leave Act (FMLA) Legislation that allows employees with at least 1 year of service to take up to 12 weeks of unpaid leave each year for the birth or adoption of a child, or to care for themselves or a sick child, spouse, or parent with a serious health condition.

Federal minimum wage The lowest amount that an employee can legally be paid for hourly work.

Fee schedule List of each service that the insurer covers and the specific amount that they will reimburse a health care provider for that specific service.

Fee-for-service The traditional model of health insurance where the health care facility receives payment for each service rendered.

Fiscal year A year structured for accounting or tax purposes.

Fixed appointment scheduling A method of assigning a set appointment time to each individual patient. Also called *stream scheduling*.

Fixed costs Expenses in the operational budget that do not change on a monthly basis.

Flowchart A tool used to organize the steps involved in a process.

Gatekeeper A primary care provider who sees the patient first to control access to other parts of the health care delivery system.

Genetic Information Nondiscrimination Act (GINA) Legislation that protects employees from discrimination based on genetic information.

Goal A statement of general purpose and desired outcome.

Graph An illustration of the relationship between two or more variable quantities.

Gross income The total income of the organization minus the costs of the goods sold.

Group plan A type of insurance policy that averages risk over a group of covered individuals.

Grouper Software used to convert diagnosis and procedure codes into Ambulatory Patient Classifications and other groupings.

Guarantor The person who is ultimately responsible for paying for health care services.

Guardian ad litem An individual who is assigned by the court to be legally responsible for protecting the well-being and interests of a ward, typically a minor or a person who has been declared legally incompetent.

Hard-to-reach population A group of individuals who may be transient, homeless, have mental illness, or have socioeconomic disadvantages and may be harder for health care professionals to reach for purposes of health care follow-up and treatment adherence.

Healthcare Effectiveness Data and Information Set (HEDIS) A performance measurement tool that allows comparison of health plans.

Health information exchange (HIE) Groups of providers whose computer systems are networked to form a secure, accessible database of patient records.

Health Information Technology for Economic and Clinical Health Act (HITECH) The portion of the 2009 American Recovery and Reinvestment Act (ARRA) that funded and mandated health information technology initiatives.

Health Insurance Portability and Accountability Act (HIPAA) Legislation protecting the privacy and security of patient health information.

Health maintenance organization (HMO) A type of managed care health insurance that seeks to reduce costs by limiting the providers and facilities from which a subscriber may obtain services.

Healthcare Common Procedure Coding System (HCPCS) Coding system created by the Centers for Medicare and Medicaid Services for use in the hospital outpatient prospective payment system.

Home health care Health care services provided in the patient's home.

Hospice care Noncurative care delivered to patients at the end of their lives.

Hospital A facility that provides medical services to the general population in the form of emergency care, critical care, intensive care, and various types of patient care requiring inpatient treatment.

Implied contract A contract that lacks a written record or verbal agreement but is assumed to exist.

Incidence The number of new cases of disease.

Incident report An administrative discovery tool used by the health care organization to obtain information about a potentially-compensable event.

Income statement A financial statement showing an organization's revenue and expenses over a certain period.

Incompetent Refers to a person who is not able to manage his or her affairs due to mental deficiency (lack of IQ, deterioration, illness, or psychosis) or sometimes physical disability; the individual cannot comprehend the complexities of a situation and therefore cannot provide informed consent.

Indemnity insurance A type of health insurance policy that pays all or part of covered services after deductibles and within the limits of the policy.

Indigent The condition of being unable to afford care.

Informed consent Voluntary agreement, usually written, for treatment after being informed of its purpose, methods, procedures, benefits, and risks.

Inpatient A patient admitted to a facility at least overnight by order of a physician.

Intermediate care facility (ICF) A health care facility that provides long-term care most often to developmentally disabled patients who do not require the degree of medical care given at a hospital or subacute health care facility.

International Classification of Disease, Tenth Revision, Clinical Modification (ICD-10-CM) Diagnosis coding system used on health care claims.

Interoperability The capacity for different computer systems to communicate, exchange data, and use the information that has been exchanged.

Interrogatory A list of questions from one party to the other in the lawsuit.

Job analysis Process by which the hiring manager identifies the skills, responsibilities, tasks, activities, training, experience, certifications, or licenses that are necessary for success in a particular job position.

Job announcement Describes the key elements of an open position within a health care organization and job expectations.

Lead time The amount of time it takes to receive an order once placed.

Lean A performance improvement philosophy that seeks to remove wastefulness from a process by constantly looking for ways to improve how things are done.

Liability A debt or other financial obligation incurred during the operation of the business.

Liable Obligated according to law or equity; responsible for an act or circumstance.

Liaison An individual assigned to communicate between multiple parties.

Libel A written remark that injures another's reputation or character.

Licensed practical (vocational) nurse (LPN, LVN) A nurse working under the supervision of a registered nurse (RN) who measures vital signs and performs some interventions.

Licensing An official permission to practice or operate.

Licensure Official permission to practice or operate.

Litigation The dispute of a matter in court.

Litigious Prone to engage in lawsuits.

Local coverage determination (LCD) Rules developed by the Medicare Administrative Contractor used to determine whether or not a service will be covered.

Long-term care facility (LTC) A health care facility that provides care on an inpatient basis to patients who are chronically ill and need extended services or treatments; commonly called a *nursing home*.

Malpractice The failure of a physician to meet the standard of care as dictated by his or her profession or the medical industry.

Managed care An insurance coverage and reimbursement structure that seeks to control costs by limiting the providers who can be seen by the patient and, in turn, discount payments to those providers.

Mandatory exclusion The result of conviction of a program-related crime, conviction related to patient abuse or neglect, felony conviction related to a controlled substance, or felony conviction related to health care fraud.

Master patient index A database containing a complete list of patients who have been treated at the health care organization.

Materials safety data sheet (MSDS) Document stating the physical properties, use, and handling of a chemical substance.

Meaningful use The set of benchmarks created under the Health Information Technology for Economic and Clinical Health (HITECH) Act to measure the capabilities of electronic health record (EHR) technology and provide financial incentives to health care providers.

Mediation A type of alternative dispute resolution involving the use of a neutral third party, called the *mediator,* to help those involved in a dispute come to a solution.

Medicaid A federal program funded by each state that pays for the health care costs of those in poverty.

Medical assistant (MA) A health professional who provides both clinical and administrative support in a health care setting.

Medical necessity Regarding insurance, the need for treatment.

Medical proxy A document that specifies who will make medical decisions for the patient and under what circumstances.

Medical record number (MRN) A unique number assigned to each patient's medical record.

Medical record An assemblage of all the medical data about an individual patient.

Medicare A federal program paying for the health care costs of those over 65 and those with certain chronic illnesses.

Memorandums (memo) Written form of communication for internal parties, often less formal and structured and includes less background information than business letters.

Merit-based Incentive Payment System (MIPS) A Centers for Medicare and Medicaid reimbursement program linking payments to the use of technology and the collection of quality data.

Minutes A summary record of what took place at a meeting.

Mission statement A written declaration of the organization's purpose and values.

Modified wave scheduling A method of appointment scheduling in which a small group of patients is scheduled at the top of an hour, with single patients also scheduled within the hour.

Morbidity Disease.

Mortality Death.

Motivation A process that evokes, guides, and sustains a behavior.

Narrative assessment In a performance review, qualitative feedback that is detailed and meaningful.

National coverage determination (NCD) Rules developed by the Centers for Medicare and Medicaid Services used to determine whether a service will be covered.

National Defense Authorization Act (NDAA) Legislation that allows employees to take 12 weeks of unpaid leave for "any qualifying exigency" that results from a call to service or active military service of a spouse, child, or parent.

Needs assessment Process used by organizations to determine priorities and "gaps" between current conditions and desired goals.

Negligence The failure to behave in the manner of a reasonably prudent person acting under similar circumstances; it falls below the standards of conduct established by law for the protection of others against unreasonable risk of harm.

Net income The total income for the company after subtracting costs of goods sold, operating expenses, taxes, shareholder distributions, and other expenses.

Net worth The amount by which assets exceed liabilities.

Nonverbal communication Communication that occurs without language, such as body posture, gestures, facial expressions, gazes, eye contact, and tone of voice.

Notice of Privacy Practices (NPP) Document listing patients' rights as mandated by the HIPAA.

Nurse A clinical health care professional trained and licensed to provide care to patients.

Objective An individual, defined, and measurable statement of an action that will achieve short- or medium-term goals.

Occupational Safety and Health Act (OSH Act) Federal legislation that promotes work safety and requires employers to ensure workplaces are free of hazards.

Office for Civil Rights The section of the U.S. Department of Health and Human Services that is responsible for the enforcement of Health Insurance Portability and Accountability Act (HIPAA) regulations.

Office of Inspector General (OIG) Federal government office that prevents fraud and abuse in Department of Health and Human Services programs.

Older Workers Benefit Protection Act (OWBPA) Legislation that prohibits employers from denying benefits to older workers.

Onboarding The process of helping new hires integrate into the organization, preparing them for job success, and becoming productive employees.

Open access scheduling A method that has no appointments at all and allows for patients to be seen as they arrive at the facility, usually on a first-come-first-serve (FCFS) basis.

Operational budget Costs related to the operation of the department, such as payroll, utilities, and supplies.

Ordinance Authoritative decree or direction; law set forth by a governmental authority, specifically, municipal regulation.

Orientation Overview of an organization for new employees, which may include organizational values, goals, objectives, policies and procedures, employee benefits, and mandatory compliance training.

Outcome The result of a patient's treatment.

Outcomes and Assessment Information Set (OASIS) Information collected on all Medicare home health patient care.

Out-of-pocket limit The most amount of money an individual will have to pay for covered medical services in a year.

Outpatient A patient who receives treatment during a visit on a single day.

Outpatient prospective payment system (OPPS) The Medicare system used to reimburse hospitals for outpatient services.

Packaging The inclusion of required minor services in a larger reimbursement grouping.

Palliative care A medical treatment to ease a patient's pain or reduce symptoms but that is not intended to cure a disease or disorder.

Par level The quantity at which supplies are reordered.

Passive candidate An individual who is not currently seeking a new position but may be inclined to consider a position if the conditions were right.

Patient portal A website on which a patient can interact and communicate with their provider; view laboratory test results; and track, monitor, and send information regarding their personal health.

Patient-centered medical home model A health care delivery model where patient care is coordinated through the primary care physician.

Payback period The length of time for the savings or revenues generated by a purchase to pay for the purchase itself.

Payer The entity responsible for most or all of a patient's bill to the provider.

Performance improvement (PI) Also known as *quality improvement (QI)* or *continuous quality improvement (CQI)*. Refers to the process by which a facility reviews its services or products to ensure quality.

Performance review A process that allows managers and employees to identify strengths and weaknesses in their job performance.

Permissive exclusion The result of lying on an enrollment application, conviction of certain misdemeanors, the loss of a state license to practice, the failure to repay health education loans, or the failure to provide quality care.

Physical safeguards Guidelines to protect physical monitoring of protected health information.

Physician A health care professional trained and licensed to diagnose and treat illnesses and disorders and to provide preventive care.

Physician assistant (PA) A clinical health care professional who provides primary care under the supervision of a physician.

Physician Quality Reporting System (PQRS) A Centers for Medicare and Medicaid reimbursement program that rewarded providers for collecting and reporting quality measures.

Physician's office An ambulatory care setting served by an individual or group of primary care providers.

Pie chart A graphical illustration of the percentage of data as they relate to a whole.

Plaintiff The person or group bringing a case or legal action to civil court.

Plan, Do, Check, and Act (PDCA) method A performance improvement method with formalized steps for improving a process.

Point of Service (POS) A type of managed care health insurance in which a patient may see certain providers in-network and pay a higher cost to see providers out of network; patients must have a referral to see a specialist.

Policy A statement that guides decision making.

Portability Refers to the first guideline of the HIPAA, which safeguards an American who is in transition between jobs by setting guidelines that health care insurance providers must follow and restrict exclusions from insurance coverage for certain reasons such as preexisting conditions in certain situations.

Potentially compensable event (PCE) An event that could cause the facility a financial loss or lead to litigation.

Practice management software (PMS) Software used to facilitate the day-to-day operations of the medical office.

Preauthorization The process of obtaining approval from the insurer for a service before the service is performed.

Preferred provider organization (PPO) A type of managed care health insurance in which a patient may see certain providers in-network and pay a higher cost to see providers out of network; some plans allow patients to self-refer to specialists.

Pregnancy Discrimination Act (PDA) Legislation that prohibits employers from discriminating against a woman who is or may become pregnant.

Premium A fixed amount paid to subscribe to an insurance policy.

Primary care The first and most basic level of treatment for injury or illness, serving as the entry point for health care consumers into the health care delivery system.

Primary care provider (PCP) A physician or other provider designated by the patient to deliver primary care and refer the patient to other specialists as necessary.

Privacy officer An individual designated to enforce the HIPAA compliance in the facility.

Privacy Rule Guidelines under the HIPAA that give patients important privacy rights to their health care information, including who can access the information and to whom it can be released.

Privileges A physician's permission to use hospital facilities to treat patients.

Procedure A description of the way tasks are to be completed or the way in which a policy is carried out.

Productivity The measure of efficiency of work, or the rate at which work is produced balanced with the time and resources spent.

Professionalism The skills, judgments, and behaviors that are expected in the workplace.

Progress note The documentation of a patient's care and response to treatment.

Project A temporary endeavor that produces a unique product, service, or process.

Project execution plan A written document that defines how the work will be accomplished for project completion.

Project management The application of processes, methods, knowledge, skills, and experience packaged together to realize project objectives.

Project manager A person who facilitates the project from beginning to end phases and coordinates all aspects in between.

Prospective payment system (PPS) A system of reimbursement in which the payment amount is determined based on the diagnosis or the treatment provided.

Protected health information (PHI) The information protected under the HIPAA regarding personal health care information that must be transmitted, retained, and destroyed in the business of health care.

Protocol A guideline for the treatment of a disease or disorder.

Provider An individual or organization that provides health services to patients.

Public-policy exception Exception to the at-will doctrine that says employers cannot fire employees for refusing to do something illegal or that would be against the best interest of the public.

Purchase order (PO) A form listing the items, quantities, and agreed prices for products or services needed from a specific vendor.

Query A tool used to clarify the provider's documentation in the patient's medical record.

Query-based exchange A type of health information exchange in which one provider can search the database of another.

Real cost The cost of an item, including the cost of all resources used to offer the good or service.

Reasonable accommodations Modifications that enable disabled individuals with a work environment or work process to allow them to perform essential job functions successfully.

Recruitment strategy The process of attracting talent to the health care organization for current job openings.

Referral A provider's request for the services of another provider, often a specialist.

Registered nurse (RN) A clinical health care professional trained and licensed to deliver interventions to promote patient well-being, including administering medications, educating patients regarding their conditions, and coordinating care.

Reimbursement The payment to the provider for health care treatments, supplies, and services.

Remittance advice (RA) Report that identifies the patient, the services that are being reimbursed, and the amount of the reimbursement.

Remote patient monitoring (RPM) A type of telemedicine in which the patient transmits physiological health data outside of a health care setting (such as at home) to a provider.

Resource-based relative value scale (RBRVS) The prospective payment system used for physician practices.

Respondeat superior Legal doctrine stating health care providers are responsible for the actions of employees acting within the scope of their employment duties.

Restitution Under criminal law, state programs that require an offender to repay money or donate services to the victim or society.

Retail care clinic A walk-in clinic that is offered onsite at a retail store, such as a large department store or pharmacy, equipped to treat uncomplicated, minor illnesses.

Retrospective audit An audit performed after a bill has been submitted to the insurance carrier for payment.

Revenue cycle The processing of health information to obtain reimbursement for health care services provided.

Revenue cycle management The gathering of the administrative and clinical information required to obtain reimbursement for health care services provided.

Revenue stream A source of income for a company.

Risk management (RM) The coordination of efforts within a facility to prevent and control inadvertent occurrences.

Scheduling matrix A tabular map of the times each provider is available.

Scope of practice The types of procedures a health care professional is permitted to perform in accordance with their licensure.

Scope of work (SOW) A written document defining the parameters of a project and what work will be completed as part of the project.

Security Rule Guidelines under the Health Insurance Portability and Accountability Act (HIPAA) regulation that set the standards for the storage and transfer of electronic protected health information.

Self-pay A reimbursement methodology in which a patient pays for his or her own health care services.

Sentinel event An unwanted occurrence that should never happen.

Shelf life The amount of time an item may be stored before use.

Shrinkage The loss of inventory.

Six Sigma A performance improvement methodology that uses a regimented, formal structure to remove defects from a process.

Skilled nursing facility (SNF) A type of long-term care facility providing subacute nursing care.

Span of control The number of employees or departments that report to an individual.

Staggered schedule The placement of providers in a variety of days and times that best meet the needs of the organization.

Stakeholder An individual with an interest in a work process or function.

Statute A law enacted by a state legislature.

Stock-out The state of being out of an item.

Store-and-forward A type of telemedicine in which images or video of a patient is recorded to be viewed by a specialist at a later time.

Strategic Human Resource Management (SHRM) The alignment of organizational strategic goals and objectives with the management of the organization's human resources.

Strategic planning The executive function of setting long-term goals for an organization and developing steps to achieve those goals.

Stream scheduling A method of assigning a set appointment time to each individual patient. Also called *fixed appointment scheduling.*

Stretch goal A goal beyond what is currently possible.

Structured interview Interviewing style in which interviewers have detailed and defined questions to ask during an interview.

Subpoena duces tecum A subpoena for the production of records or documents that pertain to a case as evidence.

Subscriber The primary enrollee of an insurance policy; known as a *beneficiary* for Medicaid recipients.

Superbill A summary of the patient's visit and charges incurred.

Survey A data-gathering tool for capturing the responses to queries. May be administered verbally or by written questionnaire. Also refers to the activity of querying, as in "taking a survey."

Table A chart organized in rows and columns to organize data.

Tax Equity and Fiscal Responsibility Act of 1982 (TEFRA) Legislation that established the prospective payment system for Medicare reimbursement.

Technical safeguards Guidelines under the Health Insurance Portability and Accountability Act (HIPAA) that safeguard protected health information through all mediums of technology.

Telehealth The remote delivery of health services using telecommunications technology.

The Joint Commission An independent, not-for-profit organization that sets standards for acute care facilities, ambulatory care networks, long-term care facilities, and rehabilitation facilities, as well as certain specialty facilities, such as hospice and home care agencies.

Title VII of the Civil Rights Act Legislation that prohibits employers from discriminating against employees based on gender, race, national origin, or religion for purposes of hiring, terminating, or determining wages/salary.

Training Teaching employees the necessary skills to perform their jobs successfully, focusing on the short-term needs of an organization.

Triage A method of sorting patients by the urgency of their needs.

Turnover The rate at which employees leave the facility and are replaced.

Unbilled charges Services and/or procedures that have been performed by the health care providers or organization but were never billed to the insurer and/or the patient.

Underinsured A term describing individuals who are covered by a health care plan but have high deductibles or out-of-pocket expenses that are not in relationship to their income level.

Undocumented charges Charges billed for services and/or procedures that were not documented in the patient's medical record.

Uniform Guidelines on Employee Selection Procedures (UGESP) Equal Employment Opportunity Commission (EEOC) guidance to assist employers in determining whether a hiring or promotions process has a disparate impact on any race, gender or ethnic group.

Uniformed Services Employment and Reemployment Rights Act (USERRA) Prohibits employers from discriminating against an employee who volunteers or is called for military service.

Unity of command The quality of a position reporting to only one supervisor.

Universal health care An organized package of benefits from the government offering access to health services and protection from financial risk.

Urgent care clinic Walk-in clinic that provides services for patients who need immediate medical care but whose injuries or illnesses are not serious enough to be seen in an emergency department.

Variable costs Expenses in the operational budget that change month to month based on the volume of activity.

Variance A deviation from the projected spending or earning in the budget.

Vendor An outside organization that provides products or services to the medical office.

Verbal communication Sharing information, thoughts, and feelings through speech.

Verdict The finding or decision of a jury on a matter submitted to it in trial.

Visit An episode of service to a patient in an outpatient setting. Also called an *encounter*.

Walk-in A type of encounter for which no appointment is required.

Waterfall (traditional) methodology A project management method that is sequential and completes one phase, including designing, producing, testing, and adjusting, before moving to the next phase.

Wave scheduling A method of appointment scheduling in which a group of patients is placed at the top of the hour and seen in the order in which they arrive.

Whistle blower One who reports illegal activities occurring within an organization to law enforcement authorities.

Workflow The sequence of processes in a medical office.

Workflow map A graphic display of the steps in a process.

Written communication Sharing information through written documents, such as emails, business letters, memorandums, and meeting agendas and minutes.

INDEX

Page numbers followed by "*f*" indicate figures, "*t*" indicate tables, and "*b*" indicate boxes.

A

AAAHC. *see* Accreditation Association for Ambulatory Health Care
AALL. *see* American Association of Labor Legislation
Abandonment, 214, 214*b*
ABN. *see* Advance beneficiary notice
Abundance mentality, 357
Abuse, 234–236, 236*b*
ACA. *see* Affordable Care Act
Accountable Care Organizations (ACO), 60, 60*b*
Accounts payable (AP), 151, 151*b*
Accounts receivable (AR), 150, 150*b*
Accreditation, 47–49, 47*b*
    documentation for, 108
Accreditation Association for Ambulatory Health Care (AAAHC), 50*t*
Accreditation Commission for Health Care (ACHC), 50*t*
Accrual basis accounting, 152, 152*b*
ACHC. *see* Accreditation Commission for Health Care
ACO. *see* Accountable Care Organizations
ACS. *see* American College of Surgeons
Act, 210, 210*b*
Action plan, 256, 256*b*, 256*f*
Acupuncture, 278, 279*f*
Acute care, 24, 24*b*
    settings, 30–31, 30*b*
ADEA. *see* Age Discrimination in Employment Act
Administrative functions, documentation for, 108
Administrative law, 214
Administrative safeguards, 243, 243*b*, 246*t*
Advance beneficiary notice (ABN), 95, 95*b*, 97*f*, 172, 172*b*
Advance directive, 94, 94*b*, 229, 229*b*, 230*f*
Advanced Alternative Payment Model, 185, 185*b*
Advanced Practice Registered Nurse (APRN), 19–20, 19*b*
Advertising channels, 322
Advocates, 311, 311*b*
Affordable Care Act (ACA), 44, 44*b*, 45*f*, 59–60, 59*f*, 253*b*
Age, structure of population for United States, 69*f*
Age Discrimination in Employment Act (ADEA), 338, 338*b*
Agency for Healthcare Research and Quality (AHRQ), 46*t*
Agenda, 292, 292*b*, 293*f*
Age-related hearing loss, 277
Agile methodology, 370–371, 370*b*
AHA. *see* American Hospital Association
AHRQ. *see* Agency for Healthcare Research and Quality
AKS. *see* Anti-Kickback Statute
Algorithm, 120, 120*b*, 120*f*
Allied health professionals, 9, 9*b*–10*b*, 22*t*–23*t*
Allowable amount, 165, 165*b*
AMA. *see* American Medical Association
Ambulance fee schedule, 168

Ambulatory care, 24, 24*b*
    settings, 24–29, 30*b*
Ambulatory Payment Classification (APC), 168, 168*b*
Ambulatory surgery center (ASC), 28, 28*b*, 29*f*
American Association of Labor Legislation (AALL), 38
American College of Surgeons (ACS), 49
American Hospital Association (AHA), 38–39
American Medical Association (AMA), 37
American Recovery and Reinvestment Act (ARRA), 124, 124*b*
Americans with Disabilities Act, 225–226, 225*b*, 226*f*
Annual educational programs, 256
Anonymous system, a compliance plan, 256
Anti-Kickback Statute (AKS), 260, 260*b*
APC. *see* Ambulatory Payment Classification
Appeal, 178–179, 178*b*
Appointments, 77*b*–78*b*, 78, 78*f*, 80*f*–81*f*
APRN. *see* Advanced Practice Registered Nurse
Arbitration, 224, 224*b*
ARRA. *see* American Recovery and Reinvestment Act
ASC. *see* Ambulatory surgery center
Assault, 211, 211*b*
Assessment piece, 96
Assets, 149, 149*b*
Assignment, 61–62, 61*b*
Assisted living facilities, 32, 32*b*, 32*f*
Associates, business, 240, 240*b*
Assumption of risk, in paying for health care, 52–55
Audit trail, 121, 121*b*, 121*f*
Auditing, 186–189, 186*f*
Audits, 186, 186*b*–187*b*
    billing, 188–189, 188*b*
    concurrent, 188, 188*b*
    external, 187–188
    internal, 187
    retrospective, 188, 188*b*
Authentication, 97, 97*b*
Automated phone calls, as marketing tool, 302, 302*b*

B

Baby boomers, 11–12, 68
Balance sheets, 149–151, 149*b*, 149*f*
Balanced Budget Act (BBA), 43–44
Bar chart, 194*f*, 194*t*–195*t*
Bar graphs, 196–198, 196*f*
Battery, 211, 211*b*
Baylor University Hospital, 39
BBA. *see* Balanced Budget Act
Bench trial, 222–223
Benchmarking method, 192–193, 192*b*–193*b*
Benchmarks, a compliance plan, 256
Billing audit, 188–189, 188*b*
Billing/claims processing, 176, 177*f*
Blind carbon copy, 287, 287*b*
Blogs, as marketing tools, 302, 302*b*
Bloodborne pathogens, 232–233, 232*b*
Brainstorming, 193, 193*b*, 194*t*–195*t*, 195*f*

Budgeting, 154–158, 158*b*
Buffer time, 81–82, 82*b*
Bundling, 168, 168*b*
Burden of proof, 223
Business associates, 240, 240*b*
Business communication, 271–296, 272*b*, 296*b*
Business letters, 287, 287*b*, 288*f*

C

CAM. *see* Complementary and alternative medicine
Capacity, 142*b*
Capital budget, 154–156
Capital expenditure request (CER), 154, 155*f*–156*f*
Capital expenditures, 154, 154*b*
Capitation, 169, 169*b*, 169*f*
CAPTA. *see* Child Abuse Prevention and Treatment Act
Carbon copy, 287, 287*b*
Care plan, 18, 18*b*
CARF. *see* Commission on Accreditation of
    Rehabilitation Facilities
Cash basis accounting, 152, 152*b*
Cause-and-effect (fishbone) chart, 194*t*–195*t*, 195*f*
CCMA. *see* Certified Clinical Medical Assistant
CDC. *see* Centers for Disease Control and Prevention
CDS. *see* Clinical decision support
Centers for Disease Control and Prevention (CDC), 46*t*
Centers for Medicare and Medicaid Services (CMS), 41,
    41*b*, 46*b*, 46*t*, 125, 254, 255*b*
CER. *see* Capital expenditure request
Certifications, 10, 10*b*, 15–16, 16*b*
    documentation for, 108
Certified Clinical Medical Assistant (CCMA), 21
Certified Medical Assistant (CMA), 21
Certified Medical Manager (CMM), 10, 10*b*
Certified Physician Practice Manager (CPPM), 10, 10*b*
CEU. *see* Continuing education units
Chain of command, 351, 351*b*
CHAP. *see* Community Health Accreditation Partner
Charge capture, 173
Chargemaster, 173, 173*b*
Charges, 165, 165*b*
Check-in, 82–83, 82*b*, 83*f*
Checklist, 194*t*–195*t*, 195*f*
Checkout, 84, 84*f*
Chief complaint, 83, 83*b*
Child abuse, 228*b*
Child Abuse Prevention and Treatment Act (CAPTA),
    227–229
Children's Health Insurance Program (CHIP), 43–44
CHIP. *see* Children's Health Insurance Program
CIA. *see* Corporate integrity agreements
Civil law, 212–214
Civil money penalties (CMPs), 248, 248*b*
Civil Rights Act, Title VII of, 331, 331*b*
Civil war, health care delivery during, 37–38, 38*f*
Civilian Health and Medical Program of the
    Department of Veterans Affairs (CHAMPVA), 41*t*
Claims, 5, 5*b*, 39, 39*b*, 173, 173*b*
Claims scrubber software, 173
Clean claims rate, 180
Clearinghouse, 240*t*
Clinic, 28, 28*b*
Clinical data, 96–98
    discharge summary of, 98
    imaging and laboratory documentation for, 98, 98*f*
    operative reports of, 98
    signatures for, 97
Clinical decision support (CDS), 120, 120*b*
Clinical documentation, 175
Clinical Laboratory Improvement Amendments Act,
    233, 233*b*
Clinical staff, 86
Cluster scheduling, 82, 82*b*
CMA. *see* Certified Medical Assistant
CME. *see* Continuing medical education

CMM. *see* Certified Medical Manager
CMP. *see* Civil money penalties
CMS. *see* Centers for Medicare and Medicaid Services
CMS-1500 paper form, 176, 177*f*
COBRA. *see* Consolidated Omnibus Budget
    Reconciliation Act
Coding, 109–111, 173–175, 174*f*, 174*t*
Coinsurance, 54, 54*b*, 163, 163*b*
Commission on Accreditation of Rehabilitation
    Facilities (CARF), 50*t*
Commitment, 142*b*
Communication, 142*b*, 274–293, 275*f*, 295*b*
    barriers in, 275–277, 275*b*
        lack of time, 276–277
        privacy, 276, 276*f*
    meetings, 292–293, 292*t*
    nonverbal communication, 283–284, 283*b*–284*b*
    special populations, 277–280
        cultural competency, 278, 278*b*
        cultural sensitivity, 278, 278*b*
        elderly patients, 277–278
        hard-to-reach, 279–280, 279*b*
        pain, in patient, 280
    verbal communication, 280–283
        patient visit, 283
        phone etiquette, 280–283
    written, 284–291, 284*b*
Community Health Accreditation Partner (CHAP), 50*t*
Community involvement, as marketing tools, 301–302
Comparative assessments, 330, 330*b*
Compensatory damages, 220
Competency, 142*b*
Complementary and alternative medicine (CAM), 278,
    278*b*
Compliance, 251–267, 266*b*
    disclosure, 263–264, 263*b*–264*b*
    documentation for, 257–258, 257*b*
    implementation, 258–259
    introduction, 252, 252*b*
    monitoring for effectiveness of, 259
    officer, 256, 256*b*
    plan, 256–257
        annually updated, 257
    policies and procedures, 256
    program, 252–259, 253*b*, 260*b*, 266*b*
        communication for, 259
        development of, 253
        effective, 253*b*
        foster a culture of, 258
        function with the right attitude, support,
            258
        office of inspector general for, 253–255, 255*b*
        regular audits for, 259
        training for, 259
        useful policies and procedures for, 258–259
    resolution process of, 264–265
Compliance auditing, 189
Compliance reporting, 227, 227*b*
Comprehensive history, 111
Computer-assisted physician order entry (CPOE), 115,
    115*b*, 125
Concurrent audit, 188, 188*b*
Conditions for Coverage (CfC), 254–255, 254*b*
Conditions of Participation (CoP), 46–47, 46*b*,
    254–255, 254*b*
Conflict
    communication in, 356
    employee engagement in, 355
    employee morale in, 356
    increased understanding in, 355
    management, 355–359, 355*b*, 359*b*–360*b*
    team cohesiveness in, 356
    team focus in, 355
    value of, 355–356
Conflict of interest disclosure form, 261*f*–262*f*

Consent
details regarding, 216–217
informed, 215, 215b–216b, 215f
for treatment, 215–217, 218b
Consistency, 142b
Consolidated Omnibus Budget Reconciliation Act (COBRA), 43
Construction phase, 368
Consumer-mediated exchange, 122, 122b
Continuing education, 11
Continuing education units (CEUs), 11, 11b, 11f
Continuing medical education (CME), 18, 18b
Continuity of care, 18, 18b
Continuum of care, 64–65, 64b, 65f, 107, 107b
Contract law, 213–214
Contraindication, 119b
Contributory negligence, 219
Control, 142b
chart, 194f, 194t–195t
Controlling, 352
Convergence, 142b
"Cookbook medicine", 57
Copayment, 54, 54b, 163, 163b
Corporate integrity agreements (CIA), 265, 265b
Cost, 142b
Cost sharing, 161–164
Cost-benefit analysis, 300, 300b
Countersignature, 97, 97b
Courtroom, inside the, 222–223
Covenant of good faith and fair dealings, 331, 331b
Covered entities, 240, 240b, 240t
CPOE. see Computer-assisted physician order entry
CPPM. see Certified Physician Practice Manager
CPT. see Current Procedural Terminology; Current procedural terminology
Credentials, 10, 10b, 15–16, 15b, 16t
Criminal law, 210–211
felony as, 211
infractions as, 211
misdemeanor as, 211
Critical path methodology, 371, 371b
Cultural competency, 278, 278b
Cultural sensitivity, 278, 278b
Current assets, 150
Current procedural terminology (CPT), 110, 110b, 175, 175b

D
Damages
compensatory, 220
exemplary, 219
general, 220
nominal, 219
punitive, 219
special, 220
types of, 219–220, 220b
Data consistency, 93b
Data presentation tools, 195–199, 196b
Day sheet, 132, 132b
Decision matrix, 198, 198b, 198t
Deductible, 54, 54b, 162–163, 162b
Deemed status, 49, 49b
Defendant, 212, 212b
Deliverable, 363–364, 364b
Demographic data, 92–94, 92t
in EHR system, 116f
Denial management, 178–179
Denials, 178, 178b, 179f, 180
Department of Health, Education, and Welfare (DHEW), 40–41, 46
Department of Health and Human Services (DHHS), 40–41, 46, 46b, 253–254, 370
Depositions, 221–222, 221b
Depreciation, 150–151
Detailed history, 111

Development, 327, 327b
DHEW. see Department of Health, Education, and Welfare
DHHS. see Department of Health and Human Services
Diagnostic facility, 28, 28b
Directed exchange, 122, 122b
Disaster management, 202–203, 203b
Discharge summary, 98, 98b
Disclosure, 263–264, 263b–264b
full description of conduct for, 264
requests for additional information of, 265
timing of a, 264
Disparate impact, 338, 338b
Diversity training, 327, 327b
Do not resuscitate (DNR) order, 94, 94b
Documentation, 90–112, 91b–92b
for accreditation, 108
for administrative functions, 108, 108b
for certification, 108
coding, 109–111
for compliance, importance of, 257–258, 257b
for licensure, 108
medical record, 91–106
for patient care, 107
for reimbursement, 108, 108b
for research, 108–109, 109b
for support of litigation, 107
types of, 106
uses of, 107–109, 107b, 109b
Double booking, 82, 82b

E
EEOC. see Equal Employment Opportunity Commission
Effective communication, 274–293, 275f. see also Communication
EHR. see Electronic health record
Elder abuse, 229
Electronic health record (EHR), 92, 114–125, 115b, 116f, 120b, 123b, 134b, 364–365, 364f
advantage of, 121
allergies in, 117f
benefits of, 115–121, 115b
challenges to implementation of, 123, 123b, 126b
challenges using, technology, 123b
contraindication in, 119–120, 120f
current medications in, 117f
demographic data in, 116f
functional, 115b
health information exchanges in, 121–123, 122b
incentives for use in, 124–125, 125b–126b
medication order in, 118f
patient history in, 117f
results, 119f
software for, 119–120
vital signs in, 117f
Electronic inventory management system, 144, 145f
Email etiquette, 284–287
attachments, 287
carbon copy and blind carbon copy, 287, 287b
closing and signature, 286
email/phone call, 285
forwarding emails, 287
message content, 285–286
proofreading, 286
reply
to all, 287
to incoming email, 285
subject line, 285, 285t
Emancipated minor, 217, 217b
Emergency Medical Treatment and Active Labor Act (EMTALA), 43, 43b
Emotional intelligence (EI), 358–359, 358b, 358f
Empathy, 359, 359b

Employee engagement, in conflict, 355
Employee morale, in conflict, 356
Employee referral program, 322–323, 322b
Employee Retirement Income and Security Act
    (ERISA), 42
Employee theft, 140–141, 140f
Employees, 319–346, 320b
    employment laws, 337–344, 345b
        based on genetic information, 340
        based on pregnancy, 341, 341b
        civil rights, 338–339, 338b
        disabilities, 339–340, 339b–340b
        discrimination, 337–341
        family leave, 341–342
        gender-pay differences, 343–344
        military leave, 343
        sexual harassment, 344, 344b
        substance addiction, 340
        wages, 343
        workplace safety, 344
    hiring of, 323–325, 325b
        interviewing, 324–325, 324f
        prescreening, 324, 324b
        selection, 325
    performance reviews of, 327–330, 327b–328b, 330b,
        337b
        assessment in, 328–330
        discussion in, 330
        evaluation form, 329f
    recruitment strategy of, 321–323, 321b, 325b
        advertising channels as, 322
        external recruitment methods as, 323, 323b
        internal recruitment methods as, 322–323
        whom to hire in, 322
    retention of, 334–337
    strategic human resources management (SHRM)
        for, 320–321, 321b
    terminations and dismissals of, 330–337, 337b
        breach of covenant of good faith and fair
            dealings in, 331
        breach of implied contract as, 331
        career growth and opportunities in, 336, 336b
        compensation and benefits in, 336
        disciplinary process as, 331–332, 331b
        discrimination in, 331
        employee turnover and retention, 333–334,
            333b
        ending employment in, 332–333, 332b
        exit interview in, 332–333, 333b
        improving employee engagement in, 334–335,
            334b, 335f
        improving employee retention in, 334–337
        legal framework in, 330–331
        organizational culture in, 336–337, 336b
        public-policy exception in, 331
        reducing absenteeism in, 335, 335b
        supportive managers in, 336
    training and development of, 326–327, 327b
        diversity, 327, 327b
        onboarding, 326, 326b
Employer-based health insurance, 40, 40b
Employment outlook, 11–12
Employment-at-will, 330–331, 330b
EMTALA. see Emergency Medical Treatment and Active
    Labor Act
Encounters, 24b
Enforcement, 248–249
Entities, covered, 240, 240b, 240t
Entitlement programs, 41, 41b
EPA. see Equal Pay Act
Epidemics, 202, 202b
Episode-of-care reimbursement, 165–169
Equal Employment Opportunity Commission (EEOC),
    323, 323b
Equal Pay Act (EPA), 343–344, 343b

ERISA. see Employee Retirement Income and Security
    Act
Ethical issues, 235–236, 236b
Evaluation and management codes (E/M) codes,
    110–111, 110b, 112b
E-visit, 132–133, 133b
Exclusion, 262, 262b
Exemplary damages, 219
Expanded problem focused, 111
Expert witnesses, 218–219, 218b
Expiration date, 138
Expressed consent, 215
External audits, 187–188
External recruitment methods, 323, 323b

F
Facilitator, 358, 358b
Facility, 86–87, 86b, 89b
    layout, 86–87, 87f–88f
Fair Labor Standards Act (FLSA), 343, 343b
False Claims Act (FCA), 235, 260, 260b
Family and Medical Leave Act (FMLA), 341, 341b, 342f
Family doctor, 25
FCA. see False Claims Act
FDA. see Food and Drug Administration
Federal government involvement, in health care
    delivery, 40–44
Federal minimum wage, 343, 343b
Federation of State Medical Boards (FSMB), 39
Fee schedule, 165, 165b
Feedback, goal, 350
Fee-for-service, 165, 165b
Felony, 211
Finance and health care accounting, 147–159, 148b,
    153b, 159b
Financial data, 94–95, 94b, 96f
Financial statements, 149–153, 149b, 153b
Finding, 223
Fiscal year, 157b
Fixed appointment scheduling, 82
Fixed assets, 150–151
Fixed costs, 157, 157b
Flexner Report, 39, 39b
Flowchart, 194f, 194t–195t, 198–199, 198b, 199f
FLSA. see Fair Labor Standards Act
FMLA. see Family and Medical Leave Act
Food and Drug Administration (FDA), 46t
Fragmented health care system, 65, 65b
Fraud, in health care, 209–237
Free-standing, 25
Front-end processes, 170–172
FSMB. see Federation of State Medical Boards

G
Gatekeeper, 25–26, 26b, 64, 64b
General consent, 215
General damages, 220
Genetic Information Nondiscrimination Act (GINA),
    340, 340b
Geographic practice cost index (GPCI), 167
GINA. see Genetic Information Nondiscrimination Act
GPCI. see Geographic practice cost index
Graph, 195–196, 195b
Gross income, 152, 152b
Group insurance, 161
Group plan, 52, 52b
Grouper, 168, 168b
Guarantor, 52, 52b
Guardian ad litem, 217, 217b

H
Hard-to-reach populations, 279–280, 279b
Hazard communication, 232
HCPCS. see Healthcare Common Procedure Coding
    System

Health care, 7
    accrediting organizations in, 50*t*
    current trends in, 57*b*–58*b*, 70*b*
    history of, in United States, 36–44, 45*b*
    paying for, 52–62, 63*b*
        insurance in, 52–55, 53*b*, 53*f*
    processes and workflow of, 75–89, 77*b*
    providers, 36–39, 37*f*
Health Care Access, Portability, and Renewability, 239
Health care common procedure coding system, 167, 167*t*–168*t*
Health care delivery, 35–71, 36*b*
    characteristics and challenges in, 64–71
        integrated and fragmented care as, 64–67, 66*b*, 66*f*
        rising costs as, 67–68
        uninsured and underinsured populations as, 68–71
    federal programs for, 41*t*
    legal and regulatory oversight in, 46–51, 51*b*
        accreditation, 47–49
        federal, 46–47
        local, 47
        professional standards, 49–51
        state, 47, 48*f*
    during 20th-century, 37, 37*b*
Health care facility, 49*b*
    liability in, 220, 220*b*
Health care fraud, 234–236, 236*b*
Health care practitioners, in 20th century, 37
Health care professionals, 15–23, 16*f*, 23*b*
    and settings, 14–34, 15*b*, 33*b*
Health care proxy, 94
Health data, 92–98
    clinical, 96–98
    demographic, 92–94, 92*t*
    financial, 94–95, 96*f*
    legal, 94
    types of, 92–98, 92*t*
Health information exchanges (HIE), 121–123, 122*b*, 122*f*
Health Information Technology for Economic and Clinical Health Act (HITECH), 124, 124*b*, 227
Health information technology (HIT), 364–365, 364*f*
Health insurance, 39–40
    basics, 161–164, 162*t*, 164*b*
    types of, 55–58
        indemnity as, 55–56, 55*b*
        managed care as, 56–58, 56*b*
Health Insurance Portability and Accountability Act (HIPAA), 43, 44*f*, 94, 128–129, 238–250, 239*b*, 253
    enforcement, 248–249
    introduction of, 239
    noncompliance, consequences of, 248–249
    portability, 239–240
    Privacy Rule, 240–243
    Security Rule, 243–247, 247*b*
    violations, 248–249, 248*b*–249*b*
Health insurer, 39
Health Maintenance Organization (HMO) Act, 41–42, 41*b*, 57–58, 57*b*
Health plan, 240*t*
Health record, 91
Health savings account (HSA), 58
Health Security Act, 43
Health services administrator, 3–13, 4*b*, 7*b*, 9*b*, 12*b*, 184*b*
    career in, 9–12
        certifications, 10, 10*b*
        continuing education, 11
        credentials, 10, 10*b*
        education, 9–11
        externships, 10
        internships, 10
        settings, 9

Health services administrator *(Continued)*
    daily activities of, 9
    definition of, 4, 4*b*
    duties of, 8–9, 8*b*, 8*f*
    employment outlook, 11–12
    role of, 6–9, 7*b*, 7*f*, 357–359
    typical visit, 4–6, 5*b*, 6*f*
Healthcare Common Procedure Coding System (HCPCS), 109–111, 175, 175*b*
Healthcare Effectiveness Data and Information Set (HEDIS), 185–186, 185*b*–186*b*
Healthcare Facilities Accreditation Program (HFAP), 50*t*
HEDIS. *see* Healthcare Effectiveness Data and Information Set
HHS, 46
HIE. *see* Health information exchanges
High-Deductible Health Plans (HDHPs), 58
High-quality care, 183–184
High-quality customer service, 308–311, 308*b*
    helpful attitude as, 308–309, 308*f*
    identifying with patients as, 309
    patient expectation in, 309, 310*f*
    patient loyalty as, 308
    patient surveys in, 309–310, 310*b*, 311*f*
    problem patients in, 310–311, 311*b*
HIPAA. *see* Health Insurance Portability and Accountability Act
HIT. *see* Health information technology
HITECH. *see* Health Information Technology for Economic and Clinical Health Act
Home health care, 33, 33*b*
Home health prospective payment system, 168–169
Hospice care, 33, 33*b*
Hospital, 30–31, 30*b*, 31*f*
Hospital outpatient prospective payment system, 168
Hospital-based ambulatory care, 24, 24*f*, 25*t*
Housekeeping, 86, 86*b*, 86*f*
Hyperlinks, 306

I
Implied contract, 213, 213*b*, 331, 331*b*
Inadvertent occurrences, 200*b*
Inchoate crimes, 211
Incidence, 108–109, 109*b*
Incident report, 200, 200*b*, 201*f*
Income statements, 151–153, 151*b*, 152*f*
Incompetent, 216–217, 217*b*
Indemnity insurance, 55, 55*b*
Indian Health Service (IHS), 41*t*
Indigent, 68–70, 68*b*
Individual insurance, 161
Information exchanges, health, 121–123
Informed consent, 94, 94*b*, 215, 215*b*–216*b*, 215*f*
Infractions, 211
Inpatients, 24, 24*b*
Insurance, 52–55, 53*b*, 53*f*
    verification, 171
Integrated delivery system, 64–65
Integrity, 357
Intentional torts, 212–213
Intermediate care facilities (ICFs), 32, 32*b*
Internal audits, 183, 187
Internal recruitment methods, 322–323
Internal/external auditing, 256
International Classification of Disease, 10th Revision, Clinical Modification, 108–109, 109*b*, 110*f*, 174–175, 174*b*
Internet reviews, as marketing tools, 303
Interoperability, 66–67, 67*b*, 121–122, 121*b*
Interpreter, 279, 280*f*
Interrogatories, 221, 221*b*

Inventory, 150
  best practices for, 145, 146*b*
  managing, 135–146, 136*b*–137*b*, 136*f*, 141*b*
    duties and responsibilities for, 137–138, 137*b*, 138*f*
    loss, 138–141, 138*b*
    tracking spreadsheet, 139*f*
  receiving, 144–145, 144*b*
Involuntary termination, 332
Ionizing radiation, 232

J

JCAHO. *see* Joint Commission on Accreditation of
    Healthcare Organizations
Job analysis, 323, 323*b*
Job announcement, 323, 323*b*
Johns Hopkins University, 38
Joint Commission on Accreditation of Healthcare
    Organizations (JCAHO), 49

L

Law
  administrative, 214
  affecting health care facility, 225–233
  civil, 212–214
  contract, 213–214
  criminal, 210–211
  overview of, 210–214, 215*b*
  tort, 212–213, 212*f*
Layout, facility, 86–87, 87*f*–88*f*
LCD. *see* Local coverage determinations
Lead time, 141*b*
Leadership, 347–361
  definition of, 348
  habits of successful managers, 353*b*
Leading, organizational management, 351–352
Lean method, 191–192, 191*b*
Lean PI philosophy, 192, 192*b*
Legal data, 94
Legal/ethical issues, 235–236, 236*b*
  in health care, 209–237, 210*b*
  in marketing, 314
LEIE. *see* List of Excluded Individuals and Entities
Liabilities, 149, 149*b*, 151
  in health care facility, 220, 220*b*
Liability insurance, 220
Liaison, 310–311, 310*b*
Libel, 212–213
Licensed Practical Nurses (LPNs), 19, 19*b*
Licensed Vocational Nurses (LVNs), 19, 19*b*
Licensing, 16–17, 16*b*
Licensure, 47, 47*b*
  documentation for, 108
Line graphs, 194*f*, 196–198, 197*f*
List of Excluded Individuals and Entities (LEIE), 262
Litigation, 107, 107*b*
Litigious society, 210, 210*b*
Live video, 132, 133*f*
Local coverage determinations (LCDs), 172, 172*b*
Local government, in health care delivery, 47
Locum tenens, 27
Long-term care facilities (LTCs), 32, 32*b*
Long-term liabilities, 151
LPN. *see* Licensed Practical Nurses
LTC. *see* Long-term care facilities
LVN. *see* Licensed Vocational Nurses

M

MACRA. *see* Medicare Access and CHIP
    Reauthorization Act
Magnetic resonance imaging (MRI) machine, 55*f*
Mailers, 303, 303*f*
Malfeasance, 218
Malpractice, 212–213, 213*b*, 218–221, 221*b*, 236*b*
Malpractice insurance, 167
  medical, 220–221

Managed care, 41–42, 41*b*–42*b*, 169, 169*b*
  insurance plans, 56, 56*b*
Mandatory exclusions, 263, 263*b*
Marketing, 297–315, 298*b*
  high-quality customer service in, 308–311, 308*b*
  legal and ethical issues in, 314, 315*b*
  needs of health care practice, 298–301, 301*b*
    identifying customers in, 299
    strategies for outpatient settings, 299*t*
    SWOT analysis in, 299–301, 299*b*, 300*f*, 301*b*
  plan, 298–299, 298*b*
  public relations in, 307–308, 307*b*
    addressing bad press, 307–308
  tools, 301–306, 306*b*–307*b*
    automated phone calls as, 302, 302*b*
    community involvement as, 301–302
    internet reviews as, 303
    newsletters and blogs as, 302
    print ads in magazines and newspapers as,
        302–303, 302*b*
    social media as, 303–304, 303*b*–304*b*
    websites as, 304–306
  "welcome to our office" packet in, 311–314, 311*b*
    introduction to medical office as, 312
    list of community resources as, 314
    medical office's financial policy as, 312
    missed appointments and cancellation policy as,
        312
    patient instruction sheets as, 313–314, 313*f*
    patient portal as, 312–313
Massachusetts Medical Society, 37
Master patient index, 106, 106*b*
Materials safety data sheet (MSDS), 232, 232*b*
Mature minor doctrine, 217
Maturity, in organization, 357
Meaningful use, 67, 124, 124*b*
Mediation, 224, 224*b*
Medicaid, 40–41, 41*b*, 41*t*, 62, 62*b*
Medical Assistant (MAs), 20–21, 20*b*–21*b*, 20*f*
Medical billers and coders, 21–22
Medical Doctor (MD), 17, 17*b*
Medical durable power of attorney, 230*b*
Medical liability, 218–221, 221*b*
Medical malpractice insurance, 220–221
Medical necessity, 96, 96*b*
  coverage, 172
Medical professional lawsuit, 221–224, 224*b*,
    233*b*–234*b*
Medical proxy, 94, 94*b*
Medical record, 91–106, 91*b*, 106*b*–107*b*
  ownership of, 98–106, 98*b*
  retention of, 99–106, 99*t*–105*t*
  types of health data in, 92–98, 92*t*
Medical record number (MRN), 92*b*
Medical schools, in 20th century, 37
Medicare, 40–41, 41*b*, 41*t*, 60–62, 60*b*, 61*f*
  part A, 61
  part B, 61
  part C, 61
  part D, 61
Medicare Access and CHIP Reauthorization Act
    (MACRA), 184–185, 185*b*
Medicare advantage, 61
Medicare and Medicaid, 254
Medicare and Medicaid EHR Incentive Program, 125
Medicare prospective payment system, 166, 166*b*
Meetings, 190–191, 292–293, 292*t*
  agenda, 292, 292*b*, 293*f*
  minutes, 292–293, 292*b*, 294*f*
Memorandums, 289–291, 289*b*, 290*f*
  body/content, 291
  distribution, 291
  formatting for, 290–291
  heading, 290–291
  mistakes in, 291*b*

Merit-based Incentive Payment System (MIPS), 185, 185*b*
MIPS. *see* Merit-based Incentive Payment System
Misdemeanor, 211
Misfeasance, 218–219
Mission statement, of strategic planning, 349
Modified wave scheduling, 82, 82*b*
Morbidity, 108–109, 108*b*
Mortality, 108–109, 108*b*
Motivation, 353–354, 353*b*
    internal and external, 354, 354*t*
MRN. *see* Medical record number
MSDS. *see* Materials safety data sheet

N
Narrative assessment, 328–330, 330*b*
National Certified Medical Assistant (NCMA), 21
National Committee for Quality Assurance (NCQA), 50*t*
National coverage determinations (NCDs), 172, 172*b*
National Defense Authorization Act (NDAA), 343, 343*b*
National Institutes of Health (NIH), 46*t*
National Integrated Accreditation for Healthcare Organizations (NIAHO), 50*t*
Nationally Registered Certified Medical Assistant (NRCMA), 21
NCD. *see* National coverage determinations
NCMA. *see* National Certified Medical Assistant
NCQA. *see* National Committee for Quality Assurance
NDAA. *see* National Defense Authorization Act
Needs assessment, 282, 282*b*
Negligence, 218–219, 218*b*–219*b*
    contributory, 219
Negligence tort, 212–213
Net income, 152, 152*b*–153*b*
Net operating income (NOI), 152
Net worth, 151, 151*b*
Newsletters, as marketing tools, 302
NIAHO. *see* National Integrated Accreditation for Healthcare Organizations
NIH. *see* National Institutes of Health
NOI. *see* Net operating income
Nominal damages, 219
Noncompliance, 260–265
Noncurrent assets, 150
Nonfeasance, 219
Nonverbal communication, 283–284, 283*b*–284*b*
Notice of Privacy Practices (NPP), 94, 243, 243*b*
NPP. *see* Notice of Privacy Practices
NRCMA. *see* Nationally Registered Certified Medical Assistant
Nurse, 18, 18*b*, 18*f*–19*f*

O
OASIS. *see* Outcomes and Assessment Information Set
Objective
    goal, 350
    signs, 96
Occupational Safety and Health Act (OSH Act), 231–233, 231*b*, 344, 344*b*
Occupational Safety and Health Administration (OSHA), 86, 231, 231*b*, 253
Office for Civil Rights, 248, 248*b*
Office of Inspector General (OIG), 46*t*, 187, 253–255, 253*b*, 254*f*, 255*b*
    audits and actions, 262–263
Officer, privacy, 243, 246*b*
Official goals, of organizational management, 349
OIG. *see* Office of Inspector General
Older Workers Benefit Protection Act (OWBPA), 339, 339*b*
Onboarding, in training and development, of employees, 326, 326*b*
Open access scheduling, 81–82, 81*b*
Operational budget, 156–158, 156*b*, 157*f*

Operational planning, 350
Operative goals, of organizational management, 349–350
OPPS. *see* Outpatient prospective payment system
Ordinance, 210, 210*b*
Organization, 26, 27*f*, 340, 340*b*
Organizational enforcement, 257
Organizational management, 347–361, 348*b*–349*b*, 357*b*, 360*b*
    conflict, 355–359, 355*b*
    controlling, 352
    function of, 348–352, 353*b*
        leading, 351–352
        organizing, 350–351
        planning, 349–350
    goal of, 349
    motivation for, 353–354
    official goals of, 349
    operative goals of, 349–350
Orientation, in onboarding, 326, 326*b*
Osteopathic Doctor (DO), 17, 17*b*
Outcomes, 184, 184*b*
Outcomes and Assessment Information Set (OASIS), 169, 169*b*
Out-of-pocket limit, 163–164, 163*b*
Outpatient prospective payment system (OPPS), 168, 168*b*
Outpatients, 24, 24*b*
OWBPA. *see* Older Workers Benefit Protection Act
Ownership, 27–28, 27*b*

P
Packaging, 168, 168*b*
PACS. *see* Picture Archiving and Communication System
PAHCOM. *see* Professional Association of Healthcare Office Management
Palliative care, 33, 33*b*
Par level, 138, 138*b*
Pareto chart, 194*f*, 194*t*–195*t*
Passive candidate, 322, 322*b*
Patient chart, 91
Patient consent form, 95*f*
Patient instruction sheets, 313–314, 313*f*
Patient portal, 77, 77*b*, 122–123, 122*b*
Patient Protection and Affordable Care Act (PPACA), 44, 253
Patient Self-Determination Act, 229–231
Patient-Centered Medical Home model (PCMH), 273, 273*b*
Patients' bill of rights, 225, 225*b*
Payback period, 154, 154*b*
Payer, 39, 39*b*, 70*f*, 161, 161*b*
Payment posting, 176–178
PCE. *see* Potentially compensable events
PCMH. *see* Patient-Centered Medical Home model
PCP. *see* Primary care provider
PDA. *see* Pregnancy Discrimination Act
Performance improvement, 182–205, 190*b*, 199*b*
    methods, 191–193
    tools, 193–199, 194*t*–195*t*
Performance review, in hiring, training, and evaluating employees, 327–330, 327*b*–328*b*, 330*b*
    assessment in, 328–330
    discussion in, 330
    evaluation form, 329*f*
Permissive exclusion, 263, 263*b*
Personal crimes, 211
Personal injury insurance, 221
Petty offense, 211
PHI. *see* Protected health information
Phone etiquette, 280–283
    answering the call, 281
    billing, 282
    closing the call, 282

Phone etiquette (Continued)
    confirming appointments, 281
    test results, 281–282
    triage and call flow management, 282–283
Physical safeguard, 246–247, 246t, 247f
Physician Assistants (PAs), 20, 20b
Physician practice expense (PE), 167
Physician Quality Reporting System (PQRS), 184, 184b
Physician Self-Referral Law, 260–262, 260b
Physician work (W), 166
Physicians, 17–18, 17b
    office of, 25–28, 25b, 26f
Picture Archiving and Communication System (PACS), 98
Pie chart, 194f, 194t–195t, 196–198, 197b, 197f
Plaintiff, 212, 212b
Plan, 96
    health, 240t
Plan, Do, Check, and Act (PDCA) method, 191, 191b, 191t
Planning, 202–203
    of organizational management, 349–350
    policies and procedures, 350, 351f
PMS. see Practice management software
Point of Service (POS), 58, 58b
Policy, 350, 351f
Portability, 239–240, 239b
Postbilling processes, 176–179
Potentially compensable events (PCEs), 200, 200b
PPACA. see Patient Protection and Affordable Care Act
PPO. see Preferred Provider Organizations
PPS. see Prospective payment system
PQRS. see Physician Quality Reporting System
Practice management software (PMS), 125–132, 125b, 126f–129f, 129f
    referral form, 129f
Preauthorization, 171–172, 171b
Precertification, 171
Predetermination, 172
Preferred Provider Organizations (PPOs), 58, 58b
Pregnancy Discrimination Act (PDA), 341, 341b
Premium, 39, 39b, 161, 161b
Presbycusis, 277
Presbyopia, 277–278
Primary care, 25, 25b
Primary care provider (PCP), 25, 25b–26b, 64, 64f
Print ads, in magazines and newspapers, as marketing tools, 302–303, 302b
Prior authorization, 171
Privacy officer, 243, 246b
Privacy Rule, 240–243, 240b, 241f, 243b, 244f–245f
Private practice, 27
Privileges, 31, 31b
Problem-focused history, 111
Procedure, 350, 351f
Processing claims, preparing for, 172–173
Productivity, 350–351
Professional Association of Healthcare Office Management (PAHCOM), 10, 49–51
    Code of Ethical Standards, 51b
Professional standards, 49–51
Professional Standards Review Organizations (PSROs), 42
Professionalism, 271–296, 272b, 274b, 296b
    dependability, 273
    patient respect, 273
    professional team collaboration, 273–274
Progress note, 83–84, 84b
Project, 363, 363b, 367b
Project execution plan, 368, 368b
Project management, 362–372, 364b
    closing of, 369
    controlling of, 368–369
    execution of, 368
    initiation of, 367, 371b–372b

Project management (Continued)
    introduction to, 363, 363b
    life cycle, 367–369, 367f, 369b
    methodologies for, 370–371
    monitoring of, 368–369
    organized, 365–366
    planning, 368
    trends in, 365b
Project manager, 365–366, 365b, 367b
    dynamic, 366, 366f
    effective communicators, 366, 366f
    expert delegator, 366, 366f
    motivational, 366, 366f
    organized, 365–366, 366f
Property crimes, 211
Prospective payment bundle, 166
Prospective payment system (PPS), 42, 42b, 166, 166b
Protected health information (PHI), 240–241, 240b–241b
    disclosures of, 242b
    privacy and security scenarios of, 242b
    protection of, 246f
Protocol, 120, 120b
Provider, 5, 5f–6f, 240t
PSRO. see Professional Standards Review Organizations
Public health insurance system, 40
Public relations, in marketing, 307–308, 307b
Public-policy exception, 331, 331b
Punitive damages, 219
Purchase order, 143–144, 143b–144b, 143f

Q
QPP. see Quality Payment Program
Quality, 182–205, 183b, 189b–190b
    measuring, 184–186
Quality Payment Program (QPP), 184
Query, 175, 175b–176b
Query-based exchange, 122, 122b

R
RBRVS. see Resource-based relative value scale
Real cost, 139–140, 140b
Reasonable accommodations, 339, 339b
Referral, 25–26, 26b, 64, 64b
Registered Medical Assistant (RMA), 21
Reimbursement, 39, 39b, 108, 108b
    methodologies, 164–169, 169b–170b
Relationship management, 358f, 359
Remittance advice, 176–178, 176b, 178f
Remote patient monitoring (RPM), 133, 133b
Research, documentation for, 108–109
Resignation, 332
Resource-based relative value scale (RBRVS), 166–167, 166b
Respondeat superior, 220, 220b
Restitution, 211, 211b
Retail health clinic, 29, 29b
Retention, of medical records, 99–106
Retrospective audit, 188, 188b
Revenue cycle, 84–85, 84b–85b, 160–181, 161b, 180b–181b
    management, 170–180, 170b
    monitoring, 179–180
Revenue stream, 151, 151b
Risk management, 182–205, 200b, 203b
RMA. see Registered Medical Assistant
RPM. see Remote patient monitoring

S
Same-day surgery centers, 28, 29f
SAMHSA. see Substance Abuse and Mental Health Services Administration
Scarcity mentality, 357
Scatter diagram, 194f, 194t–195t
Scheduling and registration, 170–171

Scheduling matrix, 78–79, 79b, 79f
Scheduling methods, 81–82, 81b
Scope of practice, 18–19, 18b
Scope of work (SOW), 367, 367b
Screening mechanisms, a compliance plan, 257
Security Rule, 243–247, 247b, 246t, 247b
Self-awareness, 358, 358f
Self-disclosure, 264b
Self-management, 358f, 359
Self-pay, 164–165, 164b
Self-reporting, 264b
Sentinel event, 190, 190b
Sex, structure of population for United States, 69f
Shelf life, 138, 138b
Short-term liabilities, 151
Shrinkage, 139, 139b–140b
SHRM. see Strategic human resources management
Site map, 304–305, 304b
Six Sigma method, 192, 192b, 193f
Skilled nursing facilities (SNFs), 32, 32b
Slander, 212–213
SNF. see Skilled nursing facilities
Social awareness, 358, 358f
Social media, as marketing tools, 303–304, 303b–304b
Solo practice, 27
SOW. see Scope of work
Span of control, 351, 351b
Special damages, 220
Staggered schedule, 78–79, 78b
Stakeholders, 258, 258b, 365, 365b
Standards of conduct, 256
Stark law, 234–235, 234b, 260–262, 260b
Statute of limitations, 99–106, 223–224
Statutes, 210, 210b
Statutory crimes, 211
Stimulus bill, 67, 124
Stock-out, 136–137, 136b
Store-and-forward technology, 133, 133b
Strategic human resources management (SHRM),
    320–321, 321b
Strategic planning, 349
Stream scheduling, 82, 82b
Stretch goals, 350
Strict liability torts, 212–213
Structured interviews, 325, 325b
Subjective section, 96
Subpoena duces tecum, 222, 222b
Subpoenas, 222, 222b
Subscribers, 52, 52b, 161, 161b
Substance Abuse and Mental Health Services
    Administration (SAMHSA), 46t
Sunshine Act, 235
Superbill, 129, 129b, 129f–131f
Supplies
    expiration date of, 138
    inventory of, 135–146
    large quantities of, 138
    management, primary and secondary goals of, 145t
    ordering of, 141–144, 144b
    receiving, 144–145, 144b
Survey, 195, 195b, 196t
SWOT analysis, in marketing, 299–301, 299b, 300f,
    301b
    opportunities and threats of, 300–301
    strengths and weaknesses of, 300

T
Table, 195–196, 195b
Target market, 299, 299b
Tax Equity and Fiscal Responsibility Act (TEFRA), 42,
    42b
Tax-related health provisions governing medical
    savings accounts, 239
TCT. see The Compliance Team
Team cohesiveness, in conflict, 356

Team focus, in conflict, 355
Technical safeguard, 246t, 247,
    247b
Technology, 113–134
TEFRA. see Tax Equity and Fiscal Responsibility Act
Telehealth, 132–133, 132b, 132f
The 7 Habits of Highly Effective People, 356
The Compliance Team (TCT), 50t
The Joint Commission (TJC), 49, 49b, 50t, 187, 187b,
    202b–204b, 253
Third-party payer, 39, 39b
Three Golden Rules of Engagement, 359
360° review, 328, 328b
Time management, 350–351, 352b
TJC. see The Joint Commission
Tort law, 212–213, 212f
Training, 326–327, 326b
    diversity, 327, 327b
Triage, 80–81, 80b
TRICARE, 41t
Truman, Harry, 40
Turnover, 321, 321b
    costs, 334b

U
UGESP. see Uniform Guidelines on Employee Selection
    Procedures
Unbilled accounts, 180
Unbilled charges, 188–189, 188b
Underinsured, 70–71, 70b
Undocumented charges, 189, 189b
Uniform Guidelines on Employee Selection Procedures
    (UGESP), 338, 338b
Uniform resource locator (URL), 306
Uniformed Services Employment and Reemployment
    Act (USERRA), 343, 343b
Unintentional tort, 212–213
Unity of command, 351
Universal health care, 43, 43b
University of Pennsylvania, 37
Urgent care clinic, 29, 29b
URL. see Uniform resource locator
USERRA. see Uniformed Services Employment and
    Reemployment Act
Usual, customary, and reasonable (UCR) rate,
    165

V
Valid contract, 214b
Variable costs, 157, 157b
Variance, 157–158, 157b
Vendors, 141, 141b–142b
Verbal communication, 280–283, 280b
Verdict, 223, 223b, 223f
Veterans Health Administration (VHA), 41t
Visits, 24b
Visual impairment, 277–278
Voluntary termination, 332

W
Waiver of liability, 172
Walk-in, 77, 77b
War Labor Board, 39
Waterfall model, 370, 370b, 370f
Wave scheduling, 82, 82b
Websites, as marketing tools, 304–306
    about us page, 305
    choosing name, 304
    contact us page, 305
    creating site map, 304–305, 304b
    designing pages, 305–306
    home page, 305
    increasing traffic, 306, 306b
    specials page, 305
    testimonials or information page, 305

"Welcome to our office" packet, in marketing, 311–314, 311b
    introduction to medical office, 312
    list of community resources, 314
    medical office's financial policy, 312
    missed appointments and cancellation policy, 312
    patient instruction sheets, 313–314, 313f
    patient portal, 312–313
Whistle blower, 331, 331b
Workflow, 76–85, 76b, 85b
    check-in, 82–83, 82b, 83f
    check-out, 84, 84f
    clinical assessment, 83–84, 83b
    revenue cycle, 84–85, 84b–85b
    scheduling, 77–82, 78b

Workflow map, 76, 76b, 76f
World War II, health insurance during, 39
Written communication, 284–291, 284b
    email etiquette, 284–287
    memorandums, 289–291, 289b, 290f
    professional and formal business letters, 287–289
        business address, 288
        closing, 289
        date of letter, 289
        greeting, 289
        main body, 289
        recipient address, 289
        signature, 289

X
X-rays, 40, 40f